Advance praise for *The Chinese Medicinal Herb Farm*

"Peg Schafer offers practical advice for anyone wanting to grow organic Chinese herbs, either in their home garden or to sell on a larger scale. There is no other book that takes on organic Chinese herb production in such an in-depth way. . . . Whether you intend to farm, or simply garden, *The Chinese Medicinal Herb Farm* is a book manifest through years of persistent sweat equity that furthers our collective knowledge of growing Chinese herbs in America, once a dream, now an ever-increasingly established reality."

—**Steven Foster,** author of *A Desk Reference to Nature's Medicine*
and Herbal Emissaries: Bringing Chinese Herbs to the West

"For the practitioner of Chinese medicine, *The Chinese Medicinal Herb Farm* is a teacher, drawing us closer to the herbs we use. For the casual gardener, it is a handbook for growing fresh Chinese herbs as part of a healthy diet. For anyone who has an interest in growing their own Chinese herbs, Peg Schafer gives us a new reason to look forward to spring."

—**Andrew Ellis,** author of *Notes from South Mountain:*
A Guide to Concentrated Herb Granules

"This is by far the most detailed and thorough book that addresses the urgent issue of organic cultivation and processing of Chinese herbs. It will have a profound effect on future land use, herb availability, pesticide burdens, and sustainability in a field that is expanding rapidly around the world. I can't stress enough how valuable and rare this information is to practitioners and users of Chinese herbal medicine. I highly recommend this book for all TCM herbalists, as well as gardeners and farmers who want to learn the art of the organic cultivation of Chinese medicinals."

—**Bill Schoenbart,** LAc, DAOM

"Peg Schafer is the best artisanal grower I know. For this book, she has distilled the knowledge of the small group who, over the past two decades, has pioneered North American production of Chinese medicinal herbs, and tested it through direct experience. This book clearly explains the whys as well as the how-tos, and delivers information into the eager hands of all perennial polyculturalists who will grow us a post-peak oil healthcare system; it is a gift to us all."

—**Jean Giblette,** owner, High Falls Gardens
and cofounder, LocalHerbs.org

"Peg Schafer, the most experienced Chinese medicinal herb grower in North America, charts a new course in Chinese medicinal plant cultivation by providing the guidance needed to grow the most important of these herbs domestically. This book offers more than just cultivation tips, but also an assurance of proper plant identification, optimal growing and harvesting conditions, freshness of materials, and the ability to access Chinese medicinals with the lowest carbon footprint possible."

—**Roy Upton,** executive director of
American Herbal Pharmacopoeia

"Peg Schafer understands in more ways than one that good health springs from the land. Herbs from the Chinese tradition perfectly complement more familiar healing plants. The concept of 'regional medicine farms' resonates so well with the growing desire to eat more locally. But of course! We are what we eat, and that includes the medicinal plants that work with our bodies to create wholeness. Every plant person will instantly recognize the gift waiting within this book—Schafer shares many astute observations of how each plant garners medicinal oomph, what she calls the vital qi (chi) of each herb. And that's the right sort of inspiration to launch any thinking gardener!"

—**Michael Phillips,** author of *The Holistic Orchard* and coauthor with Nancy Phillips of *The Herbalist's Way*

THE
CHINESE
MEDICINAL
HERB FARM

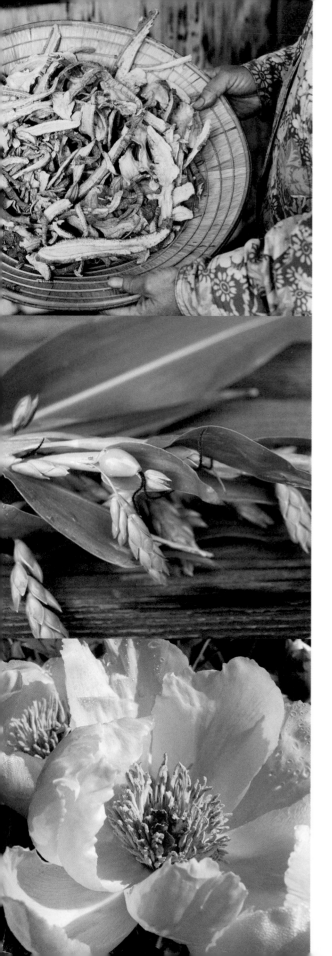

THE CHINESE MEDICINAL HERB FARM

A Cultivator's Guide to Small-Scale Organic Herb Production

PEG SCHAFER

Foreword by Steven Foster

Medicinal Use Descriptions by
Sean Fannin, CH, Dipl.CEM

Chelsea Green Publishing
White River Junction, Vermont

The information contained in this book is general in scope and not
meant as a guide to self-medication. Caution should be taken with the
introduction of any novel foods or plants. Consult a qualified medical
practitioner before using any plant for medicinal purposes.

Project Manager: Patricia Stone
Project Editor: Makenna Goodman
Developmental Editor: Fern Marshall Bradley
Copy Editor: Eric Raetz
Proofreader: Eileen M. Clawson
Indexer: Peggy Halloway
Designer: Peter Holm, Sterling Hill Productions

All photographs by Peg Schafer, unless otherwise credited.

Printed in the United States of America
First printing November, 2011
10 9 8 7 6 5 4 3 2 1 11 12 13 14 15

Our Commitment to Green Publishing
Chelsea Green sees publishing as a tool for cultural change and ecological stewardship. We strive to align our
book manufacturing practices with our editorial mission and to reduce the impact of our business enterprise
in the environment. We print our books and catalogs on chlorine-free recycled paper, using vegetable-based
inks whenever possible. This book may cost slightly more because we use recycled paper, and we hope you'll
agree that it's worth it. Chelsea Green is a member of the Green Press Initiative (www.greenpressinitiative
.org), a nonprofit coalition of publishers, manufacturers, and authors working to protect the world's
endangered forests and conserve natural resources. *The Chinese Medicinal Herb Farm* was printed on FSC®-
certified paper supplied by RR Donnelley that contains at least 10-percent postconsumer recycled fiber.

Library of Congress Cataloging-in-Publication Data
Schafer, Peg, 1962-
  The Chinese medicinal herb farm : a cultivator's guide to small-scale organic herb production / Peg Scha-
fer ; foreword by Steven Foster ; medicinal use descriptions by Sean Fannin.
      p. cm.
  Includes bibliographical references and index.
  ISBN 978-1-60358-330-5 (pbk.) – ISBN 978-1-60358-331-2 (ebook)
1. Herb farming. 2. Medicinal plants. 3. Herbs--Therapeutic use. I. Title. II. Title: Cultivator's guide to
small-scale organic herb production.

  SB351.H5S297 2011
  615.3'21–dc23

                    2011030305

Chelsea Green Publishing Company
Post Office Box 428
White River Junction, VT 05001
(802) 295-6300
www.chelseagreen.com

*In memory of Cindy Riviere and her dedication
to the cultivation of Chinese medicinal plants.*

THE HERBALIST AND THE FARMER

Inevitably a herbalist visiting the farm will say: "What?! You grow them and don't know how to use them?" Then I retort: "What? You use them and don't know how they were grown?"

Contents

APPENDICES

Foreword

In 1976, a walk through the Harvard University campus in Cambridge, Massachusetts, changed the way I looked at plants forever. At the time, I was working at the herb department at the Sabbathday Lake Shaker Community in Maine and still a teenager. A few weeks earlier I had met Dr. Shiu Ying Hu of Harvard's Arnold Arboretum when she and a friend toured the Shaker Museum at Sabbathday Lake. We became fast friends, and she invited me to visit her in Cambridge. Walking through Harvard Yard on our way to lunch, Dr. Hu pointed to various plants growing in the horticultural plantings—things such as daylilies, *Forsythia, Ginkgo,* and *Platycodon*—all the while discussing their use in Traditional Chinese Medicine. For me it was an epiphany. I had dismissed these plants as flowers or ornamentals. At the time I was solely interested in medicinal plants and herbs and could not be bothered with a mere pretty flower.

Our conversation opened up a new world of inquiry about Chinese medicinal plants in American horticulture. Since I knew the vast majority of ornamentals in American and European gardens came from East Asia, it seemed there had to be many medicinal plants among those ornamentals, and indeed there are. Simply by comparing indexes of books on Chinese medicinal plants with books on plants grown in American horticulture, in short order I compiled a list of 779 species of Chinese herbs that could be found in American gardens, and a few small grants allowed me to explore the subject deeper. Since I was engaged in growing herbs commercially on a small scale, it seemed logical that it was possible to grow what we usually include among the category of ornamental plants as Chinese medicinal herbs instead.

Dr. Hu encouraged the idea, as it was her dream, too, to see Chinese herbs grown in America. I actively pursued the project for nearly twenty years, culminating in publication of *Herbal Emissaries: Bringing Chinese Herbs to the West* (coauthored with Chinese materia medica expert Prof. Yue Chongxi—to whom Dr. Hu had introduced me in the early 1980s—and published in 1992). Now retired in Hong Kong, and enjoying her second century on the planet, Dr. Hu has lived long enough to see this dream grow into a reality. She planted the idea in the minds of others, as well, including Dr. Tso-cheng Chang, a farmer in western Massachusetts who began growing wǔ wèi zǐ (*Schisandra chinensis,* Five Flavored Fruit) in the mid 1980s. He expanded an experiment into acreage to offer fresh Schisandra juice at his family restaurant. Now he oversees many acres of Schisandra plantings and offers the fresh juice extract as a dietary supplement product. Dr. Hu had planted the seed of success. Today the idea has grown far beyond the people she knows.

In the mid 1970s one could find an acupuncturist only in a back alley or in poorly marked storefronts in Chinatowns of major cities. Today, however, more and more acupuncturists are in practice throughout North America, and not just in big cities. I live in a small town in Arkansas, population 2,000 souls, and even we have an acupuncturist. The doors of communication between the United States and China—at least in terms of alternative medicine—have opened. Information now flows back and forth. The herbal trade has increased steadily between China and the

United States with the rise of Americans who are fascinated with things such as acupuncture and herbs used in Traditional Chinese Medicine.

Sometime in the early 1990s I met Peg Schafer. She and a cadre of other Chinese herb-growing enthusiasts, whom she acknowledges in this book, had by then begun to "take the ball and run with it." Peg viewed growing Chinese herbs as a farming and business opportunity. Living in northern California she had the potential of a ready market for fresh or recently grown Chinese medicinal plants among a growing number of young Caucasian Traditional Chinese Medicine practitioners in the San Francisco Bay area. At that time, no one else was cultivating Chinese herbs on a market scale, and she was in uncharted waters.

It has not been an easy row to hoe. Undoubtedly there have been days when Peg stared in frustration at a field of weeds, while wannabe herbal hippie summer-camp apprentices lounged beneath the shade of a tree, content to commune with the weeds, rather than get up and pull them. Nor has it been easy to create a market demand for domestic herbs—even amidst the current climate of local-food activism and an increased interest in natural medicine—as most TCM practitioners still rely mainly on Chinese imported herbs. Indeed, Peg was the first person in the United States to begin growing a diversified array of herbs on a market scale and also to found a certified organic extract company using entirely domestically grown herbs. And there are still too few domestic farms to meet the ever-rising demand of practitioners. There is a need, in other words, for more domestic cultivation of Chinese herbs. Convincing young practitioners that Peg's California-grown Chinese herbs were as good as those that came from the motherland, even though their appearance may be different from what they were accustomed to purchasing, presented yet another challenge. Still, Peg was committed to her mission—more domestic cultivation and more domestic tincture production—which compelled her to push forward despite these obstacles. She had no choice, no matter what her accountant said. She was hooked.

Now, with many years' experience growing Chinese herbs, Peg, in *The Chinese Medicinal Herb Farm*, offers growers and practitioners alike practical advice for anyone wanting to grow organic Chinese herbs, either in their home garden or to sell on a larger scale. There is no other book that takes on organic Chinese herb production in such an in-depth way—*The Chinese Medicinal Herb Farm* breaks new ground. Peg offers us more than mere reference information, but the knowledge that comes from years of experience, seasoned with wisdom. Whether you intend to farm, or simply garden, *The Chinese Medicinal Herb Farm* is a book borne of years of persistent sweat equity that furthers our collective knowledge of growing Chinese herbs in America, once a dream, now an ever-increasing reality.

STEVEN FOSTER

Steven Foster is the author of seventeen titles on medicinal plants, including two books on Chinese medicinal plants.

Preface

It is early spring as I write, and it is alternately raining and hailing (as it has for a few days). I am wondering just when I will be able to get back into the field. "Hurry up and wait" is what the farm crew and I call it; eventually the weather will break, and we can rest assured that everything will—all at the same time—be in desperate need of attention. Transplanting crops, field maintenance, equipment maintenance . . . just what was it that we hit that damaged the flail mower anyway? But the seeds have been sown and nature is taking her course, a constant reminder—all in due time, all in due time.

Over the past fourteen years of cultivating Asian medicinals at the Chinese Medicinal Herb Farm, we have experimented with growing over 250 different herbs. Initially we were looking primarily for answers to seemingly simple questions: How can this seed be germinated? Will this plant grow here? If I grow it can I sell it? Does this herb have ornamental or habitat value? Now we also ask other questions: Is this an economically viable crop for the farmer? Just how do we harvest this crop? Is this herb medicinally potent if grown here?

When I decided to become a medicinal herb farmer, I figured that as I went along I'd connect with and share knowledge with others who would certainly be doing the same thing. To my surprise I've discovered that there are still very few other growers of these remarkable plants. So . . . tag—you're it!

In this book you'll find practical information not only on the cultivation of some of these unfamiliar (but important) Asian medicinal herbs, but also the descriptions of the changes taking place in current medicinal plant trade practices—and how they affect herbal quality and conservation. My goal is to create a resource that is useful to gardeners, farmers, nursery workers, and practitioners who seek detailed information on medicinal herbs. It will also be of broader interest to the acupuncture and Oriental medicine (OM) community, including students and practitioners looking to deepen their knowledge of the herbs of their chosen profession. Much of this information was largely unpublished until now. It is my hope that you will find here a tool that assists you in becoming a successful herb grower of efficacious botanicals—or a more dynamic herbal practitioner.

I welcome now the germinating seed starting on its journey, knowing it has the support and wisdom of the ever-cycling seasons. Like the seeds, I know you—the reader—can flourish, adapt, and cultivate with confidence that you have the knowledge you need to grow. I wish you great luck!

Peg Schafer
Chinese Medicinal Herb Farm
Petaluma, California
February 2011

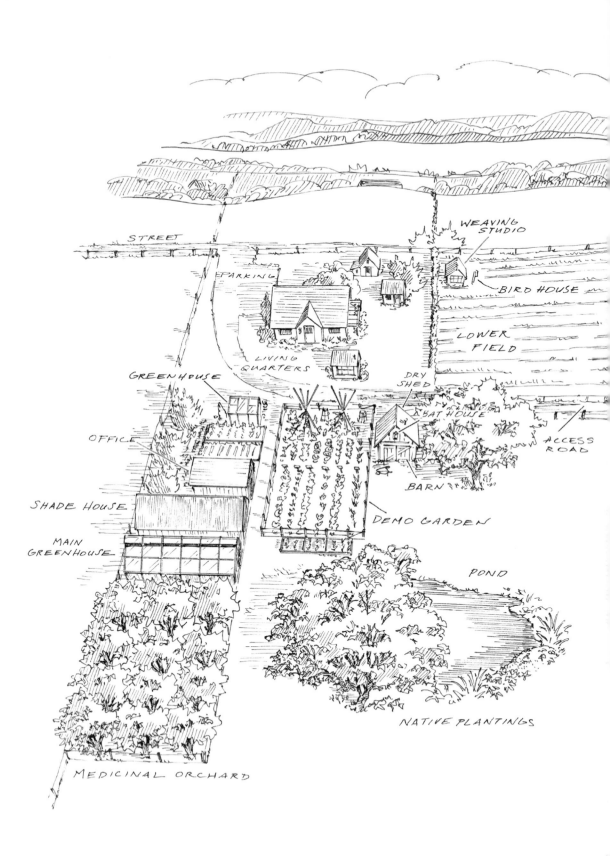

STREET

WEAVING STUDIO

BIRD HOUSE

PARKING

LOWER FIELD

LIVING QUARTERS

GREENHOUSE

DRY SHED

BAT HOUSE

OFFICE

ACCESS ROAD

BARN

SHADE HOUSE

DEMO GARDEN

MAIN GREENHOUSE

POND

NATIVE PLANTINGS

MEDICINAL ORCHARD

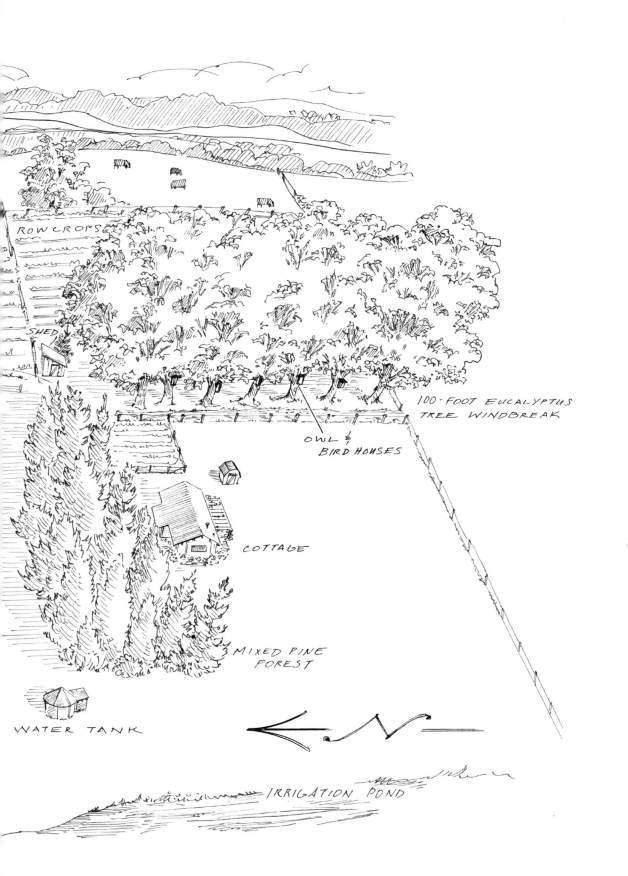

ROW CROPS

SHED

100-FOOT EUCALYPTUS
TREE WINDBREAK

OWL &
BIRD HOUSES

COTTAGE

MIXED PINE
FOREST

WATER TANK

N

IRRIGATION POND

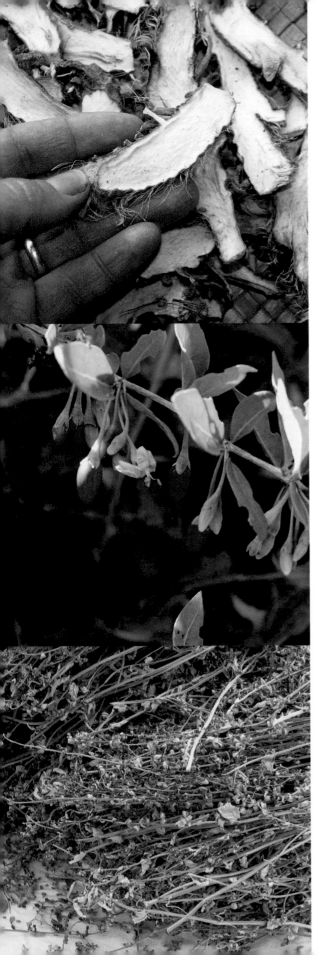

PART ONE

CULTIVATING TO CONSERVE

Connecting with Quality Asian Botanicals

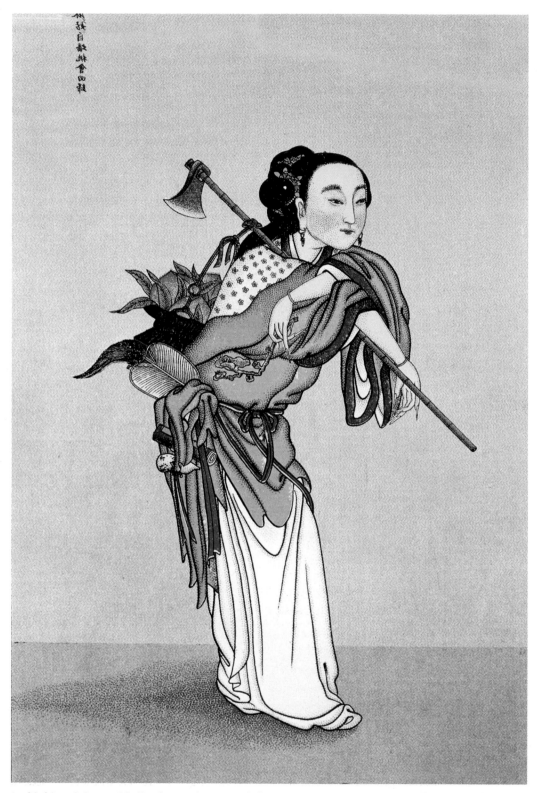

In this historic image Ma Kou is carrying recently harvested medicinal herbs. The illustration, by Father Henri Dore, is from the late nineteenth century. Photo from Bridgeman Art Library/ Private Collection/Archives Charmet CHT182703.

CHAPTER ONE

Farming to Be Part of the Solution

A holistic lifestyle has always been important to me, beginning with my childhood gardening experiences. Of all my siblings—there were five of us, and I was fourth from the oldest—I was the only one who took to gardening. In our suburban lot my father always had a vegetable garden and a huge compost pile (he was serious about that). I did the summertime watering, and I actually liked weeding and tending the tomatoes, peppers, zucchini, strawberries, and other crops that filled my father's garden beds. Then one day I saw him spraying our strawberries; from then on, we had two vegetable gardens. That childhood vegetable patch was the first of many gardens I have had the honor of tending.

My journey from raising vegetables to becoming a Chinese medicinal herb farmer started by accident—a car accident. I was not seriously injured, but I was pretty banged up. My friend Debra encouraged me to try acupuncture. After having some positive experiences with acupuncture, I started checking out Chinese medicinal herbs to see what they had to offer. Then I hit a conundrum. The herbs were helping me effectively deal with some long-term physical issues, but I had concerns about both the quality and what else (besides herbs) was in the powders I was consuming. When I shared my concerns with my wise tortoiselike practitioner, Bill Fannin, he kept inquiring why I didn't just grow my own. Always low key, and with a little *hmmm*, Bill would hand me a plant or two, saying that they were starts from his garden—and no, he didn't want any money for them.

At the time, I was a landless grower working on other people's farms, but my husband and I recently had purchased a little one-acre plot. And with a little gentle tortoise-nudging and *hmmm*, I was off growing Chinese herbs on our first little farm. I even planted a Chinese medicinal herb garden in the Fannins' backyard—which apparently never had a garden before.

Of course, the one-acre plot didn't become a farm overnight. It took two years of exploring the concept of growing Chinese botanical plants for me to feel confident that this kind of farming was doable and would be a viable market niche. I started by growing herb transplants for sale and soon found that there was a lot of interest. As I diversified into field cultivation, even more people became intrigued—just as I was figuring out that this was a much larger project and with even more potential than I initally imagined. Eventually we moved to a larger farm to further explore the potential of growing Asian medicinal herbs domestically. There are plenty of compelling reasons why growing these herbs is a good idea, not least of which is that small-scale ecological farming of herbs is a critical aspect of ensuring a high-quality supply and preventing continued loss of these herbs from their wild native regions.

EVOLVING HERBAL TRADITIONS

Traditional Chinese Medicine (TCM), with its extensive herbal focus, is more than three thousand years old; some traditions—like Ayurveda, the herbal tradition of India—are even older. In both these herbal traditions the roots, fruits, bark, leaves, flowers, seeds, and stems of specific botanicals are all utilized to address wide-ranging health problems.

Drawing on the accumulated wisdom of these and other ancient time-tested systems of medicine, Western herbal practitioners are beginning to utilize herbs from around the world. You may

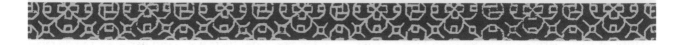

Growing Herbs as a Healing Endeavor

On a sunny day in late August, the Chinese Medicinal Herb Farm is a picture of calm. Here on a ten-acre plot of land in Petaluma, California, rows of lush dān shēn are just going to seed while green fragrant shrubs scent the wind as it blows toward Sonoma Valley. Chinese, Ayurvedic, and other Asian medicinal herbs are growing in loosely cultivated rows and flourishing under the strong sun. The blue sky, soaring hawks, and golden hills mix into a heady brew that makes visitors reconsider their occupation.

In the midst of this bucolic scene, farm owner Peg Schafer is a whirlwind. She blows in and out of the farm office, holding her work gloves in one hand and sun hat in the other as she directs interns, moves seed bins, and answers questions from visitors about her farm and educational efforts. Each day requires this kind of energy from the woman who is not only bringing quality Chinese medicinal herbs to market but also raising awareness about the plight of endangered wild medicinal herbs. Peg's business associate, herbalist Sean Fannin of Fu Tian Herbs, is present as well—serving as foil to her dynamism with quiet, measured observations from an herbalist's point of view.

Together, Schafer and Fannin are working to bring organic, locally grown medicinal herbs to the Oriental medicine (OM) community in the United States. After starting her farm in 1997 with just a few herbs, Schafer now contract grows more than forty different varieties (while keeping several hundred in the farm's collection).

Many of these herbs are processed into extracts and other products through Fu Tian Herbs.

For Schafer and Fannin, however, the reasons for farming and selling medicinal herbs go much deeper than a desire to make a profession out of personal interest. Schafer continually emphasizes that growing medicinal herbs in a sustainable manner is a healing endeavor not just for the intended users but for the plants and the environment as a whole. "Overharvesting of medicinal herbs in China and increasing use worldwide are bringing things to a crisis. We will not have enough herbs for the world," she emphasizes. "Many of the herbs in China are harvested in the wild and are not cultivated. So if we want to use these herbs worldwide we're going to have to start cultivating them."

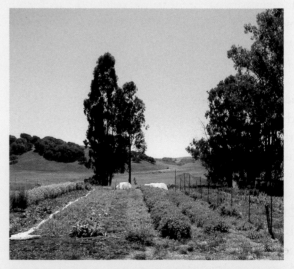

One-hundred-foot rows of mixed Chinese herbs being grown at the Chinese Medicinal Herb Farm.

notice this phenomenon in your home medicine chest: commercial herbal formulas are increasingly making the most of the world's pharmacopeias. Some commercial Western "wellness formulas" include the Chinese herbs *Isatis indigotica* or *I. tinctoria* (woad, běi bǎn lán gēn), which is used for its antiviral properties, and *Astragalus membranaceus* (milk vetch, huáng qí) and *Eleutherococcus senticosus* (eleuthero, cì wǔ jiā)—both of which are used for their immune-enhancing capabilities. Ashwagandha is one example of an herb that has crossed over from the herbal tradition of India into common usage in Western and Chinese herbalism. Ashwagandha is historically one of the most important herbs in Ayurveda, where it is considered a strengthening tonic. It has been adopted by Chinese herbal practitioners as an herb that tonifies (strengthens or supplements) without creating an undesired condition referred to as heat. Many herbalists consider the properties of Ashwagandha to be ginsenglike in quality without the associated heating qualities. Some formulas for joint health include Ashwagandha as well as turmeric (*Curcuma longa*), which is known for its anti-inflammatory action.

It makes sense that we should utilize the gathering knowledge of what nature and every cultural tradition has to offer. We can think of all these herbs as the world's medicine chest.

What Herb Consumers Want

Herbalists and medicine makers as well as herb end users want vibrant, effective, and clean medicine. Thus, they seek fresh and freshly dried Chinese herbs grown without pesticides, herbicides, and other possible contaminants. Driven by market demand and fueled by negative media reports about Chinese herbal products, progressive Chinese herbal practitioners and end users of Chinese herbs are keen to find better quality herbs.

Domestically cultivated medicinal herbs grown with integrity in healthy ecosystems exhibit a freshness and vitality that is apparent. Organoleptic, or sensory, analysis demonstrably shows the exceptional quality of such herbs— how the herb looks, tastes,

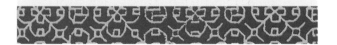

"Adopted" Chinese Herbs

Not all "Chinese" botanicals are indigenous to China; in the past thousand years or so many have been adopted from other regions. One of the most revered in China is *Panax quinquefolius* (American ginseng, xī yáng shēn), which is indigenous to the Appalachian Mountains. A few other herbs commonly used in Chinese medicine that evolved outside China include *Carthamus tinctorius* (safflower, hóng huā), *Celosia argentea* (qīng xiāng zǐ), and *C. cristata* (cockscomb, jī guān huā).

and smells indicates the vital qi (chi) inherent in the herb. A simplified definition of qi is the life force or essence that permeates the whole body and indeed the entire cosmos. Biochemical analyses of domestic herbs have clearly shown that medicinal phytochemicals required in quality products are more than accounted for.[1] (For a more thorough exploration of herb quality issues, see chapter 2.)

RISKS TO THE FUTURE OF HERBALISM

The effectiveness of Chinese herbal medicine has led to a global explosion of interest in Chinese herbs. In the United States this is partly in response to the national health care crisis. And throughout the developed world, many people are finding that serving as laboratory rats for the pharmaceutical industry is not in their best interest and are returning to an enduring and more natural healing model. For peoples that have an intact herbal tradition such as those in China and India, the high cost of pharmaceuticals often precludes their use—and herbs are the de facto

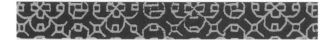

Asian Medicine

The ancient art of Asian medicine is a comprehensive health care system integrating the wholeness of the mind, body, and spirit. It encompasses, as many of you may already know, herbology, acupuncture, massage, and organized movement practices—as well as the incorporation of other methodologies of maintaining harmony. Historically the utilization of foods and herbs was the primary instrument for supporting balance and health.

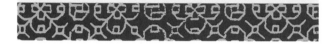

medicine of choice. This is true for many other indigenous cultures worldwide as well.

Globally speaking, if we are not careful to cultivate these herbs we are using in ever-greater quantities, there is a very strong potential that we will lose more of nature's herbal gifts to commercial or actual extinction.[2] Let's look at the market and production factors that threaten medicinal herbs.

Loss of Habitat and Unsustainable Wild-Collecting Practices

Climate change and loss of habitat are other major issues threatening the availability of these valued herbs. In China the majority of herbs are still collected from the wild; increased harvesting to meet demand is placing pressure on the natural reserves of China, and 15–20 percent of these herbs are now considered endangered.[3] See chapter 5 for a full discussion of these global problems.

Quality Concerns

As botanicals from all over the world come into U.S. markets, concerns about quality, contamination, correct identification, availability, and substitutions

of one herb for another continue to plague the herbal import industry.[4] The further afield herbs originate, the longer the supply chain—and more inherent the risks due to distance and the differences in standards and practices in herb production and handling.

Contamination is another potentially serious problem; U.S. consumers are questioning the cleanliness of crops that are not grown domestically. When a wholesale herb importer approached me about growing Chinese herbs for his business, I asked him why he was not interested in using his usual organic Chinese sources. He answered that he was indeed receiving herbs being grown organically in China; however, during routine testing they continually showed pesticide contamination. (There are many possible sources of contamination of organically grown crops, including uncontrolled pesticide drift or contaminants in the air, water, or soil.)

Rising Costs, Rising Prices

Worldwide, the cost of the majority of Chinese medicinal plants has increased sharply over the past few years. Over the next few years prices are expected to continue to rise another 30 percent.[5] Rising costs are the result of many factors. One factor is product shortages, which may result from ecological disasters, the use of herbs to treat widespread epidemics, and Chinese stockpiling practices. Other factors within China that are pushing prices higher include inflation and a growing middle class that is purchasing more and more herbs. Prices also rise as medicinal herbs are brought into cultivation because herb farming is a more costly means of production than wild-harvesting. And because labor rates are also on the rise, the costs of production of cultivated herbs will likely continue to increase. [6]

SOLUTIONS FOR CONTINUED AVAILABILITY

Despite the challenges we face in ensuring a viable future for Chinese medicinal herbs, I am optimistic about the outlook. There is hope for the continued availability of these valuable medicinal resources, especially if we look to sustainable wild-collection practices of Asian herbs coupled with the implementation of ecologically based agriculture. In conjunction with this, consumers worldwide will have to recognize the true cost and expense of producing these unique (and often long-term) crops—or farmers will not be able to afford to grow at least some of these herbs. We need to educate consumers to accept and support fair pricing reflecting the costs of production, and this is covered in more detail in chapter 4.

For cultivation as a whole to be successful in the United States *and* in China, all farmers must grow in a way that produces good quality, medicinally efficacious herbs—and create enough supply to satisfy market demand. Quantity alone is not sufficient; a reputation of poor-quality herbs will kill any potential emerging market opportunities and create further demands for wild-collected herbs.

Accessibility concerns due to extreme weather events, ecological disasters, import or export bans, or potential tariffs make it sound reasoning to spread out the risk of herb loss and cultivate in many locations. This is good news for small farmers in North America and beyond. The more farmers that choose to grow Chinese medicinal herbs in diverse habitats, the better. Chinese medicinal herbs encompass an extremely diverse set of plants with varying environmental niches. Whether you hope to grow Chinese herbs in California, Florida, or New York, you'll find plants that can thrive in your climate.

My Part of the Solution

Since 1997, my farm, the Chinese Medicinal Herb Farm, has specialized in certified organically grown Chinese, Ayurvedic, and other Asian medicinal field-grown herbs and seeds. I also happily cultivate future growers through our internship and other programs. The goal, indeed the mission, is to grow the highest quality herbs with the best medicinal value possible. Here on the farm in the coastal foothills in the northern reaches of the San Francisco Bay area, my crew and I grow sustainably—striving to produce herbs with wild qualities and in a harmony with nature that guides us and helps us feel good about what we do and how we do it. Operating partly as an experimental farm, we have grown and harvested more than 250 Asian botanicals. These botanicals are grown and harvested according to Chinese tradition. Aromatic herbs still carry their distinct scents, leaves tend to be unbroken, colors are vibrant; integrity is present.

At first we conducted multiple herb cultivation trials and recorded data for cost analysis for each herb as it applies to the methods and management at this particular farm. As this data is starting to come into focus, we are branching out into organoleptic and biochemical analysis—with the collaboration of knowledgeable individuals, schools, grant opportunities, and herb industry businesses.

Of all the many jobs I've had, this is the only one where people often thank me for what I do. It is my living, but it is also my service—my personal way of a right livelihood, trying to be part of the solution. I am grateful that I have had the opportunity, and I invite you to participate in the journey.

CHAPTER TWO

Herb Quality

This chapter is about building bridges. All who participate in Asian herbal medicine can—with an open mind—gain understanding from one another and the body of knowledge that each values. I hope you find it thought-provoking and inspiring to reach across the invisible boundaries of language and science. The world is a dynamic place, and so is the rapidly changing realm of herbal medicine.

The essence of the matter is that it does matter how and where the herbs were grown; whether wild-harvested, grown with wild qualities, or as a genetically altered herb in a conventional agricultural operation. The qualities present can be measured organoleptically or by chemical evaluation. There may be an herb industry category of "cut and sifted," but read on; the matter of herb quality is certainly not cut-and-dried.

WILD QUALITY

Most of the herbs used in traditional Asian herbal medicinal systems are still collected from wild stands in China. Why is there a demand for wild-crafted botanicals over cultivated? Herbalists understand that stresses from uneven water, nutrient availability, and insect and herbivore presence all elicit responses in the plants that amplify their medicinal value. Field-grown plants may not undergo such stresses if they are pampered too much, but research shows it is possible to simulate wild conditions in plant responses even in cultivated plants:

> Medicinal properties in plants are mainly due to the presence of secondary metabolites which the plants need in their natural environments under particular conditions of stress and competition and which perhaps would not be expressed under monoculture conditions. Active ingredient levels can be much lower in fast growing cultivated stocks, whereas wild populations can be older and due to slow growth rates and other stressors can have higher levels of active ingredients. While it can be presumed that cultivated plants are likely to be somewhat different in their properties from those gathered from their natural habitats, it is also clear that certain values in plants can be deliberately enhanced under controlled conditions of cultivation.[7]

As discussed in chapter 1, the result of long-term wild-collection practices in China is that the very survival of some herbs is threatened. The only way that Chinese herbal medicine will be able to continue into the future, while still maintaining high quality standards, is through the development of sustainable harvesting practices and the cultivation of wild-quality herbs in diverse locations around the world. Therefore, in cultivation, the goal is to attempt to reproduce the conditions found in the natural environment. Growing herbs in as natural a way as possible—with somewhat lean soils, low inputs of fertilizer and amendments, and diversified plantings—is called wild-simulated cultivation. Farmers and gardeners mimic nature by growing plants that are suited to the site or location, with the conviction that plants experience fewer problems when they grow within their comfort zone. It also means that some stress pressures are allowed. Wild-simulated cultivation has the potential to produce herbs that can be more medicinally effective than conventionally cultivated plant material. Growing herbs with wild simulation takes many forms, and it is a decidedly more hands-off approach—each growing location will have its own parameters; see chapter 3 for more information on these unique techniques.

Another key factor is polyculture, the basis for sound wild simulation. Whether forest-grown, hedgerow-grown, garden-grown, or field-grown, herbs placed in association with other plants experience synergistic environmental effects—aiding in pollination and providing diverse habitats for soil organisms, insects, and other critters.

Polycultural intercropping brings balance by way of diversification: below-ground soil biology and above-ground pollinators and other life forms all work together to enhance the whole system—including the medicinal plants. It contrasts with conventional production growing, which tends to place like species of plants together.

Concerns about Quality of Cultivated Herbs

Botanical prescriptions are traditionally linked with the original growing locations of the herbs. Historically the term *dao di yao cai*, or "authentic

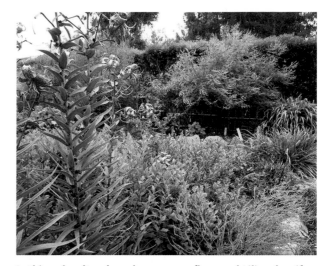

In this polycultural garden, orange-flowered *Lilium lancifolium* (Lily, bǎi hé) shares a bed with grasslike *Coix lacrymajobi* (Job's tears, yì yǐ rén) and *Chrysanthemum morifolium* (Mum, jú huā). All are suitable companions for the purple-flowered *Vitex negundo* (huáng jīng zǐ) tree at the garden's boundary.

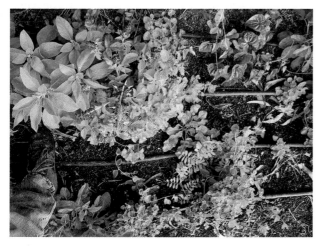

Four crops are interplanted in this bed (clockwise from top left): *Withania somnifera* (Ashwagandha), *Salvia miltiorrhiza* (red sage, dān shēn), shiny heart-shaped leaves of *Dioscorea opposita* (Chinese yam, shān yào), and *Codonopsis pilosula* (poor man's ginseng, dǎng shēn).

region medicinal products," describes this connection between herbal quality and geographical origin. An example of this would be the best quality of *Schisandra chinensis* (Five flavored fruit, wǔ wèi zǐ), considered to be from Manchuria in northeast China. However, as herbs are coming under cultivation more frequently in China, they are sometimes being farmed in locations and under conditions that differ from their endemic sites, since "as long as the nature of the *dao di* species is known, there is no reason why they cannot be reproduced in agricultural fields."[8] Growing location alone is no longer a reliable indicator of *dao di* if cultivation techniques produce only the look but not the quality of the supply. Herbs grown according to the industrial model of monocropping—where extensive fertilizers, pesticides, herbicides, or amendments have been applied—generally make for large crop yields but poor-quality medicine. Herbs are not vegetable crops—if grown luxuriously with excessive inputs, they become less potent. This, in part, may be the root of the bias against cultivated herbs—though there is some good wild-quality *Schisandra chinensis* (Five flavored fruit, wǔ wèi zǐ) being grown in the northeastern United States.

ASSESSING HERB QUALITY

Domestically produced herbs range in quality from very good to very poor, just the same as herbs from Asia. What makes the difference in the quality of an herb? Several areas must be evaluated. The first question to answer is whether the herb in question is authentic: is it in fact what it is labeled, and not either an adulterant (a "fake") or a substitution (an actual medicinal herb, but not the species labeled)? Nomenclature issues for medicinal herbs are problematic and continue to be in flux. There are diverse groups of people involved in the different fields of medicinal herbs, and each tends to hold onto their particular well-entrenched lexicon. Using botanical names is the most reliable way to identify specific medicinal plants—because generally there is only one name for a plant; however, it behooves each of us to reach across our particular field of knowledge and engage with other terminologies.

- Botanical names, which are used worldwide, are the most reliable way to reference specific medicinal herbs, but even botanical names occasionally change. For example, *Polygonum multiflora* (Fo Ti, shǒu wū/yè jīao téng) has received the new botanical moniker *Fallopia multiflora*. Both of these genus names will be used for many years to come.
- Medicinal pinyin names—which are the transliterations of Chinese characters—describe only the processed medicinal herb part itself and do not indicate specific plants; there can be one pinyin name with different regional origins describing different herbal medicines—and referring to different plants as well. One such example is shān cí gū, which can either be an orchid of the *Cremastra* or *Pleione* genuses or a different plant with completely different action, *Asarum sagittarioides*.[9] Pinyin medicinal herb names are problematic and unreliable for identification of medicinal plants due to more than one plant having the same name, exclusivity to China, and regional variability within China.
- Pharmaceutical names use some or all of the Latin-based genus and then indicate the part used. For example, Codonopsis Radix: *Codonopsis* is the genus and *Radix* indicates root. If used alone the pharmaceutical name may or may not indicate which species; the *Codonopsis* example is common and does not carry the species name—and is therefore not helpful in referencing a specific plant, of which there are a couple of standard and many more regionally commonly used species.
- Common names tend to be regional and are the least dependable of all. If one considers all the different languages and regional dialects throughout Asia there can easily be more than a dozen common names for just one medicinal plant. Asian herbal medicine is imprecise partly because Asia is vast and has a long history of regionally specific herbal medicine use—even within China itself.

Authenticity alone is not enough to guarantee quality. As herbs become scarcer, their genetic diversity—and thus their efficacy—is limited. In addition, wild herbs are sometimes collected when immature and outside of their traditional harvest times, resulting in unexpected chemical profiles or variable clinical outcomes.[10] Was the herb old enough when harvested to gather enough active compounds to impart to the end user?[11] Was the herb harvested at the correct traditional season (keeping in mind that chemical components change within the life cycles of plants), and was it harvested properly? How fresh is it? Freshness, if nothing else, has a profound effect on herb efficacy. Herbs are dried more for shipping long distances than is the custom for herbs that remain in China. Finally, chemical treatment is common for long distance shipping and preservation; sulfur is the most common treatment used for exported herbs. Sulfur, a frequent allergen, is itself considered a

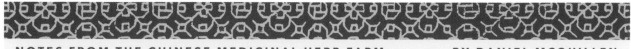

Connecting to Oriental Medicine Students

Herbalist Sean Fannin would like to see a whole superstructure of support that would link herb farmers to buyers, processors, practitioners, and finally end users. Focusing on the OM community, Fannin is working to build connections between growers like Peg Schafer and practitioners throughout the United States. "The relationship between herb growers and practitioners is starting to change. Our idea is to have a joining together of the grower, the practitioner, and the patient, so everybody is working together along the same lines—which is of course toward the individual's health, but also the health of the community and the health of the planet as a whole."

For OM students, working with living plants and the people who grow them adds an entirely new level to their appreciation of medicinal herbs. This is a crucial part of becoming a good herbalist, says Fannin. "As a student you should be around the herbs at every stage. See them in their living state. See them when they're harvested. See them when they're processed." He says that in tasting fresh herbs, you can get a better understanding of quality: "Not just the flavor but the inherent quality. When you taste it you assimilate it, and you can start to get knowledge of the herb. And you just don't

get that as much from dried herbs. You have to really chew on them!" The more you understand the herb, he adds, the easier it is to know how to apply them.

Farming with the wild is a natural—almost unavoidable—approach if the end goal is superior herbs, adds Fannin. "We look at health within the body and it's always about living in accordance with nature: having the right movements and the right nourishments. We are a microcosm of what is in nature," he stresses. Therefore, if the herbs are cultivated in accordance with nature they should have good qi and good taste, the traditional indicators of the function and quality of a Chinese medicinal herb. "And they do," he concludes.

For those students who don't have access to an herb farm, Peg Schafer offers a few tips. First, get the book *Herbal Emissaries* by Steven Foster and Yue Chongxi. Then, pick an herb of personal interest and find out the requirements for growing it—"There is a Chinese herb for every location: wet, dry, high elevation, and so on." There are vines, trees, succulents, garden-worthy perennials, and even incredibly ugly plants to choose from. Finally, start small and grow from there.

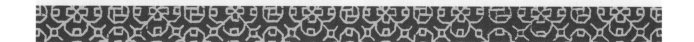

functional herb and therefore becomes an unwanted addition to anyone using the herbs. Though it is possible, I cannot verify if bulk herbs receive any treatment upon arrival in U.S. ports. Keep in mind that the distance travelled, country of origin, and the amount of regulatory compliance are all factors when assessing herb quality and supply chain risks.[12]

Traditional Physical Testing Methods

Two traditional methods of determining herb quality and potency are through physical tests of macroscopic and organoleptic analysis—i.e., using the senses to identify the characteristic values, flavors, and functions. These methods are ideal for assessing identity and quality. Organoleptic examination of the whole herb by trained herbalists is the basis of the original discovery of Chinese medicines and was further developed into the extensive methodological system that exists today. To apply organoleptics to the equation, we may ask whether an aromatic herb still carries the tastes and aromas specified by the materia medicas (authoritative reference books about the therapeutic use of medicinal substances), and thus the called-for function. Can you sense the vital qi, or potency, of the herb?

Chemical Testing Methods

In addition to the physical tests of organoleptic methodologies, the scientific approach of laboratory evaluation to determine herbal identity, the presence or lack of expected chemical components, and biological activity—as well as pesticide, heavy metal, and microbiological screening—are becoming commonplace as good manufacturing practices (GMPs) become fully integrated. These techniques are important tools, especially in an evidence-based culture; however, be aware that GMPs do not address nor consider herb effectiveness. Agricultural suppliers are not obligated by regulation to comply; but it is in the interests of growers to assist herb buyers and product makers wherever possible. There are dozens of testing procedures that can be done—including some basic and easy to manage in-house microbiological methods testing for molds, yeasts and total bacteria,

E. coli, and salmonella. For herb identification, quality, and purity, common tests include microscopy, thin layer chromatography (TLC), high performance liquid chromatography (HPLC), and gas chromatography/mass spectrometry. There are many other tests that can be used as well.

As a small grower, I cannot afford to do lab testing of the herbs I grow as it is very expensive. To my knowledge, larger growers conduct some of the nonchemically oriented tests, such as those for bacteria.

REGULATING HERBS

To promote the correct cultivation of herbs, farmers utilize certified organic (or even more stringent) guidelines, along with Good Agricultural Practices (GAPs)—standards of regulations that the Food and Agriculture Organization of the United Nations describes as "addressing environmental, economic and social sustainability for on-farm production and post-production processes resulting in safe and healthy food and non-food agricultural products."[13] At this time it should be noted that GAPs are new to the United States and China, and are not fully integrated in either country (GAPs are discussed in more detail in chapter 4). In the interim, for quality assurance, the transparency of harvest information and traceability of origin (two GAP criteria) are important safety features that U.S. cultivators should provide to buyers—along with other information, either in the form of a Certificate of Analysis (COA) or an herb specification sheet. A COA is a document that all herb manufacturers and pharmacies should be able to supply to consumers. The information provided varies according to the tests conducted. At minimum the documents should have the genus and species, origin, date and part harvested, and lot number—as well as the date tested, plant part and form of the herbal material, organoleptic and microbiological results, and pesticide as well as heavy metal figures. Identification and qualitative data are sometimes also available.

Growers can offer herb specification sheets to supply descriptive information to customers looking for transparency. Minimum information provided should be genus and species, origin, plant part and date harvested, and lot number. Occasionally organoleptic characterization as well as microbiological testing information may be available. Botanicals typically change hands many times in the supply chain from distant harvesters/farmers to domestic end users; it should be remembered that the less often this takes place, the fewer quality control issues of transparency and traceability will arise.

The best way to regulate quality and control the purity of agricultural goods is through certified organic grown products. For a farm product to be sold in the United States as certified organic, it must be inspected by a third party agency that abides by the guidelines of the National Organic Program (NOP) and grants certification. Regarding the spirit of organic production, there is room for improvement with the NOP ruling; nonetheless, currently American agricultural goods are widely known to be in much better compliance than Asian products. Heavy metals, pesticide residues, and contamination continue to be problematic with both cultivated and wild-harvested Chinese herbs. For the good of all, this is an issue that hopefully will be resolved as soon as possible, but it can be avoided by purchasing certified organic U.S.-grown botanicals when available.

There are many movements afoot as alternatives to the certified organic status gained by the NOP. A couple of reasons some of them exist are because it is felt that the NOP ruling is not holistic or stringent enough in holding to a higher standard or philosophy; others feel it costs too much money to get or maintain certification. These are valid concerns—every grower must decide for him- or herself. However, use of the wording "certified organic" or "organic" to market products is not allowed unless one is participating in the NOP program.

Genetically Modified Herbs

There is also a concern regarding the encroachment of genetically modified organisms (GMOs) currently being developed in China to alter medicinal herbs for subsequent—and unfortunately undisclosed—release into the herbal medicine trade. These

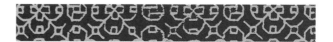

Cloned Herbs

Cloned medicinal herbs produced in China are a recent introduction throughout the world via the regular herb market channels. This practice runs contrary to the history that forms the empirical knowledge on which all Chinese medicine is based, and again brings up questions of genetic diversity and wild-simulation. Cloning is a narrowing of genetic stock and as a practice is the antithesis of the basic concept of balance and harmonious interaction with the environment. Two examples of this are *Trichosanthes kirilowii* (Chinese cucumber, guā lóu/tiān huā fěn) and *Gastrodia elata* (tiān má). Scientists have developed a method to produce these herbs through a process called tissue culture. In this process cells from a plant that has some desired quality are laboratory cultured and mass produced to make exact genetic replicas. However Frankensteinish, cloning is not necessarily an undesirable technique; the *Trichosanthes* cloned tissue culture was introduced for faster profit. Introduction of cloned *Gastrodia* is an attempt to address an accessibility issue, because *Gastrodia* is endangered in the wild. The labeling of either cloned or genetically modified herbs is not currently mandated.

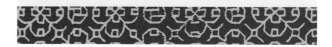

bioengineering techniques dictate gene expression, and by default will alter the nature of the herbs. Their (largely pharmaceutical originated) goal is to boost levels of what are currently thought to be the active ingredients. In the process, however, known or unknown therapeutically active compounds will be changed, simply because transgenic techniques alter basic inherited characteristics. Chinese medicine has an exquisitely refined logic that is centuries old, with an elegant system of relationships between herbs, and the question arises: do we want lab scientists to decide for us what traits are desirable (or undesirable) in our medicines? This is not to malign progress or the scientific community; in fact, the scientific principle of precaution is a good standard to apply to this virtually unknown realm.

The use of GMOs and clonal techniques contrasts sharply with traditional plant breeding and with the effort to maintain genetic stock with wild qualities. Besides the issues of restricting or adding material inputs, an important aspect of protection of wild quality entails purposefully keeping the gene pool diverse. Cultivating and selecting seed from as many plants as possible, therefore allowing for a wide variety of genetic expression (and thus chemical components) to be present, benefits both the herb user and the germplasm. As the herbs develop over generations in the same location, they take on the unique qualities of that place that impart subtle differences as expressed by the *dao di yao cai*. However, plants are not bound by national borderlines; they are dynamic and ever-changing wherever they grow in this great big world. To illustrate this point, we only need to look at the well-documented example of the cabernet grape, which when grown in Napa or Sonoma County in California will express characteristics that are slightly different from the same grape stock grown in the Bordeaux region of France.

LIKE FINE WINES . . .

So how is it that domestically grown Chinese herbs differ from their Chinese grown or wild-harvested counterparts? They are like many paradigms; the same, but different. There was a time, not long ago, that the French thought that farmers growing wine grapes in California were misguided, and that fine wine was produced only in Europe. It took a few years, but the day came when California wines surprised the old-world viticulture industry by winning international

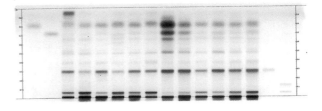

These are the results from a high performance thin layer chromatographic (HPTLC) analysis of *Salvia miltiorrhiza* (red sage, dān shēn) roots grown in different regions of the world. Work conducted by Camag, Muttenz, Switzerland courtesy of the American Herbal Pharmacopoeia, Scotts Valley, California. Image and table courtesy of Bill Schoenbart.

wine competitions. These days, California is a recognized and respected producer in the world of viticulture. Australia, South Africa, South America, and other regions are also coming into play with some distinguished high quality wines of their own. There is no reason why Chinese herbs grown outside of China cannot achieve the same level of success.

Every region and indeed every farm location has its own particular combination of air, soil composition, water, and other unique components. These qualities are expressed in the character of each harvested herb. For example, one herb that responds well to the inherent conditions at the Chinese Medicinal Herb Farm is *Salvia miltiorrhiza* (red sage, dān shēn). An analysis using high performance thin layer chromatography (HPTLC) compared some herb-specific common marker chemical profiles of root samples from my farm and several other sources. The report that accompanied the analysis concludes that "Dān Shēn (*Salvia miltiorrhiza*) can be successfully grown outside of China with organic agricultural methods. The harvested roots appear to have high levels of known bioactive compounds. This has positive implications for the environment, both in the reduction of pesticide and synthetic fertilizer usage, and in reducing pressure on Chinese agricultural land due to increased demand for Chinese herbs worldwide."[14] It continues:

> In the HPTLC analysis, Lanes 9 and 10 represent samples of Dān Shēn roots

Table 2-1. Key to HPTLC Analysis of Salvia miltiorrhiza root		
Lane #	Component	Source
Lane 1	Tanshinone I, tanshinone IIA (with increasing Rf)	
Lane 2	Dihydrotanshinone, cryptotanshinone (with increasing Rf)	
Lane 3	Salvia miltiorrhiza root	Tablet product (expired 2011)
Lane 4	Salvia miltiorrhiza root	Hong Kong herb market, 2002
Lane 5	Salvia miltiorrhiza root	Taiwan herb market, 2003
Lane 6	Salvia miltiorrhiza root	San Francisco Chinatown market, 2005
Lane 7	Salvia miltiorrhiza root	San Francisco Chinatown market, 2005
Lane 8	Salvia miltiorrhiza root	San Francisco Chinatown market, 2006
Lane 9	Salvia miltiorrhiza root	Freshly harvested and dried specimen from organic herb farm in Petaluma, California, 2007
Lane 10	Salvia miltiorrhiza root	Dried sample from organic herb farm in Petaluma, California, 2006
Lane 11	Salviae miltiorrhizae radix	Sample from analytical lab; source unknown
Lane 12	Salviae miltiorrhizae radix	Sample from analytical lab; source unknown
Lane 13	Salviae miltiorrhizae radix	Sample from analytical lab; source unknown
Lane 14	Salvia miltiorrhiza Bunge	Sample from analytical lab; source unknown
Lane 15	Salvianolic acid	
Lane 16	Rutin, hyperoside	
© 2011 Bill Schoenbart		

obtained from the Chinese Medicinal Herb Farm in Petaluma, California. They were grown with certified organic agricultural methods. Lane 9 represents roots harvested in 2007, and Lane 10 represents dried roots harvested in 2006. It can be seen that the bands representing the bioactive tanshinones and salvianolic acid are qualitatively similar to and quantitatively more dense than the samples collected from various herb suppliers (Lanes 3–8, 11–14). This indicates that the Dān Shēn roots grown locally with organic methods met or exceeded the quality of Dān Shēn roots purchased from typical suppliers of Chinese herbs. The sample from the most recent harvest showed the highest level of bioactive compounds, possibly due to its freshness, demonstrating another advantage of growing herbs locally. Future studies should use a larger number of domestic samples, and attempts should be made to acquire Chinese sample material from the most recent harvest.

CHAPTER THREE

Cultivation in the Nursery, Garden, and Field

Growing medicinal herbs is less resource intensive than producing vegetables, allowing farmers and gardeners to experiment outside the conventional models. New opportunities arise for locations and situations that are not necessarily thought of as traditional farmland. Where soils are not depleted try no-till or low-tillage techniques. Where soils are heavy with clay, consider potential opportunities for dryland farming. Where you have forest cover, try shade-loving herb interplantings. High altitude and other niche spaces might be able to support medicinal herb production—this requires gentle handling to avoid overusing the land. Whatever cultivation methods you decide to explore, remember that we are all in this for the long haul; organic, ecological, and sustainable growing techniques support a vibrant soil biology and nurture those who receive and use the plants.

This chapter is all about those sustainable techniques for growing herbs, starting right from the beginning with choosing or evaluating a site and deciding what to grow. Gardeners and beginners as well as seasoned growers will find useful information that covers all aspects of the nursery and propagation, moving into the field with soil and pest management, planting, and seasonal care right up to harvest time. There are many charts to guide you to where you want to go—quickly.

PLANNING

Everything starts with an idea, and the idea then develops into a plan. Every growing location is different; climate zones, soils, plants, cultivation techniques, and many other factors will determine the methodologies and outcomes of each garden, minifarm, urban farm, or larger operation. A grower needs patience, the ability to be observant, and the willingness to experiment—and record-keeping tools are a must. Each seed and plant has a built-in desire to grow—so you already have help! Here are some strategies to help you plan on realizing your success.

To achieve balance and more success in the garden or farm follow the path of least resistance and mimic nature. In terms of cultivation, it is to our advantage that North America and China (and some other regions of Asia) share the same general latitude and some similar climate zones. These similarities make it feasible to successfully cultivate the many varieties of Asian herbs domestically in the different appropriate climates available in the United States. A good place to start is to match your location with the growing area of China that shares the same latitude. To do this, you can use the overlay map of China and the United States in appendix B at the back of the book. Next, determine the USDA hardiness zone for the land that you will be cultivating; appendix B also includes a USDA Hardiness Zone Map and a China Hardiness Zone Map.

Now you must decide which herbs are best suited to the land in question. Over the years Jean Giblette (High Falls Gardens, New York), Joe Hollis (Mountain Gardens, North Carolina), and I have assessed the general regional adaptability of the herbs I have profiled in part 2, and the chart entitled Regional Adaptability of Chinese Medicinal Herbs is a summary. If an herb is listed for your region, that herb is potentially a good fit for your farm or garden. Plants that grow especially well in a particular region are noted in bold red letters. For example, *Anemarrhena asphodeloides* (zhī mǔ) has a large geographic distribution and indeed performs well here at the Chinese Medicinal Herb Farm. Note that this regional chart includes only four regions: the Pacific Northwest, the Southwest, the Southeast, and the Northeast. That's because Chinese medicinal herbs are not yet in cultivation in the central United States, and thus I had no one to consult with on plant performance there. Keep in mind, too, that your local climate conditions will affect what you can grow, and that not all plants marked as suitable for your region will grow equally well in your particular site and soil.

Sometimes it will also be helpful to know the general climatic conditions in China and relate them to either your U.S. growing locale or the particular herb itself. See the Climate and Precipitation Map of China in the maps section for this information. Also, the China Province Map will assist growers in relation to assessing regional suitability and forming contextual relationships with the herbs. For example, if you read that Yunnan is a major source of a certain herb of interest it is handy to know where the province is. I have this province map posted on my office wall and frequently refer to it. There are also several materia medicas that I highly recommend (some are in the recommended books list); take care to refer to the place of origin for herbs in terms of provinces.

Land and Botanical Inventories

Charts and maps, along with the individual herb profiles in part 2, are basic for determining which herbs to grow in almost any U.S. situation. The next step is to learn more about the particular characteristics of your site by conducting a land inventory. To start, take a closer look at the soil of your location. Soil survey data are available from the USDA Natural Resources Conservation Service (NRCS) for almost all of the land in the United States, either online or on paper in county libraries. The paper copies are reference materials only and have more, but potentially outdated, information. For the online version of the Web Soil Survey (WSS), see http://websoilsurvey.nrcs.usda.gov/app. It is easy to use, and the online version can be accessed by entering your physical street address (the hardcopy version requires an assessor's parcel number). This data

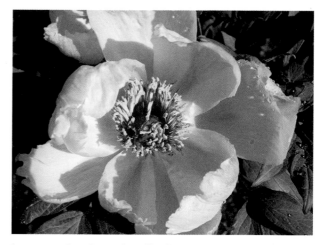

In most regions *Paeonia suffruticosa* (tree peony, mǔ dān pí) requires afternoon shade.

discloses types of soil, rainfall, drainage, and slopes— as well as other useful information.

I highly recommend professional soil testing rather than a do-it-yourself soil test kit. Farm supply companies catering to certified organic growers often offer this service, or check with your county government or extension office for a nearby laboratory. Results will take a few weeks. Make sure to inform them that you're requesting recommendations for an organic herb operation; otherwise they might recommend synthetic fertilizers in quantities targeted for the majority of growers who are cultivating vegetables, which have higher nutrient requirements—especially for nitrogen.

Once your soil analysis is underway, continue ahead with the land inventory. With clipboard in hand, make notes about the prospective growing area. Ask yourself these questions:

- Is it on a slope? If so, facing which direction? Northern facing slopes are cooler and receive less sun than southern or western facing hills. A northern facing slope isn't always a disadvantage. For example, in areas where summers may be hot, a north-facing slope may work well for growing *Paeonia suffruticosa* and *Paeonia lactiflora* (tree peony and Chinese peony, mǔ dān pí and bái/chì sháo) because peonies

Table 3-1. Regional Adaptability of Chinese Medicinal Herbs						
Botanical Name	Common Name	Pinyin	Southeast	Southwest	Northwest	Northeast
Acanthopanax gracilistylus		wŭ jiā pí	SE		NW*	NE*
Achyranthes bidentata	Oxknee	huái niú xī	SE/Invasive*	SW		
Agastache rugosa	Korean Mint	tŭ huò xiāng	SE	SW	NW	NE
Albizia julibrissin	Mimosa	hé huān pí/huā	SE/Invasive*	SW	NW	NE
Alisma plantago-aquatica subsp. *orientale*	Water Plantain	zé xiè	SE*		NW	NE
Allium macrostemon		xiè bái	SE	SW	NW	NE
Allium tuberosum	Garlic Chives	jiŭ cài zĭ	SE	SW	NW	NE
Andrographis paniculata	Kalmegh	chuān xīn lián	SE*	SW		
Anemarrhena asphodeloides		zhī mŭ	SE		NW*	NE*
Angelica dahurica		bái zhĭ	SE		NW	NE*
Angelica pubescens		dú huó	SE*		NW	NE
Angelica sinensis	Dang Gui	dāng guī	SE*	SW	NW	NE
Arctium lappa	Burdock	niú bàng zĭ	SE	SW	NW	NE
Artemisia annua	Sweet Annie	qīng hāo	SE	SW	NW	NE
Asparagus cochinchinensis		tiān mén dōng	SE	SW	NW	NE
Aster tataricus	Tartar Aster	zĭ wăn	SE*	SW	NW	NE
Astragalus membranaceus	Milk Vetch	huáng qí	SE	SW	NW	NE
Atractylodes macrocephala	Chinese Thistle Daisy	bái zhú	SE	SW	NW	
Bacopa monnieri	Brahmi	Brahmi	SE*	SW		
Belamcanda chinensis	Blackberry Lily	shè gān	SE		NW	NE
Bupleurum chinense	Hare's Ear	chái hú	SE*	SW	NW	
Carthamus tinctorius	Safflower	hóng huā	SE	SW*	NW	NE
Celosia argentea		qīng xiāng zĭ	SE	SW	NW	NE
Celosia cristata	Cockscomb	jī guān huā	SE	SW	NW	NE
Centella asiatica	Gotu Kola	jī xuě căo	SE*	SW		
Chrysanthemum morifolium	Mum	jú huā	SE	SW	NW	
Clerodendrum trichotomum	Glorybower	chòu wú tóng	SE		NW	
Codonopsis pilosula	Poor Man's Ginseng	dăng shēn	SE		NW	NE
Coix lacryma-jobi	Job's Tears	yì yĭ rén	SE*	SW		
Cornus officinalis	Dogwood	shān zhū yú	SE	SW	NW	NE
Crataegus pinnatifida	Chinese Hawthorn	shān zhā	SE	SW	NW	NE
Cyathula officinalis	Hookweed	chuān niú xī	SE	SW	NW	
Dianthus superbus	Fringed Pink	qú mài	SE	SW	NW	NE
Dioscorea opposita	Chinese Yam	shān yào	SE/Invasive*	SW/Invasive*	NW	NE
Dolichos lablab	Hyacinth Bean	bái biăn dòu	SE	SW*		
Eclipta prostrata	Eclipta	mò hàn lián	SE/Invasive*		NW	NE
Ephedra sinica	Ephedra	má huáng/má huáng gēn		SW*	NW	
Eriobotrya japonica	Loquat	pí pá yè	SE	SW	NW*	
Eucommia ulmoides	Hardy Rubber Tree	dù zhòng	SE	SW	NW	NE
Fallopia multiflora	Fo Ti	shŏu wū/ yè jīao téng	SE/Invasive*	SW/Invasive*	NW/Invasive*	
Forsythia suspensa		lián qiào	SE	SW	NW	NE
Gentiana scabra		lóng dăn căo			NW*	NE*

Table 3-1 *(continued)*						
Botanical Name	Common Name	Pinyin	Southeast	Southwest	Northwest	Northeast
Gentiana straminea		qín jiāo			NW*	NE*
Ginkgo biloba	Ginkgo	bái guǒ	SE	SW	NW	NE
Glycyrrhiza uralensis	Chinese Licorice	gān cǎo		SW	NW	NE
Gynostemma pentaphyllum	Sweet Tea Vine	jiǎo gǔ lán	SE*		NW*	NE
Houttuynia cordata		yú xīng cǎo	SE/Invasive*		NW	NE
Ligusticum jeholense	Chinese Lovage	gǎo běn	SE	SW	NW	NE
Ligustrum lucidum	Chinese Privet	nǚ zhēn zǐ	SE/Invasive*	SW	NW/Invasive*	
Lilium brownii	Lily	bǎi hé	SE		NW	NE
Lilium lancifolium	Lily	bǎi hé	SE		NW	NE
Lonicera japonica	Honeysuckle	jīn yín huā	SE/Invasive*	SW	NW	NE
Lycium chinense	Chinese Wolfberry	gǒu qǐ zǐ/dì gǔ pí	SE	SW*	NW	
Magnolia denudata		xīn yí huā	SE		NW	NE
Mentha haplocalyx	Field Mint	bò hé	SE	SW	NW	NE
Momordica charantia	Bitter Melon	kǔ guā	SE	SW*		NE
Ocimum sanctum	Sacred Basil	Tulsi	SE*	SW	NW	NE
Ophiopogon japonicus	Lilyturf	mài mén dōng	SE*	SW	NW	
Paeonia lactiflora	Chinese Peony	bái/chì sháo	SE		NW*	NE*
Paeonia suffruticosa	Tree Peony	mǔ dān pí			NW	NE*
Panax ginseng	Asian Ginseng	rén shēn	SE*			
Panax quinquefolius	American Ginseng	xī yáng shēn	SE*			NE*
Pinellia ternata		bàn xià	SE/Invasive*		NW*	NE
Plantago asiatica	Plantain	chē qián zǐ			NW	NE
Platycodon grandiflorus	Balloon Flower	jié gěng	SE	SW	NW	NE
Prunella vulgaris	Heal All	xià kū cǎo	SE/Invasive*		NW	NE
Rehmannia glutinosa	Chinese Foxglove	dì huáng	SE	SW	NW	
Rheum palmatum	Chinese Rhubarb	dà huáng			NW*	NE*
Salvia miltiorrhiza	Red Sage	dān shēn	SE	SW	NW	NE
Saposhnikovia divaricata	Siler	fáng fēng			NW	NE
Schisandra chinensis	Five Flavored Fruit	wǔ wèi zǐ	SE		NW	NE*
Schizonepeta tenuifolia	Japanese Catnip	jīng jiè	SE	SW	NW	NE
Scrophularia buergeriana	Figwort	běi xuán shēn	SE	SW	NW	NE
Scutellaria baicalensis	Baikal Skullcap	huáng qín	SE	SW	NW	NE
Scutellaria barbata	Barbat Skullcap	bàn zhī lián	SE	SW	NW	
Sophora flavescens		kǔ shēn	SE	SW	NW	NE
Trichosanthes kirilowii	Chinese Cucumber	guā lóu/tiān huā fěn	SE	SW	NW	NE
Withania somnifera	Ashwagandha	Ashwagandha	SE	SW*		
Ziziphus jujuba	Chinese Date	dà zǎo	SE	SW*		
Ziziphus jujuba var. *spinosa*		suān zǎo rén	SE	SW*	NW	NE

© 2011 Peg Schafer, Jean Giblette, and Joe Hollis

Note: Due to the great variety of U.S. climates, from mountains to seaside, this list is general in nature; consider it a starting point. Some herbs will do well in some listed areas and not in others.

Key: Asterisk indicates that the herb grows especially well in the region indicated; otherwise the herb is known to grow sufficiently well to produce crops and reproduce.

prefer cool soils and shadier locations—at least at middle to southern latitudes in the United States. On the other hand, at the Chinese Medicinal Herb Farm, where our summers tend to be cool, we can maximize the advantage of our one southern facing slope for crops that are heat loving such as *Ephedra sinica* (ephedra, má huáng/má huáng gēn).

- Are there buildings, or other objects, that may impact the growing area or provide a microclimate? If buildings are old, were they previously painted with lead-based paint? Maybe the building can provide a windbreak to shelter plants. On my farm, a big old stump rests right in the middle of a main row crop area. Our work will be a bit easier someday when that stump finally rots away.
- Consider the water source. Is it well water, pond, or chlorinated city water (all of which can be tested), or is rainfall the only option? The source will often determine the type of irrigation system employed.
- Does the soil drain well? To find out, dig a two-foot-deep hole and fill it with water. Wait for it to drain and fill it with water again. Does it drain in an hour or two, indicating that the soils are well-percolating, or does it just sit there—illustrating a lack of drainage?

After you've evaluated those aspects of your site, examine the plant life in more detail by taking a simple botanical inventory.

- What is already growing on-site? List the plants. If a plant is unknown, clip a portion of it, in flower if possible, and take it to a local nursery, master gardener, or other local horticultural educator for identification. To ensure that your sample will be durable, make an impromptu herbarium sample and apply plant to paper with wide

clear tape. Regional weed guides or books are frequently available either online or at a local bookstore. My favorite for the Western United States is *Weeds of the West* by Tom Whitson, which includes great photos and descriptions of several (invasive) Chinese medicinal plants. Don't forget to make note of trees or a forest with interplanting potential, as well as plants that pose invasive root issues.

- Is there any vegetation at your location that could be wild-harvested for medicine? Some Chinese medicinal herbs are not indigenous to China, and others were introduced to the United States long ago and may be free for the collecting. Refer to the Potentially Invasive Chinese Herbs chart later in this chapter to explore the potential.
- Are the on-site plants predominantly native or introduced? One important reason to make records is to take note of any plants that could genetically contaminate any seed stock you save and potentially render future herbs unsuitable for medicine.

Take special note of any sites on your land that are infested with noxious or invasive weeds. The soil biology in such areas may be compromised and the land difficult to cultivate. These are soils that may have been overgrazed or overused. Is there wide representation of different families or are there only a few kinds of plants present? There are several books on the market that describe specific plant indicators of soil types and soil health.

Deciding What to Grow

One of the most important questions you'll need to answer is which herbs to grow, especially if the plants are unfamiliar to you. Start by doing some research, and consider three things about each plant. First is the suitability of the herb—how well it will thrive where you plan to grow it without it becoming invasive. The second is the ease of harvest and cleaning or drying. Lastly, is there a viable market for the herb? (Each herb profiled in part 2 has a viable market.) Do your research first, but keep in mind that some of these questions can only be answered through growing trials—as described later in this chapter.

As you do your research, you'll discover that sorting out the identity of some Chinese herbs is a taxonomic nightmare. This problem is due in part to early U.S. introductions of plants from China that were labeled with pinyin medicinal names instead of the scientific binomial. People then made the leap—sometimes in the wrong direction. One example I experienced was seed that had been sold as *Baphicacanthus cusia*, but which grew out to be *Isatis tinctoria*—both are source plants of bǎn lán gēn. Sometimes the mix-ups involve plants with different cultural conditions. There are other herbs currently making the rounds that are incorrectly named. Often *Rehmannia elata* is erroneously labeled as dì huáng (which is actually *Rehmannia glutinosa*)—and unfortunately, *R. elata* does not appear to be medicinally viable. Doubly sad, as it is much easier to grow! Plants labeled as sān qī are also in cultivation, shared by well-meaning people excited about growing an important Chinese herb; most frequently the plants turn out to be *Anredera cordifolia*, an adulterant, instead of *Panax notoginseng*. It is best to be watchful as unfortunately there are many such examples.

If your growing location's cultural conditions are optimal for a large selection of herbs and the choices need to be effectively limited, consider growing herbs that together make traditional therapeutic formulas or ones that are important and commonly used. Every year, I continue to ask herbal practitioners what they use the most and what would they buy or be interested in.

Another important factor to keep in mind as you make plant choices is to choose seed or stock that is unselected—i.e., most like the wild, and thus imbued with diverse genetic traits that equal a diverse action or function for the end user. Stock that has been developed for selected traits usually have Latin names with their cultivar names following them (appearing in single quotation marks). For example, *Platycodon*

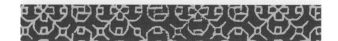

Letting the Land Decide What to Grow

Conversely, perhaps it will be your land itself that will set your limits for herb cultivation. Is it a niche of high mountain, or subtropical, or otherwise unique in nature? If so, targeting herbs that other locales cannot carry, or those considered at risk—which tend to reside in marginal environments—is certainly a marketable opportunity. Some of these endangered herbs are CITES (the Convention on International Trade in Endangered Species of Wild Fauna and Flora) listed (see chapter 5). These unique growing situations will not look like a fence-to-fence conventional agricultural operation; forest interplanting and desert/high altitude farming are more subtle and require a deeper partnership with nature. The stressors of each ecosystem and its UV exposure, weather, soil biology, visiting herbivores, and all the other environmental attributes lead to the expression of medicinal components in the herbs themselves. Farming in atypical locations such as forests and deserts usually requires more land and more time to produce a marketable crop. Farming methods should be low impact, requiring fewer inputs of time and materials. Above all, respect must be paid to these sometimes fragile places.

grandiflorus 'Apoyama' is a variety developed for its short stature—it will not fall over when in bloom like the species stock. There are many hybrids (the offspring produced by genetic combination of dissimilar species or varieties) and many beautiful Chinese herbs that were introduced to the nursery trade as ornamental plants. Among these are the popular ornamentals chrysanthemum, honeysuckle, dianthus, heavenly bamboo, and balloon flower. Many of these were developed for decorative rather than medicinal traits, so be wary of cultivating them for medicine as their genetics are unknown.

When buying seed or planting stock for your garden, nursery, or farming operation, your best bet for finding medicinal stock as opposed to ornamental material is to go through a vendor that is selling to this market (see appendix C at the back of this book for specific vendors). There is still some suitable material to be found in the general nursery trade. Notations in this regard are included in the individual herb profiles. However, it is still a buyer-beware situation—occasionally general nursery stock is sold without indicating it is a cultivar.

It is also best to check the state and federal noxious weed lists to avoid cultivating any pernicious weeds. The USDA NRCS Website http://plants.usda.gov/java/noxiousDriver hosts these noxious weed lists. Remember that the state and county agricultural officials maintain the right to fine growers that cultivate listed noxious weeds. Always monitor the cultivated herbs for qualities that may allow them to become weedy, and curtail their cultivation so as not to introduce an invasive plant.

Conducting Plant Trials

A growing trial is simply a pilot study or a comparison of one method to another, or one variety or species to another. A good place to start is to trial up to fifteen different herbs in your first season. Then build on the successes by adding new herbs each season. Make the trial plan diverse; grow some annuals (usually easiest and fastest), some perennials, and some longer-term perennials and tree crops. Group your production beds, blocks, gardens, or hedgerows by similar cultural (sun, water, and length of growing time) and harvest requirements; see the Harvest chart toward the end of this chapter. This makes for ease of access, especially for a large-scale trial, and will allow you to replenish the soil effectively and efficiently afterward. The size of the trials should

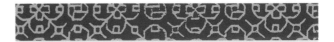

Plant Type Terminology

As a quick review, annuals are plants that live their whole life cycle in one season and can be either warm- or cold-season (hardy) annuals. Biennials spend their first season in vegetative growth and their second getting down to the business of reproduction. Perennials, either herbaceous or woody, live for more than a year (sometimes reproducing in the first year). Don't forget about shrubs and trees—plants that tend to need a longer time frame to produce a crop but which also tend to be the ones that yield for long periods of time and are the lowest maintenance.

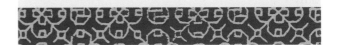

be large enough to be able to effectively measure the outcomes; fifty or one hundred plants would be good. Sometimes reality interferes with your plans—germination of your trial plants may be less than ideal, or you are limited to backyard gardening space constraints. Do what you can.

Common variables to test by running a trial include sun exposure, water and nutrient allotments, interplanting with different crops, and trellising and other training techniques. Then, of course, there are the harvest trials of timing and technique. Two factors I always try to determine through trials is (1) how little interaction can I get away with to produce a viable crop and (2) how few inputs are necessary—just how hands-off can I be?

I've conducted many trials over the years at the Chinese Medicinal Herb Farm. For example, in one trial I investigated how a row crop cover (I used a reinforced white spun bonded polyester brand Agribon) might affect an *Ocimum sanctum* (sacred basil, tulsi) crop. The reason I wanted to conduct this trial is that tulsi, an annual, is endemic to the warm humid areas in and around India—decidedly different from my relatively cool coastal northern California summers. My reasoning was that row crop covers can increase the ambient moisture and heat around a crop. For this trial, we transplanted several hundred greenhouse-started plants into the field and then covered half with the cover; water and other components were equal. We found that the covered crop did produce more volume and weight as a fresh crop, but the crop dried down more by ratio than the smaller but stout uncovered crop. In other words, one pound of fresh material from covered plants yielded a smaller quantity of dry material than one pound of fresh material from uncovered plants. The covered crop was flawlessly beautiful, but it was soft and flaccid and lacked vital qi. Even though temperatures were probably warmer under the cover, the volatile oils were stronger in the exposed tulsi. The only tool I needed for that test was my nose. Other factors contributed to the decision not to use the row cover in future plantings, too. Agribon costs money to purchase and install, frequently gets damaged by high winds, and is not a recycled or recyclable product. I've included the crop-specific information I've gleaned from such trials in the herb profiles in part 2.

A database is a useful tool for evaluating plant trials, and I find that a database is also an essential tool for evaluating changes and modifying my crop management methods. Two kinds of databases are helpful: one to track and manage information and the other to perform spreadsheet calculations. A simple general purpose database might include the following fields:

- Accession number. When you start growing out seed from a source, give it a number, tied to your operation.
- Plant name. Make this the botanical or scientific name.
- Common name. Easy reference.
- Family name. This may aid in cultivation if information is scarce on the genus or species.

- Sown. This field will have all the dates sown for the particular accession.
- Pinyin. This name will come in handy for cross-referencing and interacting with practitioners.
- Date. When the accession was received, quantity of seed or stock, and a physical description.
- Type. Is the accession an annual, perennial, tender perennial, tree, or vine?
- Notes. In this field record transplant dates, if something is deciduous and when it breaks dormancy, when seed was collected and from how many plants, and so on.
- Germination. This field covers days to emergence from sow date, percentage of germination, light or dark requirements, if and what stratification is needed, and best sow dates.
- Field spacing. Listed in spacing by the foot.
- Season to harvest. This field contains the time from transplant to harvest and season of year for harvest as well.
- Harvest. Weight fresh, either per plant or per hundred-foot row.
- Ratio of fresh to dry weight.

There are Asian herbs that grow in just about every environmental situation, and the information gathered in the planning and trial plots will lay the groundwork for success in each unique growing location. Gather your resources, gumption, and spirit—and enjoy your botanical journey.

SEED STARTING AND PROPAGATION

Sowing seeds is kind of magical: put little brown specks in soil, add water, and get a bunch of plants—flowers, fruits, trees, vegetables, and medicine if you please. Propagating by seed continues the evolutionary process by remixing genetics through sexual reproduction. Seed sowing (and subsequent seed saving) is the best method for adapting crops to a specific growing site, which is what I prefer to do here

Table 3-2. Cultural Needs of Chinese Medicinal Herbs								
Botanical Name	Harvest Portion	USDA Zone	Sun	Part Sun	Shade	Drought Tolerant	Aquatic Plant	Direct Seed Candidate
Acanthopanax gracilistylus	Root Bark	5–10	x	x				
Achyranthes bidentata	Root	8–10	x					
Agastache rugosa	Herb	5–11	x					x
Albizia julibrissin	Flower/Bark	8–10	x			x		
Alisma plantago-aquatica subsp. *orientale*	Root	4–10	x				x	
Allium macrostemon	Bulb	8–11	x			x		
Allium tuberosum	Seed	5–11	x					
Andrographis paniculata	Herb	8–11	x	x	x			
Anemarrhena asphodeloides	Rhizome	3–9	x	x				
Angelica dahurica	Root	4–9	x					
Angelica pubescens	Root	8–9	x					
Angelica sinensis	Root	6–9		x				
Arctium lappa	Seed/Root	4–10	x			x		x
Artemisia annua	Herb	4–9	x			x		
Asparagus cochinchinensis	Root	5–10		x				
Aster tataricus	Root	2–9	x					
Astragalus membranaceus	Root	4–10	x			x		x
Atractylodes macrocephala	Rhizome	7–11	x			x		x
Bacopa monnieri	Herb	9–11		x	x		x	
Belamcanda chinensis	Rhizome	4–9	x	x		x		
Bupleurum chinense	Root	2–10	x	x				
Carthamus tinctorius	Floret	All	x			x		x
Celosia argentea	Seed	All	x					x
Celosia cristata	Flower	All	x					
Centella asiatica	Herb	7–11		x	x		x	
Chrysanthemum morifolium	Flower	6–9	x					
Clerodendrum trichotomum	Leaf	7–10	x					
Codonopsis pilosula	Root	2–11		x				
Coix lacryma-jobi	Seed	2–11		x	x		x	x
Cornus officinalis	Fruit	4–9	x					
Crataegus pinnatifida	Fruit	6–9	x			x		
Cyathula officinalis	Root	7–10	x					
Dianthus superbus	Herb	3–9	x	x				
Dioscorea opposita	Root	5–9	x			x		
Dolichos lablab	Seed	9–11	x					x
Eclipta prostrata	Herb	All		x	x			
Ephedra sinica	Herb/Root	2–9	x			x		
Eriobotrya japonica	Leaf	8–11	x	x				
Eucommia ulmoides	Bark	5–10	x					
Fallopia multiflora	Root/Stem	5–10	x					

Table 3-2 *(continued)*								
Botanical Name	Harvest Portion	USDA Zone	Sun	Part Sun	Shade	Drought Tolerant	Aquatic Plant	Direct Seed Candidate
Forsythia suspensa	Fruit	5–9	x					
Gentiana scabra	Root	3–9	x	x				
Gentiana straminea	Root	5–9	x	x				
Ginkgo biloba	Seed/Leaf	3–10	x					
Glycyrrhiza uralensis	Root	3–10	x			x		
Gynostemma pentaphyllum	Herb	7–9		x	x			
Houttuynia cordata	Herb	5–9	x	x	x		x	
Ligusticum jeholense	Root	4–9	x					
Ligustrum lucidum	Fruit	7–11	x	x	x	x		
Lilium brownii	Bulb	6–10	x			x		
Lilium lancifolium	Bulb	4–9	x			x		
Lonicera japonica	Flower	5–11	x	x		x		
Lycium chinense	Fruit/Root Bark	3–10	x			x		
Magnolia denudata	Flower Bud	6–11	x					
Mentha haplocalyx	Herb	5–9	x					
Momordica charantia	Fruit	All	x					x
Ocimum sanctum	Herb	All	x					x
Ophiopogon japonicus	Tuber	6–10		x	x			
Paeonia lactiflora	Root	3–8	x	x				
Paeonia suffruticosa	Root Bark	5–9		x				
Panax ginseng	Root	3–8			x			
Panax quinquefolius	Root	3–8			x			
Pinellia ternata	Tuber	5–9		x	x			
Plantago asiatica	Seed	All	x	x	x			x
Platycodon grandiflorus	Root	2–10	x					
Prunella vulgaris	Herb	4–9		x				x
Rehmannia glutinosa	Root	4–9	x					
Rheum palmatum	Root	4–9	x					
Salvia miltiorrhiza	Root	6–9	x			x		
Saposhnikovia divaricata	Root	3–9	x					
Schisandra chinensis	Fruit	5–9		x	x			
Schizonepeta tenuifolia	Herb	All	x					x
Scrophularia buergeriana	Root	4–9	x					
Scutellaria baicalensis	Root	4–9				x		x
Scutellaria barbata	Herb	7–10		x				
Sophora flavescens	Root	6–10	x					
Trichosanthes kirilowii	Fruit/Root	5–9	x					x
Withania somnifera	Root	8–11	x			x		x
Ziziphus jujuba	Fruit	6–11	x			x		
Ziziphus jujuba var. *spinosa*	Seed	3–9	x			x		

at the Chinese Medicinal Herb Farm. Start with good seed, collect good seed, and evolution will continue its journey on your farm.

Vegetative methods, such as plant division and cuttings, produce genetic clones and are best for retaining unique traits such as fruit characteristics in *Lycium chinense* (Chinese wolfberry, gǒu qǐ zǐ/dì gǔ pí). The different propagation techniques are dependent on the individual plant in question and have advantages and disadvantages in fitting in with production at each unique farm or garden.

Growing Structures

If you aspire to grow herbs in a serious way, you will need a nursery with a greenhouse and shade house; if not right away, then certainly by your second year of production. Otherwise, your choices of what to grow will be limited. Although many herbs can be direct seeded into either a garden or farm field, others will not crop successfully unless started early under cover to expand their growing season. I was lucky enough to start out with a greenhouse, although it was nothing fancy—an old chicken coop. My handy-husband-who-can-build-or-fix-anything (or Andrew, as he is more commonly known) pulled off the plywood and applied polycarbonate glazing—and then installed plumbing, ventilation, and electricity. The greenhouse we have now serves us—and the plants—better. This one is also a polycarbonate semiautomated greenhouse; it measures 1,000 square feet with a companion shade house that is 800 square feet (but really should be 1,200 square feet to suit the needs of the farm). This space can work well for about three acres of crops. Beware of small greenhouse kits as they can be very expensive and tend not to function as well, with rapid heating and cooling vacillations; try working with plans and components and build your own. At one point said husband pointed out that I could have a new vehicle or the greenhouse—my twelve-year-old car is still working just fine.

The bottom line, of course, is that there are as many nursery models as there are locations and growers; each one needs to be designed according to the resources available. The minimally outfitted nursery will have a well-vented greenhouse (polyethylene or polycarbonate) with fans providing horizontal airflow, a shade house, and a work area with water and electricity. The shade house should have a waterproof covering so the amount of water going into the pots can be controlled; this is rarely found (but easily made or retrofitted), but I find this an essential feature for growing herb starts. A covered shade house (or a cold frame) will keep the herbs from sitting in wet pots; it will also keep precipitation from leaching water-soluble nutrients out of the potted media. In cold climates greenhouse heaters are necessary, as are insulated north walls. Dual-wall greenhouses can save on heating costs, as can heat sinks such as large vessels of water; the gathered heat from the sun is stored and then released when the air temperature dips below that of the heat sink. On a small scale, zone heating with electric heating mats can provide localized warmth under pots or flats. For colder regions, options include radiant heat via heated water cables under benches (or in-floor in a benchless greenhouse) or the popular, but less energy efficient, large space heating units. For these forced air heaters it is advisable to install a simple convection tube to evenly disperse the heated air throughout the greenhouse space. Shade in the greenhouse is necessary as well, provided by either internal or external structures—or the use of a sprayed-on shade compound. In cold winter areas remove greenhouse or shade house exterior shade cloths in fall, as they can hold heavy snow loads and cause structural damage.

Many growers clear all of their plant stock out of the greenhouse by summer, and the house remains empty until late summer or fall when cooler temperatures return. But if you plan to use your structure in the summer or where overheating is an issue, you'll probably need to install a fan and pad evaporative cooling system. Generally speaking, temperatures over ninety degrees are injurious to potted stock.

It's best to irrigate by hand in a greenhouse, unless the greenhouse is over two thousand square feet or if only a few different varieties are being grown. Herbs are very diverse in their watering needs, and in a

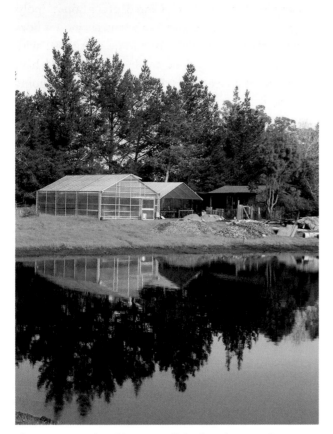

The nursery at the Chinese Medicinal Herb Farm; the greenhouse is on the left, shade house on the right, and media and compost amendments under tarps and bark mulch in the foreground. This dual-wall polycarbonate greenhouse with horizontal airflow fans, internal shade structure, and automated ridge vent makes a versatile growing space.

small space there is often not enough room to create separate watering zones.

Nursery Media

The media you use for seeding and propagation should mimic nature and be biologically active. Commercial medias are not only expensive but use a limited number of ingredients. Some of these are originally of unknown quality, so the material is sterilized—killing all life, the good with the bad. If commercial media is your only option, inoculate it with a couple of handfuls of local soil. Make sure media is premoistened before use to facilitate the proper absorption of water. When moist, media should still crumble in the hand but not be dripping wet.

Media that is created on-site can be vastly superior to purchased germination mix. Compost is the backbone of the recipe we developed at the Chinese Medicinal Herb Farm. The role of quality compost (described in more detail below) is vast, offering stable long-term nutrition and soil structure, plant immunity, organic matter, and a home for the soil web community.

Our time-tested formula utilizes coir (or *coco-peat* as it is sometimes known), which is coconut husk fiber and a by-product of coconut processing. It is produced primarily in Sri Lanka, India, and Mexico. Coir retains water and air and breaks down slowly. We use it in place of traditional peat moss, which should be avoided because it most frequently comes from ancient peat bogs in Canada. Thousands of years are required to produce what can be harvested in a matter of days—decidedly not environmentally friendly.

Coir must be thoroughly leached, since most of it has a high salt content. Leach ahead of time. I place coir bales in an old bathtub (garbage cans work well too) to thoroughly soak for a day or so; place a heavy object on top of the bale to keep it submerged. Then I drain the water and soak two more times. Another option is to leave the bales outside for several good soaking rains. Perlite, a superheated, mined volcanic mineral, is important for maintaining aeration in the mix. Premoistening perlite before you mix up a batch of media will prevent the release of lung-irritating dust. Another by-product that's come on the market recently is partially boiled rice hulls. These may be a suitable substitution for perlite; be sure to conduct trials before using rice hulls extensively.

Here's a rundown of the rest of the ingredients and the role they serve:

- Conditioned fir or pine bark, a by-product of the logging industry, provides light-weight water-holding capacity and media structure.
- Rock powder provides a basic slow-release elemental fertilizer.

- Fertilizer should be organic in origin and macronutrient balanced; a blend formulated for timed release will help ensure that nutrients are available at all times until the fertilizer is utilized.
- Oyster shell provides calcium; you can substitute rock phosphate or another calcium source if another product is locally available.
- Kelp meal is high in trace minerals that assist in nutrient uptake.
- Mycorrhizal powder is a combination of naturally occurring fungal organisms that work in symbiosis with plant roots, helping them take up water and nutrients more efficiently.

I alter my basic recipe, which is suitable for the average needs of most herbs, for certain specific plants. Examples are *Ephedra sinica* (ephedra, má huáng/ má huáng gēn), preferring the addition of 10–20 percent sand; *Astragalus membranaceus* (milk vetch, huáng qí), requiring extra drainage with the addition of 10 percent sand or rock; and *Glycyrrhiza uralensis* (Chinese licorice, gān cǎo), preferring the addition of a little extra calcium.

Seed-Starting How-To

There are many seeding systems, but what works well for the majority of herbs are deep, large wooden flats where there is enough mass so that wild crops do not have to conform to limited allotments of water and space. The ideal boxes are 15 inches by 15 inches by 6 inches deep with many holes or slots for drainage in the bottom. This mass also allows for a reservoir of nutrients so fertilization and watering are not an issue. Annuals are quick and easy; sow them in small cell packs or the large flats. Seeds of longer-term crops or tree seedlings often need to grow in the deep flats for a period of time before being transplanted—sometimes up to two full years for *Paeonia* or *Asparagus*. These will need some supplemental feeding once or twice a year with a long-lasting, slow-release granular fertilizer. Because many botanicals

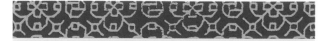

Chinese Medicinal Herb Farm's Basic Bark-Based Media Mix

Some nurseries use separate germinating and transplant medias but we use this recipe for both applications. This time-tested nursery potting media recipe can be mixed in a large wheelbarrow using a shovel, or you can increase the whole recipe and mix the materials in a pit or on a tarp. Some people use an old small cement mixer to mix media.

You'll find the ingredients available bagged in small amounts at garden centers and farm supply businesses. If you need large quantities, pick up materials or arrange to have them delivered from landscape supply companies.

5 gallons compost (homegrown and screened to a ½ inch)
5 gallons coir, thoroughly leached of salt and fluffed
5 gallons perlite (premoistened)
5 gallons sifted fir bark (screened to a ¼ or ½ inch)
½ cup granite dust / rock powder
½ cup balanced slow-release organic fertilizer
¼ cup oyster shell
¼ cup kelp meal
Dash of mycorrhizal fungal powder

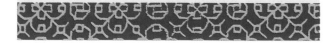

are wild and unselected, they have ongoing or variable germination times, or cultural requirements to fulfill before they will germinate (as explained later in this chapter). If there is no germination information available on a plant you want to grow, look to

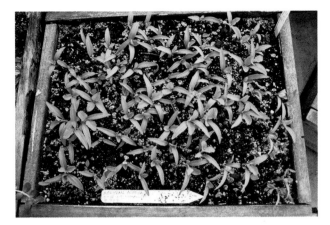

Big wooden flats work great for starting medicinal herb seedlings. Label each flat with genus and species, date sown, and lot number.

the genus or family affiliation for clues to the best methods of propagation. For example, the genus *Crataegus* is a common western herb that has a lot of information written about it. So I extrapolated that the more uncommon eastern variety used in Asian medicine *Crataegus pinnatifida* (Chinese hawthorn, shān zhā) is probably also a multicycle germinator like its cousin—giving me a place to start in germination trials.

Use plastic nursery labels and mark them in pencil, not permanent marking pens—which turn out to be not so permanent. I advise making not one but two labels for each flat. Label information should include genus and species (not pinyin), date of sowing, and origin of seed with the lot number (the unique number that comes on each package of seed, which is assigned to each batch for later tracing if needed). Place the labels in opposite corners of the flat.

Seed Sowing and Potting Up

The individual herb profiles in part 2 offer specific seed sowing information. As a rule of thumb, however, seed can be sown roughly two times the depth of the diameter of the seed. Tamp gently, water in well, keep moist, and (assuming the creek doesn't rise) germination occurs. Try mixing very fine seed with sand to facilitate even sowing. Water thoroughly using a mist nozzle or by placing the seeded flat in a shallow container of water. The idea is to water very gently to avoid washing all seed to one corner

of the flat. After germination, thin the seedlings to give them room to grow as individuals. The first set of leaves that appears is the cotyledons; seedlings are too young at this stage to be transplanted. Then comes the first set of true leaves; seedlings can be potted up after the second set of true leaves appears. When transplanting the young plants into pots, take care to gently lift the plant from below with a small tool. Hold the leaves with the hands, and avoid handling the stems or roots; some herbs (such as the *Gentiana* genus) are quite delicate. If you handle them roughly, they will be injured, and they will die—and then you'll have to dump the whole flat on your compost pile. Transplant young seedlings into small pots, either the two- or four-inch size. When potting up, do so incrementally to just the next size pot. Almost without exception, containerized stock does much better with this method than transplanting a small plant into a large pot. Usually plants are still in the greenhouse at this stage and will need to be hardened off before they go out into the cold, cruel world. To harden off, bring the plants into the shade house when a period of mild weather is expected and then after another week or two outside the shade house to give them full exposure, to acclimatize them to the outside conditions of temperature and wind. This process should take two to three weeks before the plants are ready to go into the field, assuming that the planting day is mild.

Seeds That Need Special Treatment

Chinese medicinal herb seed is closer to the wild than most vegetable seed, which over time has been adapted to germinate easily and predictably. Seed of wild plants sometimes has nature's built-in survival systems: chemical germination inhibitors, stratification (exposure to a cold period) requirements, or multicycle germination (usually warm and cold cycles to ensure that winter really is over and germination will not fail, which would result in the extinction of the species).

The easiest way to encourage seeds that require stratification to leave their slumber and germinate is to sow them in deep flats and expose the flats to the

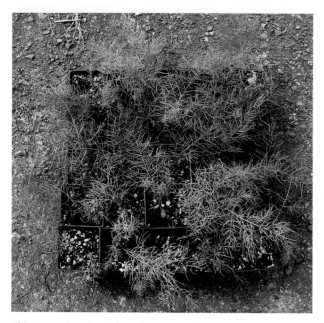

This recently potted flat of *Asparagus cochinchinensis* (tiān mén dōng) will be ready for planting out soon.

winter elements of temperature variations, snowfall, and rains, letting the action wear on the seed naturally. Protect from excessive moisture and precipitation, or the seed may rot. Generally I leave flats outside fully exposed to the weather, unless there are many rainstorms in a row (in this area of California we receive thirty to fifty inches of rain in a mere five winter months) that would keep the seed flats wet—whereupon I move them into the shade house. The shade house has a rain cover but no walls so it is cold and dry. This outdoor technique works well for cold-winter climates as well—the seeds freeze and thaw in cycles—just like seeds would in nature. Cover seeded flats with inverted black plastic nursery flats to keep critters (mainly cats and raccoons) out.

Alternately you can condition seeds in the refrigerator. My preferred refrigerator treatment process is to soak the seed for a few hours, then pour off the water and place the seed in a moistened (but not wet) fabric square. Fold the square of fabric with the seed inside and place the fabric pouch in a baggie surrounded by washed moist (not wet) sand. Make sure to label the baggie with genus and species, date treatment started, and when it ultimately needs to be taken out of the refrigerator. Do not close the plastic

bag fully—let it breathe—and look weekly to make sure the sand is still moist. Start checking the seed for signs of germination after three weeks of cold treatment, as seed frequently germinates at variable times; seed generally remains in the cool conditioning (artificial winter) for two to three months. If the seeds start to germinate, remove them, keep them moist, and bring them up to room temperature for thirty minutes or so before sowing. After the cold treatment time period is reached, sow all ungerminated seed. Some examples of cold-stratification and multicycle germinators are *Asparagus cochinchinensis* (tiān mén dōng); *Crataegus pinnatifida* (Chinese hawthorn, shān zhā); *Eucommia ulmoides* (hardy rubber tree, dù zhòng); *Panax* spp.; and *Schisandra chinensis* (five flavored fruit, wǔ wèi zǐ). The herb profiles in part 2 describe individual germination requirements.

Some seed is dependent on light or dark conditions for germination; this can be achieved with less or more media covering the seed. A few examples of light dependent germinators are *Angelica* spp., such as *Angelica pubescens* (dú huó) or *Angelica dahurica* (bái zhǐ); *Scrophularia buergeriana* (figwort, běi xuán shēn); and many *Gentiana* spp.

Some seeds have hard seed coats that need to be nicked to begin the germination process. This is called scarification. Depending on the seed size and shape, various tools such as sandpaper, files, rough stones, and nail clippers are all serviceable; I tend to use sandpaper. Gently remove some of the hard testa or seed coat so the seed will be able to take on water; do not go into the softer and oftentimes white endosperm (food storage part of the seed). Examples of plants that are frequently scarified are *Astragalus membranaceus* (milk vetch, huáng qí); and the *Glycyrrhiza* spp. (licorices).

Sowing Seed with Unknown Germination Requirements

For seed that has a reputation of being difficult or has some unknown germination requirements, sow on the surface and cover with media or sand from very thinly at one end of the flat to a depth of two to three times the thickness of the seed at the other end. If the plant is endemic to the northern climes, sow in the fall and expose the seeded flats to winter; if endemic to warm regions, spring sow and place in a warm greenhouse. Some seeds are short lived and should be fresh and planted in their first or second season or they may no longer be viable. Examples are *Angelica* spp., *Allium* spp., or *Acanthopanax gracilistylus* (wǔ jiā pí). Still others need to stay fresh and moist until they are sown, such as *Ginkgo biloba* (ginkgo, bái guǒ).

If seed (that was not old and was kept protected from moisture and heat changes before sowing) sown in a flat doesn't germinate readily, don't toss it into the compost pile. Sometimes you have to wait a long time for seed to be ready to germinate. Keep watered and be patient, and more often than not they will come of their own accord. As an experiment I managed to get three consecutive spring germinating flushes out of one sowing of *Bupleurum chinense* (hare's ear, chái hú) seed. Now that's an example of untamed seed!

Vegetative Propagation

Vegetative or asexual reproduction of plants yields an exact genetic copy of the mother plant. Some examples of these processes are division, cuttings of stems or roots, and layering (the herb profiles in part 2 include specific suggestions for vegetative propagation where applicable).

Of the various vegetative methods, division is one of the easiest and is suitable for plants that have expanding clumps. Simply dig up and divide; each new plant will need to have roots and crown material. *Mentha haplocalyx* (field mint, bò hé), which readily hybridizes with other mints, is a good choice for division; I keep a knife on the potting bench for this purpose. *Bacopa monnieri* (brahmi) and *Centella asiatica* (gotu kola, jī xuě cǎo) are two other plants that are commonly divided. In the field after harvesting I dig out two-inch plugs of both of these tropical herbs, transplant them into large wooden flats, and place them in the greenhouse to overwinter. By spring planting time they have filled in the

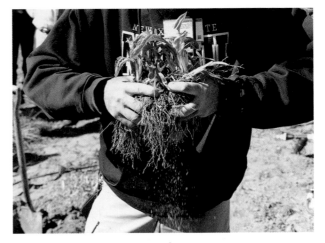

To vegetatively divide *Aster tataricus* (tartar aster, zǐ wǎn) dig roots up with a digging fork, pull the roots apart, and they are ready to replant.

flat and get cut up like a sheet cake, dividing them again back into the field. They are tender perennials and will not reliably overwinter—even in our USDA hardiness zone 9.

Stem cuttings work well for many woody plants. Take hardwood cuttings in fall or semihardwood (more flexible) cuttings in summer: cut pencil-thick stems with four or five leaf junctions, and remove the lower foliage. Prepare a deep wooden flat with a cutting media of perlite or sand, use rooting hormone on the stems if desired, and place the stem upright in the media with at least two leafless leaf junctions covered. Water, keep warm, and mist frequently. Please note that certified organic rooting hormone may not be available. When irrigating cuttings I often use water in which willow stems have been soaking. Any kind of willow, taken in any season, will serve the purpose. Just cut up stems and put in a watering can kept full of water; twenty-four hours ought to be enough time for the water to be imbued with the natural rooting hormones. After a few weeks the willow stems will start to root themselves, and I just try to keep them somewhat fresh—and from growing out of the can.

Root cuttings taken in spring can also be successful with some varieties of plants. Choose strong-looking roots. Make cuts across the root (not lengthwise), and place the cuttings just under the surface of the media in a pot or flat. Place in a greenhouse on a heat mat. For all cuttings provide a liquid fertilizer once the plants start to grow, as the media offers no nutrition. There are many good liquid nutrient products available, but I like to use Maxicrop for this purpose, as it contains kelp, a known plant stimulant, with the addition of Biolink 3-3-3 fertilizer. You can also use this product as a foliar spray or apply it to the media.

Layering is another vegetative technique suitable for plants that are adventitious; in this case, above-ground stems are able to form roots at leaf nodes where they touch soil. Use U-shaped irrigation pins to hold the stems in place either on the surface of the soil in the garden or into a pot near the mother plant until rooting has occurred, then separate them from the mother stock and transplant. Two examples are *Forsythia suspensa* (lián qiào) and *Lycium chinense* (Chinese wolfberry, gǒu qǐ zǐ/dì gǔ pí), which both root—and a little too easily—whenever their stems come in contact with moist soils.

Monitor the nursery daily and be familiar with the plants. Record everything—take photos and label them! I keep a photo journal of all the growing areas on the farm. I find this visual record helpful when planning for the future and for catching extra details, or verifying features such as time and color of bloom, plant size, or if an herb is deciduous. There is little information out there in relation to many of these herbs, so I encourage you to record all the information you can.

Nursery Diseases and Pests

To prevent pest and disease problems in the greenhouse, shade house, and nursery beds (where seedlings as well as permanent motherstock grow) strive to develop a balanced organic system where stock is regulated naturally. Monitor frequently to look for and eliminate small issues before they become big problems. Preventive measures are the key: maintain a clean and uncluttered nursery and encourage natural predators. Although the vast majority of insects are not pests, in the modified environment of the nursery, imbalances occur more easily than outside in a natural setting.

Humidity, especially in the greenhouse, is good for plants and unfortunately also for the diseases that evolved with them. Solutions? Ceiling-mounted horizontal airflow fans and a quality pot media are both extremely important in producing trouble-free plants. The infectious plant diseases of fungi, bacteria, and viruses can be some of the more challenging potential nursery problems. Damping off is a common fungal disease that causes emerging seedlings to collapse and die. Once present it is hard to get rid of. Another fungal disease is botrytis, which shows as a grey mold on leaves and stems. To avoid both of these diseases, keep air moving and use a quality potting media. Virus issues occasionally affect greenhouse crops, causing a variety of symptoms such as yellowing leaves and wilting due to vascular problems; there is no cure for virus diseases. Thankfully Chinese herbs tend to have strong immune systems partly due to their diverse genetics. For persistent diseases on specific host plants in the nursery, consider their removal—as in the trash can. Sometimes it is easier to start over and not let the pathogen have the opportunity to infect other plants.

Monitor closely to catch pest problems before they spread. In the spring the most common pest you're likely to encounter might be one of the many colors of plant-sap-sucking aphids. The green peach aphids are the most ubiquitous—but there are also black, orange, and white colors as well; the different varieties are usually host specific. If I find an outbreak, I tend to spray an insecticidal soap. Whiteflies can be problematic, especially in wet soil conditions; to avoid whitefly infestations, use larger seeding vessels so you can water deeply and less frequently. Later in the season, usually when the humidity is low, thrips and two-spotted spider mites can crop up. These pests pierce plant cells to suck out plant juices. Most often the damage they cause is minor, but they—as well as aphids—can be vectors of disease. Scale can also be problematic on woody motherstock plants; when I find them I first look for ants, which farm them for their honeydew—then I exclude or trap the ants. I follow up by spraying horticultural oil on scale. Each region and location will vary as far as its specific flora

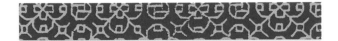

Greenhouse Biocontrols

I am a lazy grower, so every spring I buy lacewing larvae from an insect laboratory. They are the best general predators and will help maintain a pest-free nursery if introduced into the nursery in spring before infestations begin. They are delivered on a schedule every two or three weeks for two to three months in the early spring. Please do not buy lady beetles (ladybugs) unless they are lab grown because they are often harvested from the wild. Also note that adult lady beetles are not very effective predators; they sell mostly because they are cute.

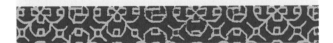

and fauna; but for each operation the most successful pest control programs include understanding the life cycle of the insect or pathogenic disease. Separate any plants that are infested or infected, or look unwell, from the rest of the population. Always be vigilant and isolate any stock coming from off-site for six months or more and monitor for any signs of trouble.

MANAGING YOUR SOIL

Herbs that are grown in lean soils with even, stable nutrition availability grow slow and strong. Biologically active healthy soils, managed with cover crops and compost, will enable the soils to grow quality medicinal herbs while discouraging potential pests from staking claims. While all growers need to follow basic agricultural tenets of seasonal crop rotation and maintain a balance of soil nutrients, medicinal herb growers have it easier because the crops we grow require fewer inputs and our actions are lighter on the land.

I do advise testing your soils yearly and taking different samples from areas that have had different soil management techniques or from soils that look or behave differently from other farm or garden soils. Follow the sample collection recommendations from whichever laboratory you will use. The results will guide you in providing a balanced soil management and fertilization plan.

Cover Crops

Cover crops feed the soil, compared to fertilizers, which feed the plant. If the soil is healthy, the plant crops are healthy. Permanent crops, cover crops, and perennial plantings keep soil biology alive by feeding the soil food web, bringing balance. Besides improving soil structure, cover crops prevent or lessen water and wind erosion and also loosen compacted soils. They are usually a combination of legumes and grasses. For the even nutrition that is needed in herb cultivation, I have found that a cover crop combination with yields higher in organic matter—the building grasses rather than nitrogen-fixing legumes—works best. The organic matter will yield the most food for vital soil organisms in the long run. Premixed soil-building seed blends are formulated for vegetable production and have a higher ratio of legumes to grasses. I use a mix of legumes and grasses to create the desired ratio of 40:60 that I find does best for the land (and crops) I work. When to plant and which particular seeds to sow are regionally specific; inquire with local suppliers and county farm advisors.

At the Chinese Medicinal Herb Farm I sow most of the cover crops in fall. The blend I use for the soils on this farm is usually a combination of oats and yellow mustard for the organic matter portion and bell beans and vetches for the nitrogen share. In fall after crops are harvested I lightly rototill with the tractor and sow whole blocks of land broadcasting the seed by hand. With one variety I seed lightly going from, say, west to east, covering the whole area; then to get good overall seed density and coverage I sow the same variety lightly crosswise to the first direction, which would be north to south. Different seeds have different weights, making combined broadcast sowing have potentially spotty results; so I broadcast each variety of seed singly. Then I simply run over the seed with the wide tractor wheels; this makes good contact between the seed and soil. This technique works on a small scale; larger areas will require different equipment. If I have timed it right the winter rains come tumbling down to germinate the seed and the cover crop grows all winter.

The John Deere 4000 series I use is a light (under-three-thousand-pound) tractor; its lightness is good for relatively less compaction issues—problematic with our heavy clay soil. However it has less power and has a smaller bucket, making it less suitable for bigger jobs. It is common to have more than one tractor on-site; local farmer-friends with larger tractors are helpful, too!

If you have enough land available for longer term rotations, grow your cover crops to maturity, whereupon they will become carboniferous; the durable organic matter created will offer stable slow-release nutrients for seasons to come. This of course means growing the cover crops past the green manure stage that most farmers turn under as a high nitrogen crop. When a cover crop needs to be cut down, I attach a flail mower and make a couple of passes over the crop to chop it up. After that, I usually use a disk or tiller to incorporate the crop material while it is still green. After that, the land needs to rest for two to three weeks, to let the cover crops break down before planting anew. It is best to keep plants growing on the land, as long periods without cover starve the soil life; so if it is not wintertime and I have harvested out an area, I will sow a summer cover crop—usually buckwheat. It keeps the soil biology active, provides weed competition, and offers nectar for beneficial insects. It is a fast-growing crop, so it doesn't tie up the land but simply tides it over till I am ready for the next action. The rate or speed of breakdown of all cover crops will partly depend on temperature: several weeks is common. If herb crops are planted into a field that has not mellowed, the decaying cover crops will rob any new starts of nitrogen. Wait for the soil biology to achieve balance before planting. We

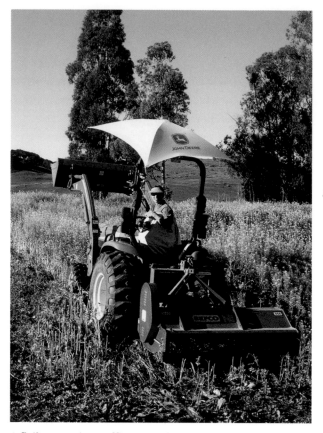

A flail mower is an efficient tool to take down a cover crop. Photo courtesy of Andrew Jacobson.

always utilize a cover crop between herb plantings, whether short or long term.

Making Quality Soil-Building Compost

Every operation should have an active composting process, as a vital amendment source. On-site cured compost (compost that has been pasteurized by heating to 150–180 degrees and is fully broken down, looking and smelling like soil) is a key component of soil fertility.

We use farm plant waste for our compost ingredients. We stockpile it until there is sufficient volume (ten to fifteen square feet) that it will heat up when we add a fresh influx of a large amount of something green (full of nitrogen), such as freshly mowed grass. We water the pile to keep it moist—but not wet. The larger the volume of composting material the easier and longer it stays hot. I try to turn an actively composting pile (with the tractor bucket) once every week or two for a minimum of five weeks to keep it active. The best way to turn the pile to expose all ingredients (such as weed seeds) to the pasteurizing effects is to rotate the material from inside to outside. At any one time we usually have several piles at different stages. I keep the compost piles covered with tarps to exclude weed seeds and prevent rain from leaching out water soluble nutrients such as nitrogen. I use compost thermometers to monitor compost temperatures.

Using Purchased Compost

Most purchased compost is rarely ready to use when first delivered and is often poor quality. If you must bring in outside compost, buy from a reputable company, purchase in the fall, and sequester it under a tarp until spring when it will be ready to use. If delivered compost comes off the truck smelling of ammonia and is steaming hot, it has not finished the composting process. If it is ordered early in the spring, it may have been made in a hurry due to seasonal demand. Conversely, purchased compost that's been subjected to heavy winter or spring moisture may be leached of its nutrients.

Application of Compost

I apply compost either in the fall before sowing a cover crop or at planting time in spring. For fall application, I apply the compost by loading my tractor bucket with compost and driving over the application area, dumping a steady stream out of the raised bucket. My goal is to apply a layer about a half to one inch thick. Next I till in the compost along with any additional nutrients such as rock powders. After that, the area is ready to plant. If an area is especially rich in clay and lacking in structure, or is nutrient poor after a fall root crop is harvested, I may vary my method. My helpers and I put compost down into the space from where the roots were removed, dig it in deep with digging forks, replace the soil above, and then sow the cover crop. For the addition of compost with spring planting I use either the tractor bucket or wheelbarrow.

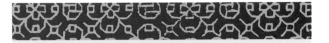

Small-Scale Composting

Good quality composting can be achieved in a space as small as four cubic feet. That is the smallest a compost pile should be to allow for enough volume to generate enough heat to pasturize the compost. On-site nonwoody green waste, kitchen scraps, and coffee grounds are high in nitrogen; these ingredients, along with a larger portion of dry material and frequent turning, will help keep the compost pile at the desired temperature of at least 150 degrees. If the compost smells bad it may be either too wet or have too much nitrogenous material. A less active process that still yields quality compost is a cold technique where the aforementioned ingredients are simply layered and not turned; make sure to bury kitchen waste into the pile to avoid attracting rodents. This method takes longer to obtain usable material but will speed up—with added nutrients as well—with the addition of red composting worms. These red wrigglers are often available at home and garden stores, gardening centers, or by mail order. I do not recommend putting weeds with maturing seed heads into a cold compost pile as they oftentimes do not rot and may return to the garden along with finished compost. It is helpful to have two bins, both protected from precipitation—one for active composting and the other ready to use. Simple wire hardware mesh with half-inch holes wired in a circle or shipping pallets wired together are, in my opinion, better than the expensive, plastic, hand-turned units commercially available.

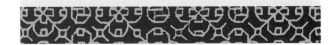

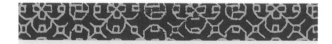

Animal Manure and Herbs

Add animal manures only sparingly to soil and only after it has been actively composted. Animal manures are very rich. Excess use generates widely fluctuating nutrient availability (which is not the foundation of the uniform availability and slow release of nutrients that grow efficacious herbs).

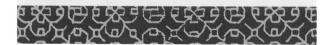

Working with the Soil

When to rototill or otherwise work the soil is a learned activity. Sandy soils are more lenient and will sustain less damage if worked when wet than clay soils. The right time to work the soil is when it is moist but not wet; dig with a shovel straight down into the soil and turn it out. If the soil retains the shape of the shovel, or especially if the soil is shiny where it contacted the shovel—as is common with clay soils—wait until it dries out more. In the clay-rich areas at the Chinese Medicinal Herb Farm, it seems like there is only half a day when the soil is right for working in the spring.

If soil has good tilth and is ready to work, it should crumble when turned out of a shovel. When soil is ready to till, you may use a walk-behind tiller (for up to one acre) or a tractor-mounted rototiller (or, of course, any other soil-preparation tool you choose). Work the land as lightly as necessary to achieve your planting goal. For example, overworking clay soil can lead to the notorious clay pan layer; imagine eight inches of fluffy soil atop a hardened layer made by a tractor repeatedly beating clay at the same depth. This hard subsurface layer is almost impervious to water. These soils can be opened by ripping with tines or chisels—a fall task. In the old days some farmers used to dynamite to fracture these layers—and with our clay soils, there are days that I actually muse on this over-the-top technique. Sandy soil does not have this problem; however, predominantly sandy soils lack structure as much as heavy clay lacks structure and need the addition of compost just as much as clay-predominant soils. Sandy soils tend to need fertilizing more frequently (use half strength twice as often) because it doesn't hold nutrients as readily as clay soil.

PLANTING

Many Chinese herbs are well suited to incorporation into existing landscape and ornamental settings and, for the more edible types of herbs, the family vegetable garden. The interplanting of medicinal herbs and row cropping are also viable methods of producing crops.

Designing Planting Areas

Keeping in mind the importance of maintaining wild quality (defined in chapter 2) of medicinal herbs, you'll want to avoid monocrop plantings; instead explore diversified cropping systems (polyculture). Two possible ways of laying out gardens are by

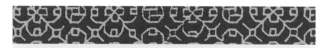

Organizing Crop Areas

We organize our growing beds into blocks of like needs for sun, irrigation, and how long it takes the crop to reach harvest stage—as well as by the season of harvest. In some blocks of long-term perennial beds the soil will not be disturbed for years except for weeding. Soil management is more intensive for annual crops—or perennials that we treat as annuals. In the course of less than a year, we may plant a cover crop, incorporate it, then plant an herb crop, harvest it, and sow another cover crop.

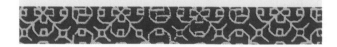

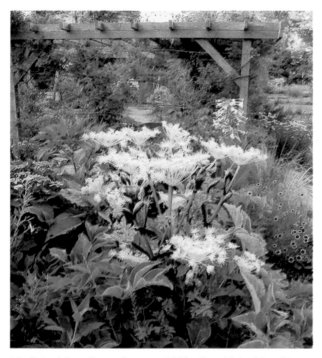

Medicinal *Angelica pubescens* (dú huó)—with its big white flowers—as well as tobacco and dye plants reside gracefully in this ornamental garden.

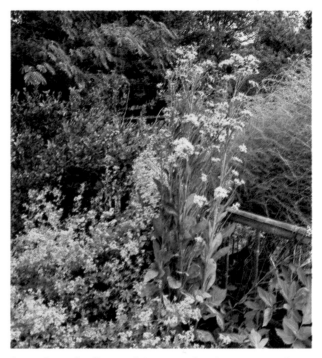

Pretty lavender-flowered *Aster tataricus* (tartar aster, zǐ wǎn) along with other Asian medicinals makes an attractive demonstration garden at the Chinese Medicinal Herb Farm.

the cultural needs of the plants or by their medicinal function. The former is more common for production gardens and the latter is often favored by practitioners and the public because function-designed gardens serve well as teaching gardens, ornamental theme botanic gardens demonstrating herb use. Function-designed gardens are, however, not always the most efficient in terms of gathering the harvest. And after you've planted an herb garden, don't be surprised if some of the herb progeny move themselves around, choosing their own positions to fit their needs.

Growing medicinal herbs in containers does not necessarily yield the best medicine; the available qi is limited and the connection to the ecosystem is interrupted. However, there are reasons for potted propagation: control of invasive species, if potted material is the only option for apartment dwellers, as a spirit plant to be kept nearby, or for ornamental display. Potted herbs will require more frequent fertilization; the media recipe given earlier in this chapter is an excellent potting soil. Avoid growing out medicinal herbs in plastic containers (like kiddie pools

or storage tubs), due to the possibility of chemicals leaching into the crop—or choose plastics that are FDA rated for food storage. For species that respond well to containerization see table 3-3 and part 2.

Many of the Asian herbs also produce stunningly beautiful potted ornamental flowers or long-lasting cut flowers. The peonies, lilies, mums, and *Forsythias* are among the most famous of the medicinal cut flowers. The individual plant profiles in part 2 will have specific information.

Diverse plantings should be the goal even when planting on a farm scale. If you plan to plant more than a quarter of an acre of any one herb, consider breaking up the planting with blocks of other species of crops in between. If the crops have similar cultural requirements and the same harvest schedules, you will save on time and organization and it will be easier to mechanically work the land. For example, I frequently include in the same blocks (but different rows or beds) *Salvia miltiorrhiza* (red sage, dān shēn) and *Scutellaria baicalensis* (baikal skullcap, huáng qín) because they share the same cultural requirements and are harvested in about

Table 3-3. Ornamental Uses of Medicinal Herbs						
Genus	Species	Common Name	Pinyin Name	For Beds and Borders	For Growing in Containers	For Cutting
Acanthopanax	gracilistylus		wǔ jiā pí		x	
Agastache	rugosa	Korean Mint	tǔ huò xiāng	x	x	x
Albizia	julibrissin	Mimosa	hé huān pí/huā	x		
Alisma	plantago-aquatica subsp. orientale	Water Plantain	zé xiè		x	
Allium	macrostemon		xiè bái	x		
Allium	tuberosum	Garlic Chives	jiǔ cài zǐ	x	x	x
Andrographis	paniculata	Kalmegh	chuān xīn lián		x	
Anemarrhena	asphodeloides		zhī mǔ	x	x	
Angelica	dahurica		bái zhǐ	x		x
Angelica	pubescens		dú huó	x		
Artemisia	annua	Sweet Annie	qīng hāo	x		x
Asparagus	cochinchinensis		tiān mén dōng	x	x	
Aster	tataricus	Tartar Aster	zǐ wǎn	x	x	x
Atractylodes	macrocephala	Chinese Thistle Daisy	bái zhú	x	x	
Bacopa	monnieri	Brahmi	Brahmi	x	x	
Belamcanda	chinensis	Blackberry Lily	shè gān	x	x	x
Bupleurum	chinense	Hare's Ear	chái hú	x	x	
Carthamus	tinctorius	Safflower	hóng huā	x		x
Celosia	argentea		qīng xiāng zǐ	x	x	x
Celosia	cristata	Cockscomb	jī guān huā	x	x	x
Centella	asiatica	Gotu Kola	jī xuě cǎo	x	x	
Chrysanthemum	morifolium	Mum	jú huā	x	x	x
Clerodendrum	trichotomum	Glorybower	chòu wú tóng	x	x	x
Codonopsis	pilosula	Poor Man's Ginseng	dǎng shēn	x	x	
Coix	lacryma-jobi	Job's Tears	yì yǐ rén	x	x	x
Cornus	officinalis	Dogwood	shān zhū yú	x		
Crataegus	pinnatifida	Chinese Hawthorn	shān zhā	x	x	
Dianthus	superbus	Fringed Pink	qú mài	x	x	x
Dioscorea	opposita	Chinese Yam	shān yào	x	x	
Dolichos	lablab	Hyacinth Bean	bái biǎn dòu	x		x
Ephedra	sinica	Ephedra	má huáng/má huáng gēn		x	
Eriobotrya	japonica	Loquat	pí pá yè	x		
Eucommia	ulmoides	Hardy Rubber Tree	dù zhòng	x		
Forsythia	suspensa		lián qiào	x		x

the same length of time, which is two or three years. Keep plot maps to refer to the crop history of each bed or block.

In moving past the trial phase, there is an economy of scale that will be different for each growing situation. Experimentation will find the sweet spot. Keep track of these details and it will become clear which crops require 10, 20, or 30 percent extra plant stock at planting time to reach the targeted yield. Unexpected variables can be numerous: roaming feral pigs, accidental underwatering or overwatering, employees who misunderstand instructions . . . the list goes on.

Genus	Species	Common Name	Pinyin Name	For Beds and Borders	For Growing in Containers	For Cutting
Gentiana	*scabra*		lóng dǎn cǎo	x	x	
Gentiana	*straminea*		qín jiāo	x	x	
Ginkgo	*biloba*	Ginkgo	bái guǒ	x		
Gynostemma	*pentaphyllum*	Sweet Tea Vine	jiǎo gǔ lán	x	x	
Houttuynia	*cordata*		yú xīng cǎo	x	x	
Ligusticum	*jeholense*	Chinese Lovage	gǎo běn	x	x	
Ligustrum	*lucidum*	Chinese Privet	nǚ zhēn zǐ	x		
Lilium	*brownii*	Lily	bǎi hé	x	x	x
Lilium	*lancifolium*	Lily	bǎi hé	x	x	x
Lonicera	*japonica*	Honeysuckle	jīn yín huā	x	x	x
Lycium	*chinense*	Chinese Wolfberry	gǒu qǐ zǐ/dì gǔ pí	x		
Magnolia	*denudata*		xīn yí huā	x		
Mentha	*haplocalyx*	Field Mint	bò hé	x	x	
Momordica	*charantia*	Bitter Melon	kǔ guā	x		
Ocimum	*sanctum*	Sacred Basil	Tulsi	x	x	
Ophiopogon	*japonicus*	Lilyturf	mài mén dōng	x	x	
Paeonia	*lactiflora*	Chinese Peony	bái/chì sháo	x	x	x
Paeonia	*suffruticosa*	Tree Peony	mǔ dān pí	x	x	x
Pinellia	*ternata*		bàn xià	x	x	
Plantago	*asiatica*	Plantain	chē qián zǐ	x	x	
Platycodon	*grandiflorus*	Balloon Flower	jié gěng	x	x	x
Prunella	*vulgaris*	Heal All	xià kū cǎo	x		x
Rehmannia	*glutinosa*	Chinese Foxglove	dì huáng		x	
Rheum	*palmatum*	Chinese Rhubarb	dà huáng	x		x
Salvia	*miltiorrhiza*	Red Sage	dān shēn	x	x	x
Saposhnikovia	*divaricata*	Siler	fáng fēng	x	x	
Schisandra	*chinensis*	Five Flavored Fruit	wǔ wèi zǐ	x	x	
Schizonepeta	*tenuifolia*	Japanese Catnip	jīng jiè	x		
Scrophularia	*buergeriana*	Figwort	běi xuán shēn	x		
Scutellaria	*baicalensis*	Baikal Skullcap	huáng qín	x	x	x
Scutellaria	*barbata*	Barbat Skullcap	bàn zhī lián	x		
Sophora	*flavescens*		kǔ shēn	x	x	
Trichosanthes	*kirilowii*	Chinese Cucumber	guā lóu/tiān huā fěn	x	x	
Withania	*somnifera*	Ashwagandha	Ashwagandha	x		
Ziziphus	*jujuba*	Chinese Date	dà zǎo	x		

Planting How-To

During planting season, keep a keen eye on weather conditions to avoid hot or windy spells that might desiccate seedlings. As much as feasible, plant at times when the seedlings will not be stressed; early or late in the day is often the best. Thoroughly water transplants the day before and after planting. Avoid the use of chlorinated water for irrigation; it is not life enhancing. Protect seedlings further, if necessary, with row crop covers or shade cloth, since temporary shade can ease transplant shock. Row crop cover can also protect should frost or wind threaten, or if

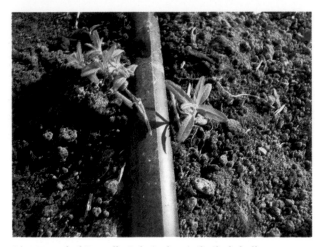

Direct-seeded *Scutellaria baicalensis* (baikal skullcap, huáng qín) makes long straight roots. Sown next to in-line emitter T-tape irrigation.

planting time is close to the summer equinox. At that time the sun will be too strong for most young plants. Directly seeding into the field is a good method if a greenhouse is not available (though I like to direct seed as it saves on greenhouse labor). Direct seeding works well for some annuals or perennials that will be grown for several seasons. If using in-line emitters be sure to sow in the morning when it is still cool, and when you will be watering—because as the day warms up the plastic expands and the emitters move from the seed locations.

For critical, rare, or valuable stock hold some back in the nursery, or plant in two different locations altogether as an "insurance policy" to guard against total loss. But even if the worst happens and some dieback occurs, many herbs are quite durable and can manage just fine and return with gusto. I know from experience that wind or heat top kill can be taken in stride by *Dioscorea opposita* (Chinese yam, shān yào), *Codonopsis pilosula* (poor man's ginseng, dǎng shēn), and *Lilium* spp. (bǎi hé) to name a few. Note that these examples are durable root crops; always gauge the risk with individual crops as there is a permanent point of no return (plant death) if conditions are too stressful. If a crop isn't looking its best and needs a boost as it is getting established, but certainly well before harvest time, fertilize with a fish and seaweed combination, humic acid, or compost tea foliar feed. Spray on the foliage, top and bottom,

in the morning before the heat of the day accumulates or the wind picks up.

Extending Further Afield

Sometimes you may want to use special management techniques in order to coax varieties of plants that might not otherwise grow well in your region into production. For example, if an annual crop needs a longer warm season than you can expect in your location, start the crop extra-early in a heated greenhouse. Some tender perennials need only a year and a half of growth before harvest. For example, if you live in a cold climate, you can still grow some of these herbs by fall-sowing these tender perennials in your nursery, overwintering them in a greenhouse, and planting them out in the spring.

I often modify the environment to provide shade and humidity to more closely match an herb's native environment. There are plenty of options: you can

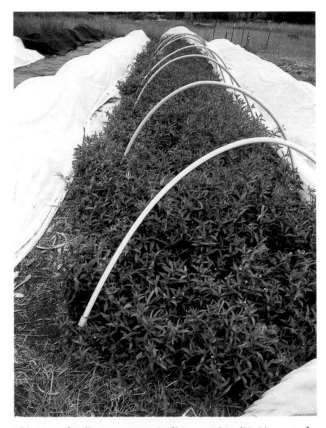

This row of *Eclipta prostrata* (eclipta, mò hàn lián) is part of a whole block of crops that we grow under Agribon row crop cover to provide shade, humidity, and warmth.

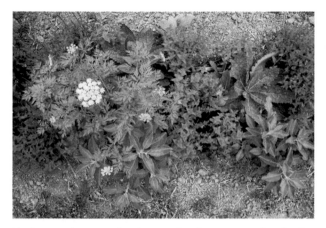

Herbs growing together harmoniously—an example of polycultural intercropping. White-flowered *Cnidium monnieri* (shé chuáng zǐ) is a seed crop, low-growing *Rehmannia glutinosa* (Chinese foxglove, dì huáng) is a root crop, pretty blue-flowered *Scutellaria barbata* (barbat skullcap, bàn zhī lián) is an herb crop, and *Withania somnifera* (ashwagandha) is a root crop.

heat or cool a crop by using row crop covers, in-field high tunnels, or other materials. You don't have to have a greenhouse or in-field hoophouse, but then the herb varieties you can grow will be more limited. Concentrate on multiyear crops that can be directly seeded into the field.

For added protection from weather or insects, temporarily cover a newly transplanted or seeded bed with a row crop cover. The Chinese Medicinal Herb Farm resides in a relatively mild climate so we cover only a few crops for sun or wind protection, and we always wait to plant until after the threat of frost. If your climate is more extreme, row crop covers will be an even more useful tool.

For the most efficient use of cropping space, intercrop herbs within the row, such as planting annuals around young longer-term crops. An example would be a large multiyear or long-term crop planted in the middle of a long row—the edges of the bed will not be needed by the large crop for another year or two. Planting the edges with a shorter-term crop makes the most of the space. We have employed this strategy—with the large crops being many of the shrubs *Acanthopanax gracilistylus* (wǔ jiā pí) and *Sophora flavescens* (kǔ shēn) flanked by the quick-to-harvest smaller crops *Atractylodes macrocephala* (Chinese thistle daisy, bái zhú), *Prunella vulgaris* (heal all, xià

kū cǎo), and *Ocimum sanctum* (sacred basil, tulsi).

The Harvest chart will help determine which crops to plant near each other for the coordination of harvesting. The type of plant and portion used will aid in planning field row crop blocks or interplanting strategies—for example, a crop where the fruits are used in the first season, say, *Dolichos lablab* (hyacinth bean, bái biǎn dòu) interplanted with a root crop of *Angelica pubescens* (dú huó). The hyacinth beans will be fall collected and the *Angelica* root will be dug in late fall or winter—good companions.

SEASONAL CARE

Oftentimes wild-quality herb crops are fertilized and watered sparingly, creating stress and increasing the phytochemical profiles. These herbs are often smaller than herbs grown in pumped-up soils, but the qi is there—the aromas, tastes, and medicinal strength shine through in organoleptic as well as laboratory chemical assays. Now we just have to sell the crops by the qi and not by the pound!

Having said that, most of the herbs will need some supplemental nutrients and water—as well as monitoring for pests and diseases. If you have reliable summer rainfall, you'll probably be able to bypass the cost, labor, and trouble of irrigating. Those of us in the arid west should use drip irrigation instead of overhead watering. Drip irrigation is much more water efficient, and we all need to use as little as possible of this finite resource. Where growing areas are flat, T-tape is the most cost-effective choice for in-line emitter irrigation. If there is any amount of slope, pressure compensating emitter irrigation is necessary—or all the water will end up at the bottom of the run. Pressure compensating in-line emitter line is more expensive. I've used several brands, and all have worked reasonably well.

Herbs require less fertilizer than vegetables and more simple fertilizers as well, such as rock dust. This is good news: low inputs also keep labor and supply costs down. Besides rock dusts or powders (also known as granite dust), I use a time-release 7-5-7 from California Organic Fertilizers. But any fertilizer that

Table 3-4. Harvesting Information at a Glance

Botanical Name	Type	Harvest Portion	Season of Harvest	1st Season	2nd–3rd Season	4th Season	Years to Harvest
Acanthopanax gracilistylus	Shrub	Root Bark	summer or fall			x	
Achyranthes bidentata	Perennial	Root	fall or spring		x		
Agastache rugosa	Perennial	Herb	summer	x	x	x	
Albizia julibrissin	Tree	Flower/Bark	summer and fall				5/5
Alisma plantago-aquatica subsp. *orientale*	Perennial	Root	spring through fall		x		
Allium macrostemon	Perennial	Bulb	fall or spring		x		
Allium tuberosum	Perennial	Seed	fall	x	x	x	
Andrographis paniculata	Tender Perennial	Herb	summer	x			
Anemarrhena asphodeloides	Perennial	Rhizome	fall or winter		x	x	
Angelica dahurica	Biennial or Perennial	Root	fall	x			
Angelica pubescens	Biennial or Perennial	Root	fall or winter	x			
Angelica sinensis	Perennial	Root	fall		x		
Arctium lappa	Biennial	Seed/Root	summer and winter	x	x		
Artemisia annua	Annual	Herb	summer or fall	x			
Asparagus cochinchinensis	Perennial Vine	Root	winter			x	
Aster tataricus	Perennial	Root	fall or spring		x		
Astragalus membranaceus	Perennial	Root	fall or spring			x	
Atractylodes macrocephala	Perennial	Rhizome	fall or winter	x	x		
Bacopa monnieri	Tender Perennial Ground Cover	Herb	summer	x	x	x	
Belamcanda chinensis	Perennial	Rhizome	fall or spring		x		
Bupleurum chinense	Perennial	Root	fall or spring		x	x	
Carthamus tinctorius	Annual	Floret	summer	x			
Celosia argentea	Annual	Seed	fall	x			
Celosia cristata	Annual	Flower	summer or fall	x			
Centella asiatica	Tender Perennial Ground Cover	Herb	summer	x	x		
Chrysanthemum morifolium	Perennial	Flower	fall	x	x	x	
Clerodendrum trichotomum	Shrub	Leaf	summer				3
Codonopsis pilosula	Perennial Vine	Root	fall		x		
Coix lacryma-jobi	Tender Perennial	Seed	fall	x	x	x	
Cornus officinalis	Tree	Fruit	fall				5
Crataegus pinnatifida	Tree	Fruit	fall				5
Cyathula officinalis	Perennial	Root	fall or winter		x		
Dianthus superbus	Perennial	Herb	summer or fall	x	x		
Dioscorea opposita	Perennial Vine	Root	fall	x	x		
Dolichos lablab	Annual/Perennial Vine	Seed	summer or fall	x	x		
Eclipta prostrata	Annual	Herb	summer or fall	x			
Ephedra sinica	Perennial	Herb/Root	fall and winter		x		
Eriobotrya japonica	Shrub	Leaf	year-round				3
Eucommia ulmoides	Tree	Bark	spring				15–20

Botanical Name	Type	Harvest Portion	Season of Harvest	1st Season	2nd–3rd Season	4th Season	Years to Harvest
Fallopia multiflora	Perennial Vine	Root/Stem	fall and winter		x		
Forsythia suspensa	Shrub	Fruit	fall				5
Gentiana scabra	Perennial	Root	fall or spring			x	
Gentiana straminea	Perennial	Root	fall or spring			x	
Ginkgo biloba	Tree	Fruit	fall				5
Glycyrrhiza uralensis	Perennial	Root	spring or fall			x	
Gynostemma pentaphyllum	Perennial Vine	Herb	summer or fall	x	x	x	
Houttuynia cordata	Perennial Ground Cover	Herb	summer or fall	x	x	x	
Ligusticum jeholense	Perennial	Root	fall		x		
Ligustrum lucidum	Shrub	Fruit	fall				5
Lilium brownii	Perennial	Bulb	fall or winter		x		
Lilium lancifolium	Perennial	Bulb	fall or winter		x		
Lonicera japonica	Perennial Vine	Flower	spring or summer		x	x	
Lycium chinense	Shrub	Fruit/Root Bark	fall and winter		x	x	
Magnolia denudata	Tree	Flower Buds	spring				7–11
Mentha haplocalyx	Perennial Ground Cover	Herb	summer	x	x	x	
Momordica charantia	Annual Vine	Fruit	fall	x			
Ocimum sanctum	Annual	Herb	summer	x			
Ophiopogon japonicus	Perennial Ground Cover	Tuber	summer		x		
Paeonia lactiflora	Perennial	Root	summer or fall			x	
Paeonia suffruticosa	Perennial	Root Bark	fall			x	
Panax ginseng	Perennial	Root	fall				6–7
Panax quinquefolius	Perennial	Root	fall				5
Pinellia ternata	Perennial Ground Cover	Tuber	summer	x	x	x	
Plantago asiatica	Perennial	Seed	fall	x	x	x	
Platycodon grandiflorus	Perennial	Root	spring or fall		x		
Prunella vulgaris	Perennial	Herb	summer	x	x		
Rehmannia glutinosa	Perennial Ground Cover	Root	fall	x	x		
Rheum palmatum	Perennial	Root	winter		x		
Salvia miltiorrhiza	Perennial	Root	fall or spring	x	x	x	
Saposhnikovia divaricata	Perennial	Root	fall or spring		x		
Schisandra chinensis	Perennial Vine	Fruit	fall			x	
Schizonepeta tenuifolia	Annual	Herb	summer	x			
Scrophularia buergeriana	Perennial	Root	winter		x	x	
Scutellaria baicalensis	Perennial	Root	fall or spring				
Scutellaria barbata	Perennial	Herb	summer	x	x	x	
Sophora flavescens	Shrub	Root	fall		x	x	
Trichosanthes kirilowii	Perennial Vine	Fruit/Root	fall and winter		x		
Withania somnifera	Perennial	Root	fall	x	x		
Ziziphus jujuba	Tree	Fruit	fall				3+
Ziziphus jujuba var. *spinosa*	Tree	Seed	fall				3+

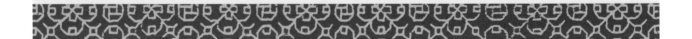

NOTES FROM THE CHINESE MEDICINAL HERB FARM   BY DANIEL MCQUILLEN

Cultivating "Wild-Quality" Herbs

It's an intern day at the Chinese Medicinal Herb Farm, and Peg Schafer is sitting down just long enough to share a short lunch with her interns and explain the process of growing herbs. She repeats the terms "cultivating wild quality" and "farming with the wild" like mantras. The terms, she says, describe the method of re-creating natural, semiwild conditions for cultivated plants. Primarily, this means growing herbs that are not "pushed," or grown with a lot of fertilizer. This yields smaller plants but, according to Schafer, higher concentrations and diversity of active medicinal components.

The technique also means not growing herbs too lushly or deflowering plants in order to artificially increase root size. The grower allows natural pressures, even if those pressures mean insect pests and hungry herbivores. "I let deer browse on some herbs, as long as they don't take all of it!" Schafer laughs. All of this helps create herbs that are closer to what is found in the wild.

Learning how to reliably grow medicinal herbs naturally and organically has been the biggest challenge of Schafer's endeavor: there are few experts and fewer books, even from sources in China. "I do a lot of thinking outside the box," she says. "For example, there's nothing written in English about harvest methods and processing for many of these herbs. So, I experiment, run trials, grow something out, then I talk with my connections: researchers, botanists, herbalists from China. Finally, I look closely at the finished product." After a decade of farming, experimenting, networking, researching, and educating, Peg says, "I'm still very much a beginner—it is a more-you-know the less-you-know kind of thing."

is a balanced formula permitted in organic production is a good choice; apply it at one-quarter to one-half the strength recommended on the label. One way to ascertain a product's organic status is to look for the Organic Materials Review Institute (OMRI) logo on the package label. Not all manufacturers are willing to go to the expense to be OMRI listed, but their products may certainly be allowed, so check with your organic certifying agency for approval. All fertilizer labels, by law, state the percentage of the three major macronutrients needed by plants: nitrogen (N), phosphorus (P), and potassium (K). Naturally derived formulated products will also contain traces of micronutrients. If a product does not have the N-P-K ratios on the front label it is a soil amendment, not a fertilizer. It may very well be a good product, but it contains the macronutrients in too small a percentage to be legally considered a fertilizer.

Pests and Diseases

Instead of bats in the belfry do you have deer in the *Dolichos lablab*? Gophers stealing plants and foxes stealing gophers in gopher traps? Frequently monitoring for pests is another aspect of the growing operation. It turns out that many Chinese herbs are rather

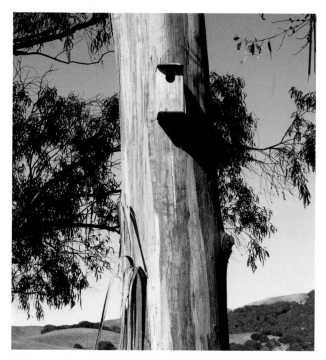

This screech owl box, one of several at the Chinese Medicinal Herb Farm, is a popular nesting site; place them near but not in the growing area that you'd like rodent-controlled.

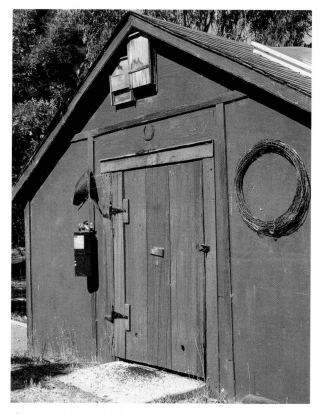

These two bat condos house many farm-friendly bats. Every day, we find a *lot* of evidence of their nighttime foraging— maybe next time we will not place bat houses directly over the barn door!

strong tasting, are an unappetizing grey-green, or are strong smelling—such herbs are eschewed by critters. But even when a plant suffers pest damage, the news is not all bad. As animal or insect pests eat part of a plant, the plant mobilizes a cascade of chemical responses to guard itself . . . which is efficacious medicine in the making!

Biological controls for animal pests include cats (not recommended in sensitive ecosystems); they eliminate a number of small herbivores, but they usually avoid the rototilling insectivore moles. Dogs are good deterrents for deer, hedgehogs, raccoons, armadillos, and other large pests. I recommend putting up nesting boxes for predatory birds; they are your great ally in rodent management. We have a lot of gophers and voles; they excessively impact production, and we trap them effectively with Cinch brand and mouse traps, respectively; the mouse traps are baited with oatmeal mixed with peanut butter. The tonic herbs are some of the most appealing to the gophers— *Astragalus membranaceus* (milk vetch, huáng qí), *Codonopsis pilosula* (poor man's ginseng, dǎng

shēn), *Ophiopogon japonicas* (lilyturf, mài mén dōng), as well as *Saposhnikovia divaricata* (siler, fáng fēng). Deer are a major pest in many areas, especially in the eastern states. Jean Giblette from High Falls Gardens in the Hudson Valley region of New York reports that deer like *Lilium* spp. (lily, bǎi hé) so much that they dig up and eat the bulbs. Among some of the other herbs that deer also consume—east or west—are *Acanthopanax gracilistylus* (wǔ jiā pí), *Crataegus pinnatifida* (Chinese hawthorn, shān zhā), *Dioscorea opposita* (Chinese yam, shān yào), and *Forsythia suspensa* (lián qiào). We have not fenced our entire field; instead we exclude pests from individual crops with fencing, bird netting, or a floating row crop cover. Where deer pressure is too great to successfully grow herbs, Jean Giblette mentions that a single-strand electric fence—baited with peanut butter and powered by a solar battery—will give a shock on their tongue so they learn to stay away, but that is only

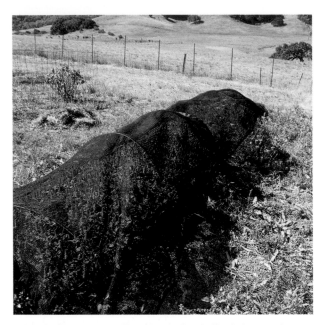

When in flower, *Prunella vulgaris* (heal all, xià kū cǎo) is attractive to browsing deer; this is an example of an exclusionary technique.

effective for light predation. A several-strand, ten-foot-high deer fence is her best recommendation. Another fence system that works is two four-foot-tall parallel fences set four feet apart. But ultimately deer are browsers and they do persevere—and so must we if they take more than their share. Pests and diseases are very regional; your local resources may have the best tactics for managing the pests in your area.

Ideally in a balanced system, insects and diseases are kept in check with immunity instilled by healthy soils and benevolent management practices. As part of facilitating this environment I recommend encouraging beneficial insects. Diversified hedgerow plantings as well as insectaries (nectar-producing plants that attract and feed adult beneficial insects) invite beneficial insects not only to dine but to stay and start families. Many of these nectar-rich foods are from the Umbel family, and mixes of their seed are regionally specific. Because they are so effective we grow blocks of insectaries throughout the growing areas, some as small as one hundred square feet and others twice that size. Check with your local farm supply operation for the best local or native mix. Lacewing larvae are the most effective general predator.

Japanese beetles are problematic in the eastern

United States. Jean Giblette uses pheromone traps (two per acre) to lure them to a bait plant area. She also uses *Dioscorea opposita* (Chinese yam, shān yào) as a trap crop, lets the beetles chew it until their season is over (mid-July to mid-August), and then cuts down the shredded vines. Jean notes that they prefer Asian species to North American if available: "They hit *Dioscorea opposita* and *D. nipponica* very heavily, but leave the *D. villosa* alone. They also eat *Schisandra chinensis* (five flavored fruit, wǔ wèi zǐ) leaves, but not enough to affect fruiting." In the morning while temperatures are still cool Japanese beetles can be shaken from the plants onto a tarp and then drowned in soapy water; alternately the concentration of beetles can be sprayed with a neem-containing product.

Because of the genetically diverse backgrounds of Asian herbs, diseases are thankfully not that common. Occasionally viral, bacterial, or fungal pathogens will present a wide range of symptoms. I have seen *Saposhnikovia divaricata* (siler, fáng fēng) infected with aster yellows; even though the foliage was slightly misshapen the plants produced

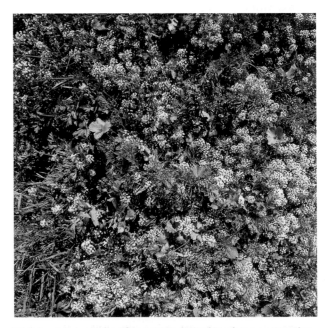

This insectary at the Chinese Medicinal Herb Farm contains nectar-rich foods for adult beneficial insects to encourage them to stay and reproduce—and they do! This regional mix contains alyssum, California poppy, tidytips, phacelia, coriander, and other plants from the Umbel family.

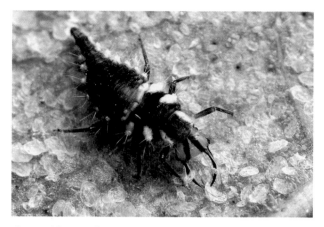

The workhorse of general predators, this green lacewing larva is dining on whitefly nymphs. Photo courtesy of Jack Dykinga.

respectable flowers, seed, and roots. (Since aster yellows is transmitted by sucking insects such as leafhoppers, it would have been wise for me to remove and destroy the infected material.) If the problem is unknown, consult with local nurseries, someone from a master gardener program, or a local agricultural advisor. Do not compost diseased plants as the disease may survive to reinfect more plants.

Weed Management

Sooner is better when it comes to taking action to minimize weed growth. Preparing a "stale seed bed" can control young weeds before you even plant out a crop. This is how it works: two to three weeks after tilling soil in the spring, weeds brought to the surface by the tilling will germinate. These fragile starts can be quickly flamed without disturbing the soil, leaving a competition-free area ready to plant. There are many models of flamers on the market; wear safety glasses and be very careful when using! Always have a hose nearby turned on (with a shut-off valve) and frequently look back over your shoulder to check for any smoldering material. In times of drought do not use flamers at all.

Mechanical weeding, by hoe or tractor, is best done while the weeds are still young and before they set seed. During the (almost) daily monitoring of the growing grounds, weeds are something I keep an eye out for. Early in the season I try to remove thistles before they set seed, digging to literally get to the

root of the problem. Weeds are definitely a problem on most farms: open the soil and it is an invitation for opportunistic plants—weeds. My main goal in relation to weeds is to keep the worst offenders from proliferating—usually by cultivation or removal. Another method I use is to keep the soil covered with plants that I do want—this outcompetes the weedy plants I don't want. Another goal is to make sure that they do not contaminate any herb harvests, so some crop areas will receive more weeding than others. Since we receive almost no rainfall for five months, if there is no input of water there are few weeds—another reason for drip irrigation.

I recommend the use of an organic mulch such as wood chips around trees and compost around other plants. Mulch suppresses weeds, and it also slowly feeds the soil food web and helps control erosion. Thick sheet mulch can be used to repair deficient or weedy soils; this can be piled up to a foot deep and placed on overlapped wet newsprint or cardboard (with any plastic tape removed). This may need to be in place for several years. If you are using wood chips it is best to use on-site material (locally we have sudden oak death, and oak root fungus can be brought in on infected material).

Soil solarization is an option to kill weeds and weed seeds and is most successful in the summer or fall in regions that are hot. The process involves covering moist, leveled soil—cleared or mowed of large weeds—with clear plastic sheeting. It is essential to weigh down the edges of the plastic to have good soil contact for maximum heat penetration; leave in place for a minimum of four weeks. Solarization is a useful technique to eliminate established lawns or difficult-to-eradicate weeds and pathogens, but the heating process will also kill beneficial soil organisms. Solarization is not effective for bindweed control.

Weeds sometimes have the potential to heal the land. For example, thistles bring up nutrients from below and their taproots eventually create air and water channels, softening compacted soils and bringing aeration and tilth. You will find that wild-farming techniques are at odds with clean cultivation, meaning that some weeds are allowed. However, do take care to remove invasive and noxious weeds to keep them from spreading or contaminating crop harvests. If you use overhead irrigation or live in an area with reliable summer rainfall, you can keep the soil covered by growing permanent or semipermanent cover crops in the paths between crop rows. Some of these crops are nitrogen producing and will also reduce wind-borne and waterborne soil erosion.

MANAGING INVASIVE PLANT RISK

While dealing with weeds is an expected part of growing, we need to distinguish between "ordinary" weeds and invasive weeds. Noxious or invasive weeds are unwanted opportunistic plants that are persistent and compete with other plants for sunlight, nutrients, water, and other resources. These much maligned plants—oftentimes rightly so—are site specific and take advantage of comparable biomes or regional climates that share the same latitudes and moisture availability, and often similar temperature ranges, as their home environments. Unfortunately in some regions, some Asian herbs can be weedy. The Climate and Precipitation Map of China in appendix B illustrates China's general weather patterns. This map illustrates the rainfall and temperature patterns that can be compared to your own growing grounds—not only for the goal of cultivation but for recognition of potential invasive qualities. Regions that have wet summers and mild winters are most conducive to successful invasive plant colonization. The following Potentially Invasive Chinese Herbs chart is a summary of those Asian herbs that have exhibited invasive qualities in at least one location in the United States.

For just about every ecological niche that exists, there is an Asian herb that can thrive in those conditions. The potential problem is that plant placement can be significant in terms of biodiversity displacement. Always remember that it is easier and less expensive to prevent invasive plant introductions than it is to try eradicate them once they have taken hold. Please be responsible when choosing which herbs to grow. Look for plants that will grow well in your bioregion and conditions, but be aware that plants have the potential to become invasive in settings that match their native growing conditions. Monitoring for invasive qualities is essential. The risk is dependent not only on the plant in question and the environment, but also the human element and the management conditions applied.

Noxious or Invasive Plant Characteristics

Common qualities of successful invasive plants include:

- ability to reproduce both asexually (by roots or stems) and sexually (seed)
- capability of rapid growth
- ability to adapt to a wide range of habitats
- deep roots
- proficiency at flowering and successful heavy seed producer
- effective seed dispersal techniques
- resistance to grazing pressures
- established history of overly persistent growth

Frequent methods of dispersal are by wind, water, and animal—but as you can imagine, introductions into new areas often occur in conjunction with human activity.

A rather underappreciated quality of some invasive weeds is their ability to heal compromised and overused soils. One of the most noxious, persistent weeds is *Pueraria montana* (kudzu, gé gēn), which was originally imported into the United States to control erosion—and it does that, perhaps too well. Like many legumes it is an initial colonizer, thriving in abused or exposed soils lacking in biodiversity. Like kudzu, many opportunistic plants take footing in overworked soils that have been left open due to human activity, fire, or geologic events.

Assessing Potentially Problematic Plants

Monitor any new plant, Asian herb or otherwise, for qualities that may make it invasive in your region. Take special care not to plant potential weeds into

Table 3-5. Potentially Invasive Chinese Herbs

Botanical Name	Common Name	Pinyin Name	Botanical Name	Common Name	Pinyin Name
Abutilon theophrasti	Velvet Leaf	qǐng má zǐ	Lobelia chinensis	Chinese Lobelia	bàn biān lián
Achyranthes bidentata	Oxknee	huái niú xī	Lonicera japonica	Honeysuckle	jīn yín huā
Agrimonia pilosa	No common name	xiān hè cǎo	Lycium chinense, L. barbarum	Chinese Wolfberry	gǒu qǐ zǐ/dì gǔ pí
Ailanthus altissima	Tree of Heaven	chūn gēn pí	Lycopus lucidus	Bugleweed	zé lán
Albizia julibrissin	Mimosa, Silk Tree	hé huān pí/huā	Malva verticillata	Farmer's Tobacco	dōng kuí guǒ, dōng kuí zǐ
Allium tuberosum	Garlic Chives	jiǔ cài zǐ	Mentha haplocalyx, M. arvensis	Field Mint	bò hé
Ampelopsis japonica	No common name	bái liàn	Morus alba	Mulberry	sāng bái pí, sāng yè, sāng shèn zǐ, sāng zhī
Arctium lappa	Burdock	niú bàng zǐ	Nandina domestica	Heavenly Bamboo	nán tiān zhú
Artemisia annua	Sweet Annie	qīng hāo	Peganum harmala	African Rue	luò tuó péng
Artemisia argyi	Moxa	ài yè	Perilla frutescens	Shiso	zǐ sū yè, zǐ sū zǐ, zǐ sū gěng
Artemisia japonica	No common name	mǔ hāo	Periploca sepium	Chinese Silk Vine	xiāng jiā pí
Artemisia princeps	Japanese Mugwort	kuí hāo	Persicaria orientalis	Kiss Me Over the Garden Gate	chuān liǎo zǐ
Aster tataricus	Tartar Aster	zǐ wǎn	Phellodendron amurense	Amur Cork Tree	huáng bǎi, huáng bò
Bacopa monnieri	Brahmi	brahmi	Pinellia ternata	No common name	bàn xià
Bassia scoparia	Summer Cypress	dì fū zǐ	Plantago sp.	Plantain	chē qián zǐ
Broussonetia papyrifera	Paper Mulberry	chǔ shí zǐ	Polygonum aviculare	Common Knotgrass	biān xù
Celastrus orbiculatus	Chinese Bittersweet	nán shé téng guǒ	Polygonum cuspidatum	Japanese Knotweed	hǔ zhàng
Cinnamomum camphora	Camphor Tree	zhāng nǎo	Polygonum multiflorum	Fo Ti	shǒu wū, yè jiāo téng
Cirsium spp.	No common name	xiǎo jì, dà jì	Portulaca oleracea	Purslane	mǎ chǐ xiàn
Clerodendrum bungei	Rose Glory Bower	chòu mǔ dān	Prunella vulgaris	Self Heal, Heal All	xià kū cǎo
Cnidium monnieri	Monnier's Snow Parsley	shé chuáng zǐ	Pueraria montana	Kudzu	gé gēn
Coix lacryma-jobi	Job's Tears	yì yǐ rén	Rosa x rugosa	No common name	méi guì huā
Commelina communis	No common name	yā zhí cǎo	Scrophularia buergeriana	Figwort	běi xuán shēn
Cuscuta sp.	Dodder	tǔ sī zǐ	Siegesbeckia pubescens	No common name	xī xiān cǎo
Dioscorea opposita	Chinese Yam	shān yào	Thlaspi arvense	Field Pennycress	sū bài jiang
Dipsacus sp.	Fuller's Teasel	xù duàn	Toona sinensis	Toona Tree	xiāng chūn
Eclipta prostrata	Eclipta	mò hàn lián	Tribulus terrestris	Puncture Vine, Caltrop	cì jí lí
Fallopia multiflora	Fo Ti	shǒu wū/yè jīao téng	Trichosanthes kirilowii	Chinese Cucumber	guā lóu/tiān huā fěn
Firmiana simplex	Chinese Parasol Tree	wú tong zǐ	Vaccaria hispanica	Cow Cockle	wáng bù liú xíng
Forsythia suspensa		lián qiào	Xanthium sp.	Cockleburr	cāng ěr zǐ
Glechoma longituba	Ground Ivy	lián qián cǎo			
Glycyrrhiza uralensis	Chinese Licorice	gān cǎo			
Houttuynia cordata	No common name	yú xīng cǎo			
Inula japonica	Japanese Elecampane	xuán fù huā			
Isatis tinctoria	Woad	bǎn lán gēn, dà qīng yè			
Koelreuteria paniculata	Goldenrain Tree	luán			
Leonurus spp.	Motherwort	yì mǔ cǎo			
Ligustrum lucidum	Chinese Privet	nǚ zhēn zǐ			

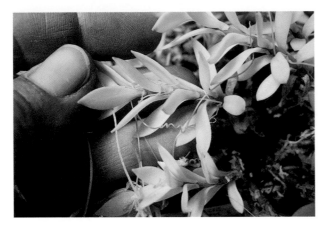

Cuscuta spp.—the orange thread-looking thing—is listed as a noxious weed and is indeed a very invasive parasite. The host of this one is *Sedum sarmentosum* (chuí pén cǎo)—it randomly showed up in our nursery. I promptly cut it away and it has not returned.

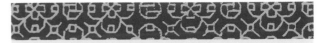

Noxious Weed Lists

Your county's agricultural commissioner extension office will have noxious weed lists and information on locally persistent plants. Please note that they also occasionally exercise their authority to fine growers who cultivate listed noxious plants. The USDA Natural Resources Conservation Service (NRCS) offers state and federal noxious weed lists at http://plants.usda.gov/java/noxiousDriver.

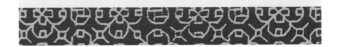

fragile ecosystems, or in or near open wetlands or waterways—the dispersal methods are too difficult to control and the potential risk to biodiversity is high. Examples of Chinese medicinal plants that can become weedy by aggressive opportunistic roots in many bioregions are *Aster tataricus* (tartar aster, zǐ wǎn) and *Glycyrrhiza uralensis* (Chinese licorice, gān cǎo). Stems that layer and root give *Forsythia suspensa* (lián qiào), *Lycium chinense* (Chinese wolfberry, gǒu qǐ zǐ/dì gǔ pí), and *Fallopia multiflora* (fo ti, shǒu wū/yè jiao téng) invasive qualities in many regions or where soils are moist. Some plants are prolific reseeders, such as *Coix lacryma-jobi* (Job's tears, yì yǐ rén), which is self-sowing primarily in the moist warm regions of the southern United States; *Artemisia annua* (sweet annie, qīng hāo) also self-sows readily in most regions. It is interesting to note that in Chinese medical theory the very quality of environmental persistence in an herb is the same quality that lends the plant its medicinal efficacy.

Economic Opportunities

Where invasive medicinal plants have been previously introduced, colonies have spread, and populations already persist as uncultivated stands, opportunities for wild collecting exist. Some populations are dense enough that wild-harvesting is economically viable—without the efforts and costs of cultivation. However,

the environmental conditions need to be unpolluted: ensure that no harvest occurs in areas near roads or from soils that are of questionable cleanliness. As always it is important to verify plant identity, and keep good records as to origin, date, and location of harvest. Photograph whole plants and specific parts, or scan plants or plant parts for future identity and assurance of authenticity. The Flora of China has a free online Website (http://www.efloras.org) where one can scientifically key out different floras; there are line drawings as well. Once again, always question the authenticity of Chinese herbal plant material because there are so many plants in circulation that may have either hybridized or been incorrectly identified in the first place.

Preventive Measures and Methods of Control

We all need to take a proactive approach to curbing potentially weedy botanicals. In the field, use broad buffer zones of at least twenty-five feet around block-grown herbs that spread by underground running stolons and roots. Monitor this space and disk, rototill, or use a chisel tine to control escapees. This technique is effective for *Glycyrrhiza uralensis* (Chinese licorice, gān cǎo) and some of the perennial

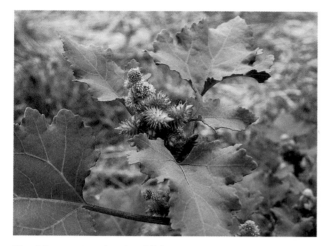

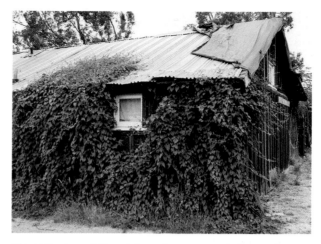

Xanthium strumarium (cockleburr, cāng ěr zǐ) is a noxious weed. Cockleburr has seeds that irritate furred creatures; it grows as an annual around our irrigation pond. When we first started harvesting it for medicine, there was about two hundred pounds per year; now we only have about fifty pounds per year.

This *Fallopia multiflora* (aka *Polygonum multiflorum*, fo ti, shǒu wū/yè jīao téng) was planted on the other side of this barn and has grown under and over it in a summer drought region. It has been cut back repeatedly but will probably never be eradicated from this site.

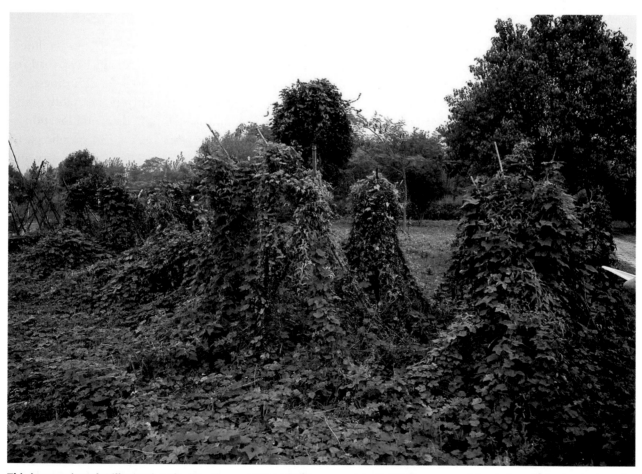

This impressive plot illustrating the invasive qualities of *Dioscorea opposita* (Chinese yam, shān yào) was found on a tour of a Chinese herb company farm in Anhui province, eastern China.

Artemisia spp. as well. Deadhead (remove the flowers) from plants that aggressively reseed such as *Isatis tinctoria* (woad, běi bǎn lán gēn) and *Siegesbeckia pubescens* (xī xiān cǎo). Remove plants where experience, information, and monitoring show them to be too opportunistic and aggressive. It will probably take multiple assaults to be successful, but it beats introducing a new scourge.

To control the spread of plants already growing on-site, good management is essential: methods such as pruning, digging, mowing, and rototilling are effective. Also consider the use of physical barriers; if a landscape client would like to have a planting of *Mentha haplocalyx* (field mint, bò hé) in their garden I often plant it in a five-gallon pot and then sink the pot halfway into the garden. Try modifying the irrigation regimen to create inhospitable conditions. Don't forget the option to employ the technique of very heavy sheet mulch. Flaming is a useful tool when seedlings are young, especially for dicots, but it should be handled only by trained staff that possess a cautious nature; many destructive fires have been started by careless operators. Always have water readily available and never flame in hot, dry, or windy conditions.

Maintaining your organic status also can require careful management strategies. Certified organic operations must comply with regulations concerning a variable property boundary setback tolerance if synthetic chemicals are being applied on neighboring properties. Check with your certifying agency for explanations of rules, rights, and assistance if needed. And of course, never be the one to plant potentially problematic plants along a shared boundary line.

CHAPTER FOUR

The Harvest and Marketing

Harvesting can be rewarding and daunting all at the same time. There are usually time constraints so we have to keep on track. At the Chinese Medicinal Herb Farm, a typical harvest of *Scutellaria baicalensis* (baikal skullcap, huáng qín) happens in late November. The morning is cold as we head out into the field with our shovels and harvest bins in hand-pulled carts. Our winter rains have begun, and our clay soils are too wet to drive over with the tractor. In block H row 3 the H3 wooden stake marker says this seed was direct-sown into the field on May 20th, three years previous. Three hundred "spots" were sown where I turned on the in-line drip emitter irrigation to mark just where to place the seed; I count and we should get 270 plants—not bad, 90 percent. After a quick woo-woo session of invoking good medicine for all who will be using the crop, we dig in to unearth bright yellow, 1½-foot-long, Medusa-like roots—the crowns indicated by brown twigs telling us where to look. The sun is out now, but that is not what makes us warm; a banter of jokes and spells of quietude meter the steady rhythm of movement. After we've dug about 20 pounds, one of us takes the roots down to the washing area and puts them in a bin prefilled with water to soak while setting up the power washer and screen-topped table. The one crew member places some of the crop on the table and sprays as gently as possible to remove any clinging soil. The yellow roots become even more yellow as they come clean—then off into a clean harvest bin. Another person has set up the cutting station; the next step is removing the root crowns. Then the roots are cut—parallel slices a quarter-inch thick, cutting from the crown end down to the tip of the roots. More *Scutellaria* comes out of the field, and there's a steady stream of root and water and slicing until the end of the day yields 122 pounds of fresh root. Not bad: nearly half a pound per plant. The winter sun is low, and there is less bantering as the wash stations are themselves washed and we are all ready to be done for the day. Lot number 112610H3SB. Tomorrow we have H4 to tackle—I think I will try out the new waterproof boots.

HARVESTING MEDICINE

Throughout the growing season, it pays to think ahead to the harvest. Consider when and how you'll achieve the desired end product, and monitor your crop frequently with this in mind. As harvest time draws near, contact the buyer and confirm that they still want the crop and exactly at what stage they want it harvested. Confirm whether the buyer wants the product fresh or dried, as well as what form they would like (whole, powdered, diagonally sliced, pitted, and so on). If it is a fresh product, find out exactly *when* and *how* they want it to be shipped.

One week before harvest, make sure that the crop is freely accessible and that there are no weeds that might contaminate the harvest or otherwise make the process more difficult. If herbs are to be dried, make sure the drying room is clean and ready to receive the crop.

All herbs should be washed either before or after harvest—unless it is a floral crop. For crops that won't be washed after harvest, plan ahead to rinse the crop in the field a day or two before harvesting. The plants should be dry when harvested, or they won't dry or ship well. To rinse field crops to rid them of dust and impurities (especially the white ones gifted from above by birds), hose them off as standing plants in the field. Use potable water only, with a directional or variable nozzle sprayer to wash all plant parts to be harvested.

The day before harvest, prepare the wash station, collect harvest vessels and any tools that may be needed, secure any extra help necessary, and check the weather forecast. If a big rain is in the forecast it might be prudent to reschedule a harvest—especially if the crop is to be dried on the farm or if the harvest is a same day air shipment. On the day of harvest, start early so you can collect in an unstressed manner. It may take longer than imagined—workers may not arrive, or the temperature may come up (or down) and adversely impact the crop. There has been more than one occasion where the temperature climbs faster than workers can pick. For example we had a crop that was to be sold fresh—*Agastache rugosa* (Korean mint, tǔ huò xiāng). We started picking leaves and stems early in the morning, but the temperature started soaring and soon it was ninety degrees. Even though we were moving the crops into the refrigerator on a regular basis, the plants were transpiring moisture through the leaves faster than they could uptake moisture from their roots, resulting in wilting leaves. We had no choice but to quit harvesting, because wilted leaves do not usually recover.

Leaves and Flower Harvesting

Leaves get rinsed off in the field a day or two before harvest or after harvesting. Rinsing leaves while they are in the field yields dry leaves which are superior for either drying or shipping. It is on a case-by-case basis whether leaves are rinsed before or after harvesting. For example, the leaves of *Centella asiatica* (gotu kola, jī xuě cǎo) will always need to be rinsed after harvest as they grow right on the ground. Flowers tend to be the most fragile harvestable plant parts and do not usually get rinsed. Both ideally get collected right after the dew has dried but before they heat up.

The wash station can be as simple as freshwater access and large tubs. More convenient are multiple stainless steel sinks or troughs alongside farm-sized

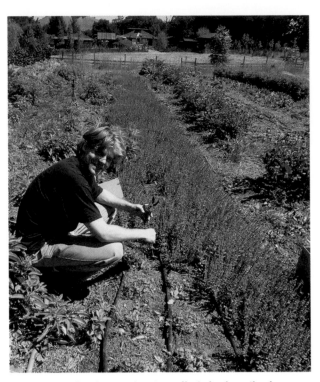

Intern Kurt Baker harvesting *Scutellaria barbata* (barbat skullcap, bàn zhī lián).

salad spinners. Crops that have clinging soil need to be rinsed multiple times to ensure that no soil remains and, as usual, inspected for any hitchhiking weeds, or other potential contaminents. To keep well, the crop (especially leaves) will then need to be rid of surface water by draining and spinning—and then immediately placed in cold storage until shipment, or put into the drying room. Remember, if the herb is to be sold fresh and wilting begins, it is too late: the crop will not recover. Refrigerate leaf or flower that is to be sold fresh immediately after processing. We put the clean material into clean baskets or shallow trays to cool down quickly. There is more leeway for dried product, since wilting is the first step in its drying process, but it should still be moved quickly into the drying room. At the Chinese Medicinal Herb Farm we can harvest and process roughly one hundred pounds of leaves to be ready to ship fresh, or put to dry, per person per day.

Root Harvesting

Roots are more durable and often harvested when temperatures are cool or cold. Common harvest times are late fall, early winter after the roots have gone dormant, or in early spring before new growth emerges. Check the individual herb profiles or the Harvest chart in chapter 3 for specific harvest times. Unless there is heavy rain or snow, weather should not be a problem. Tools of choice are shovels or tractor-mounted modified potato diggers. For the scale of our operation, we do most of the harvesting of roots by shovel. It's necessary to wash roots after you dig them. On a small scale a power washer with different settings is most helpful—but be careful not to spray so hard that you remove root bark, because it is usually considered part of the product. The roots are spread out on a wood- or metal-rimmed half-inch screen "table" we devised and are sprayed, turning as necessary, to rid the crop of soil. After harvesting, according to Good Agricultural Practices (more on GAPs below), always keep the harvest off the ground and in clean containers—which also are not on the ground. Another small-scale method is to place roots in a mesh bag and agitate in water. The roots will rub against each other and scrub themselves clean; place similar-size roots together for best results. Repurposed washing machines can work well. For batches over several hundred pounds a root or barrel washer can be very helpful.

It is common practice to soak roots before washing to loosen the soil, but do this for only a short period of time, a few hours at most—or the water-soluble medicinal constituents may be lost. Fresh roots are usually sold whole or as close to whole as is feasible.

Bark and Seed Harvesting

Although root crops comprise the bulk of Chinese herbs, barks and seeds are also used. Wash barks with a power washer before harvesting, on the tree or as whole cut logs—it is much faster. Each tree gives up its bark differently. I have used draw knives, hand saws, and pry bars with hammers. If I were harvesting a lot of bark I would look into specific logging tools that are designed for removing bark from trees.

Harvest seeds early in the day for fresh sale. If the

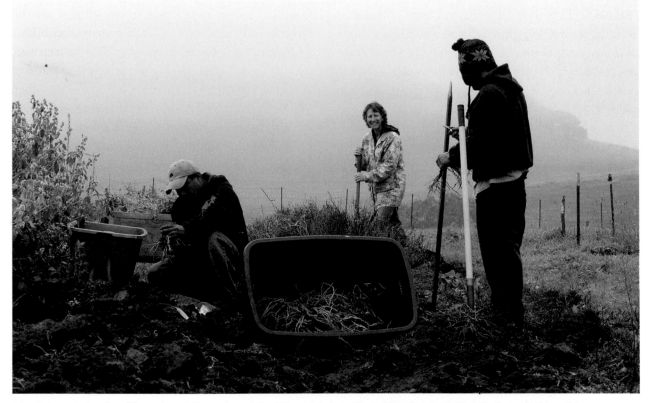

Digging roots is most often a late fall or winter job; this crop is *Scutellaria baicalensis* (baikal skullcap, huáng qín).

seed is to be dried further, harvesting later in the day often gets the drying process off to a good start. Chamomile or blueberry harvesting rakes are sometimes helpful for seed collection if the ratio of seed diameter to rake tine openings is correct. If seeds do not separate easily from the maturing flowers, I often harvest and dry whole flower heads, which will then release the seed as they dry. To further clean the harvest, use seed cleaning screens and winnow if necessary (I describe the winnowing process later in this chapter).

As with any cleaning (or other farm) process, the skill and experience level of the operator makes all the difference in terms of how efficiently the process is completed. A quicker person with less mechanization is probably faster than a slower person with fancier tools.

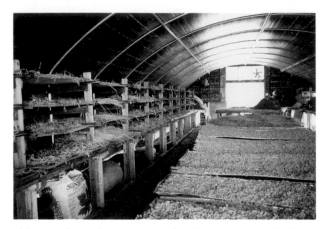

This greenhouse is repurposed for the summer as a drying shed by covering the polyethylene with black plastic. The doorway serves as the intake vent and the outtake vent is an exhaust fan–giving a lot of space.

DRYING HERB CROPS

For herbs that are to be dried, always start the drying process as soon as possible after harvest. The best quality dry herbs look like the fresh herbs, only dry. If leaves were green when fresh they should be green dry, and flowers should retain their live floral hues. All plant parts should smell fresh and look vibrant.

Setting up a Drying Area

Drying areas can be as small and simple as a food dehydrator, or as large as a building. Your operation will need an operable drying setup of appropriate size in the first season. There are many renditions but the requirements are the same: lots of air movement provided by fans in a dry, dark, warm space. Intake vents that are low on the building on the windward side and outlet vents placed high on the opposite side are recommended. Dehumidifiers and heaters can increase efficiency, especially when drying roots in the winter time. At the Chinese Medicinal Herb Farm we have repurposed a 20-by-15-foot building as a drying shed. This size services two acres of herbs as long as harvests are staggered. We installed a wire apparatus near the ceiling for hanging bunched herbs still on their stems as well as movable racking

for bench drying of loose herbs. The wire on the ceiling is set one foot apart, and the benches for drying are also set up with a foot between racks.

The Drying Process

For bunching herbs together use rubber bands. The bands will contract and continue to hold the herbs together as they dry. If you're spreading herbs on racks, layer them thinly, or be prepared to turn them frequently. Cut or grade or size the herbs so that they will dry in about the same amount of time.

When I put a batch of herbs in the drying room, over a day or so I raise the temperature slowly. Temperatures for drying leaves, flowers, seed, and fruit generally should not exceed 100 degrees; roots and barks should be no more than 120 degrees. Turn several times a day to facilitate even drying. Dry herbs thoroughly. I test for moisture by breaking and cutting stems and roots and opening whole flowers or any part that is dense. Do not overdry them or they will lose their integrity; leaves can turn to powder, flowers can lose their petals. Overdried herbs will not hold as well in storage, either.

STORING DRIED HERBS

Herbs keep best in as whole a form as possible; store herbs whole and further process when the herb is needed or ordered. Dry bunched herbs are too big to

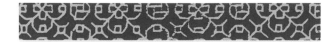

Open Air Drying

Many old texts will mention drying outside in the open air. I do not recommend this practice. Sunlight rapidly degrades the herb and the product can reabsorb moisture at night—and birds might leave their droppings.

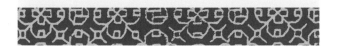

store on-stem and will need to be garbled or riddled to reduce their size or separate the leaf from the stem. We use framed stainless steel screens of different gauges positioned over bins for this task. With a flat hand, simply roll the bunched herb against the screen—the leaves will fall through the holes into the bins. When the stem is traditionally included in the herb we often hold the bunch upside down and move it back and forth over the screen so that the leaves and stems break off and fall into the bin together.

Some buyers ask for "cut and sift" (herb particles all of uniform size); tea companies and retail stores often request this. You can use the same screens, or seed screens, to prepare cut and sift herb product.

Ask for specifics before accepting any contracts. A hammermill is a size-reducing machine and is an ideal tool for producing herbs of differing sizes. (This is a different tool from the powdering machines for herb encapsulation.) Hammermills for plant material are not that easy to come by—nor are they cheap; look for a secondhand machine. The investment depends on the market segment one is after—you might consider one after a few years of production.

Assign a traceable unique lot number to each harvest and record weights before and after drying. There are many complicated systems for lot numbering of harvested herbs. In light of transparency I want people to know when our herbs were harvested, so my lot number is comprised of the date harvested, location, and the first two letters of the genus and species. For example, 113010E2WS means November 30, 2010, from block E in bed 2 and the herb is *Withania somnifera* (Ashwagandha). This number is recorded in the farm database (mentioned in chapter 3), which interfaces with the documents that I need to submit for my organic certification. Lot numbers appear on all dried herb package labels as well.

Store herbs in bins with tight fitting lids, or use large, thick, recloseable plastic bags. Large glass jars are good for storing a small amount of herb. Be sure to label all containers with the herb name and lot

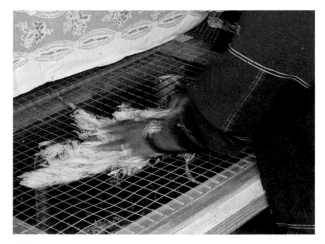

Riddling *Artemisia argyi* (moxa, aì yè) on a one-inch screen is a good way to break the leaves off the stem material.

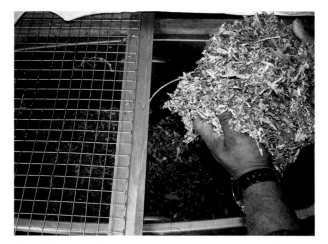

The riddled product from the previous picture—the fragrance is strong!

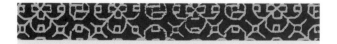

Herb Processing or Pao Zhi

Many Chinese herbs have specific processing methods beyond simply drying, and they are an important consideration when deciding what to offer in this emerging market. At the Chinese Medicinal Herb Farm we have been utilizing the information on traditional processing from industry experts and conducting experiments. We have some interesting results, such as *Rehmannia glutinosa* (Chinese foxglove, dì huáng) roots steamed in rice wine; *Fallopia multiflora* (fo ti, shǒu wū/yè jīao téng) root cooked with black soybeans; and *Pinellia ternata* (bàn xià) tubers, cooked with ginger and alum. Feedback from respected industry experts has been promising. A book for growers and clinicians on traditional Chinese processing techniques, *The Farmers' Pao Zhi Manual: Processing and Preparation of Chinese Herbs,* is due to be released soon by herb grower Jean Giblette of High Falls Gardens (published by High Falls Foundation).

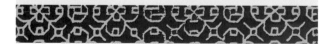

number. At the farm we have an ideal storage space: a north-facing room that is dark, stays cool and dry year-round, and is rodent proof.

Generally dried leaves, flowers, fruit, and seed have a storage life of one year, and roots and barks two years. Monitor stored herbs every few weeks for insect or rodent activity. For each herb sold, a retention sample should be held back for several years so that if there is ever a question of identity, there is a reference. The sample amount should be roughly half a pound—enough to be able to run several kinds of laboratory tests.

SHIPPING FRESH OR DRY HERBS

Once your crop is ready for the customer, you'll need to pack it properly for shipping. Shipping fresh herbs requires thorough chilling before packing. We do most harvesting and shipping on Mondays so herbs will have all week to reach their destination, and less of a chance of languishing over the weekend when the pace of transit slows. Ultimately the shipping method depends on the distance, the time of year, and the crop in question; discuss this ahead of time with the buyer. Since it is traditional for the buyer to pay shipping, they will indicate how fast they want it to be sent. However, if the herb is a fresh leaf or flower crop being shipped while the weather is warm or hot, I always recommend shipping overnight by air—or if the buyer is local, delivering the same day; otherwise, I can't guarantee the quality. I place small prefrozen plastic water bottles in the shipping containers with the crop. Wrap the bottles with a few sheets of newsprint to protect the crop (which is in plastic bags) from locally freezing, and tape them to the side of the shipping container so they don't bludgeon the herb. Don't use gel-type ice packs, because they could contaminate the crop if a shipment is damaged; also, they are not recyclable. Dry herbs (thankfully) do not need to be expedited.

COLLECTING AND SAVING SEED FOR SOWING

Another kind of harvesting is saving your own seed for replanting. Seed saving makes sense from a sustainability perspective—and for certified organic growers, it may become an essential practice. Certified organic rules are more restrictive than in the past, stipulating that seed grown for organic production is itself certified organic. There are other good reasons to grow your own seed, too: the genetics become acclimatized to the location (evolving to suit the niche), seed freshness and the quality of the genetics are known, and the price per plant volume can't be beat. Seed harvesting is usually a later-season activity, when seed has reached its maximum dry weight on the plants.

Plants are pollinated by wind, insect, animal, or

bird—or they self-pollinate. A certain amount of planning must take place to ensure that any seed collected is true to type (same intended genus and species) and not the result of accidental cross-pollination. Cross-pollination occurs most usually within a species, by wind or insect, so the isolation distance needed to ensure true seed can be miles. Wind-pollinated plants evolved before there were insects to do the pollination task, so these plants tend to not be very showy—grasses are one example of wind-pollinated plants—and it is possible that pollen granules can be carried several miles to achieve pollination. Showy flowers attract insects, birds, or bats to do their bidding; bees can cover one to three miles a day spreading pollen and fertilizing flowers. There are many methods to avoid heritable contamination: examples include deadheading one of the varieties that will (alas) be blooming at the same time, isolation by distance, use of screened cages, or growing for maturity at different times. If using screened cages, the screen must be small enough that pollinating insects cannot pass through; move the screens between the (hopefully only two) varieties, alternating every other day so the insects can do their pollinating work. *Seed to Seed* by Suzanne Ashworth is a great book, indispensible for anyone interested in saving seed. Please see appendix C for more information.

Seed Cleaning

Once seed has been collected, I spread it out in a shady area or inside to let it dry out a bit before cleaning it of any extraneous material. Seed cleaning screens are great tools for processing dry seed. I first use a screen larger than the seed to remove stems, leaves, and anything else large—and then a screen smaller than the seed to remove dust, dirt, and small bits of unwanted material. To further clean the seed I put it in a bowl and blow gently across the top of the seed. Or I winnow the stock using a fan, a large tarp, and a ladder. I set up the fan behind the ladder and turn it on. Then I climb the ladder and slowly pour the seed onto the tarp. The heavy, denser quality seed will fall straight down and the lighter material (chaff) will blow further away. This works best if the sizes or

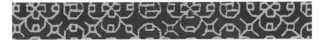

Tips for Seed-Saving Success

- The best quality seed is collected from as large a population of plants as is feasible, contributing a wide spectrum of genetics. I have found that of the crops we grow, 200 plants will produce better quality seed than 20 plants (though sometimes this may be all that one has to work with). Larger plantings bestow the best opportunities not only for healthy vigor but species survival.
- If you notice a drop in vitality in a population of seed that you've been saving for a while, especially from a small population, you may need to reinvigorate it with fresh genetics. Intentional crosses, which increase gene flow, keep stock strong. Be certain to keep track of these crosses.
- Grow open pollinated seed, as hybrid offspring will have unknown genetics—not a good idea when growing medicine.
- When growing plants for seed, rogue out any weak-looking, diseased, or pest-affected plants before they have a chance to contribute their genetics during pollination.

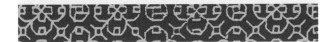

weights of the seed and unwanted material are different. Traditionally, winnowing is done with the aid of wind, but wind is variable enough that results are spotty and it takes a lot more time.

Wet processed seed, usually from a wet fruit such as *Withania somnifera* (Ashwagandha) or *Acanthopanax gracilistylus* (wŭ jiā pí), is cleaned with water. The process entails mashing the fleshy seed in water by hand or in a food processor fitted with a plastic blade and rinsing several times. After separating the pulp from the seed, add more water

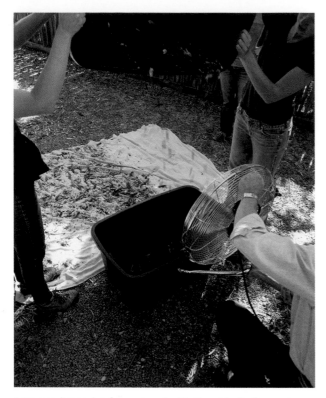

Interns winnowing heavy seed with the aid of a fan and large bins.

keep moist (but not too wet or the seed will rot). Avoid areas with gas appliances, as natural gas is known to inhibit seed germination. After one week check daily for germination (this may take two or three weeks). This technique works for the majority of seed. For multicycle germinators, try this variation (but keep in mind that the seed must be ultra-fresh): Place the moist seeded towel in the refrigerator for two to three weeks—do not let it dry out. Then bring it into the seventy-degree room and follow the process as with typical seed.

SELLING WHAT YOU GROW

One reason the Chinese Medicinal Herb Farm is certified organic is I am leveraging this as a marketing tool. A segment of my market is makers of products such as extracts, dietary supplements, teas, and so on, and those buyers that offer certified organic products require certified organic ingredients. The county of Marin, where our farm resides, is also a third party certifier similar to California Certified Organic Farmers (CCOF)—this is unusual, is fiscally farmer friendly, and effectively supports local growers and ranchers. I highly recommend obtaining organic certification because it will expand and diversify your sales opportunities. There are other ecologically minded designations as well, and many of these organizations have holistic philosophies and more stringent guidelines. Though many ecological designations do not first require one to be certified organic (through the USDA National Organic Program), the Demeter Biodynamic Certification does. The different methods of organic certification can be costly; but in this niche sector, in my opinion, foregoing certification is a marketing error.

and float the pulp and any floating seed off to be discarded. The floating seeds are dead (take a look, there are no embryos)—heavy live seed usually sinks.

For the best viability, all seed will need to dry to a low moisture content. Use a lot of dry air movement and do not heat seed over ninety degrees, since some seed can sustain damage. Store the seed in a cool, dry, dark location that has little temperature variation. An old industry standard formula holds that the temperature plus relative humidity should not exceed one hundred.

If seed is of questionable quality or you want to check on the viability, conduct a simple germination test. When I do this I lay out a few sheets of heavy paper towel, moisten them, and line up the seed to be tested in a row of ten, twenty-five, or fifty toward the top of the sheets. I then fold over the rest of the towel from the bottom, roll the whole sheet laterally, moisten again, and hold lightly with two rubber bands. Then I put all this in an open jar in a warm location (seventy degrees is ideal) out of the sun and

Domestically grown Chinese herbs have a noticeably higher cost of production than herbs imported from China. Reasons for this include higher wages, higher land costs, more environmental precautions, and little crop support via traditional regional agricultural farm advisors or research assistance (which used to be spearheaded by our land grant colleges). However, domestically grown herbs also have significant advantages in the marketplace, such as undeniable herb quality, freshness, and the growing trend of US buyers choosing to support local economies. All of the advantages and disadvantages are what make Asian herbs a niche market. There is also a collective awakening to issues of global habitat conservation as well as fair trade and social livelihood issues. As growers, we can conserve through cultivation by simply making these herbs available and lessening the impact of wild-collecting practices in China. But we need to cultivate in a way that simulates wild quality, so that the herbs exhibit strong medicinal potency, thereby creating a demand. The qualities that domestic crops express are benefits that need to be highlighted by transparency in the supply chain. And I find that consumers are increasingly choosing domestically grown medicinal herbs. For further discussion of transparency see the Regulating Herbs section in chapter 2.

Growing a Market

When I was starting my farm, one of the big challenges I faced was figuring out which herbs to grow—not only from a cultivation standpoint, but from a marketing perspective. Who would buy my herbs, and which ones would they want? So I embarked on a little basic market research. I contacted virtually all the local practitioners to introduce myself, making cold calls and following up with a letter. I inquired which herbs they used in their practice and whether they would be interested in purchasing anything in particular. From there I embarked on a threefold approach: I started growing individual herbs that were in demand, herbs that I could find seed for (there were fewer resources fifteen years ago!), and the combination of herbs that made complete traditional formulas. However, I have found that no one bioregion, here or in China, can grow all the herbs that OM practitioners need to make formulas.

If you're just getting started, you can try my homegrown marketing approach—but I would suggest that nowadays there are much more efficient and less limiting means of approaching a more diversified market. Buyers, in all markets, want convenience and

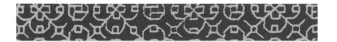

Diversified Operations

Before I grew Asian botanicals I worked on vegetable farms. Although the cultural treatments can be quite different, choosing the right crops can benefit your operation. There is a wide assortment of Asian herbs that can maximize unused marginal land, either incorporated as an intercrop or straight-on row cropping. Perhaps you have land that has a shady slope, or is excessively wet or dry for most other plants. Intercropping in between vineyard or orchard rows or planting into a woodlot may be opportunities. Crop selections that utilize different planting or harvest schedules, spreading out the seasonality of the work, can keep valued workers employed—or distribute your own work schedule. Some Asian herbs, especially the food herbs, are increasing in popularity and can be grown alongside and treated like many other common vegetables. A few examples of Asian herbs that can fit well into a vegetable operation with a general regiment of water, sun, and fertilizer are *Ocimum sanctum* (sacred basil, tulsi), several types of onions (*Allium* spp.), *Dolichos lablab* (hyacinth bean, bái biǎn dòu), and *Momordica charantia* (bitter melon, kǔ guā). For shrubs and trees, hedgerows at the field margins are ideal for habitat and pollination value as well as conducting trials and may be a good source of longer range revenue. There are many Asian crops to explore for niches to diversify your operation.

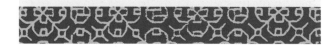

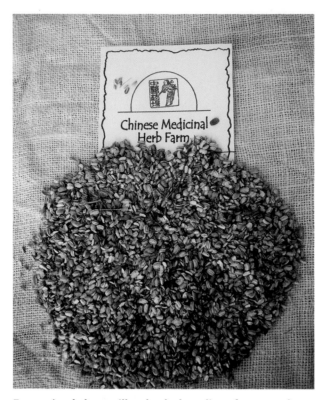

Even a simple logo will make the branding of your product more effective.

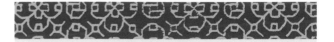

Setting Prices

Pricing structures for medicinal herbs differ with the markets. The profit margins are very tight; after all, it is agriculture—and this market is still in the fledgling stages of development. Collecting information that will enable you to figure out your costs of production for each herb you grow will be key for pricing. After conducting your trial crops, you will have preliminary postharvest handling figures available to plug into your growing database to help calculate your herb pricing. The numbers will change as you gain experience with the individual crops and production processes. I start with my best guess and change herb pricing—up or down—as I move through production year to year. We sell out of what we can grow every year—the market is there. It helps to have some agricultural experience and be a person who thinks outside the box— and a dose of entrepreneurial spirit is always useful medicine.

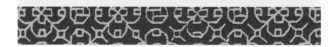

one-stop shopping—they are busy people. Marketing with a collaboration of growers offering a diversified array of herbs to practitioners in their region has a lot more synergy and power than an individual grower trying to sell a few herb varieties. Advertising to local practitioners that "our group of growers is selling nine root, eight leaf, and four flower and bark crops"—now that has promotional weight. For herbs that are not possible to grow locally, cooperation between regions will be the win-win solution. There is tremendous potential, and I believe that cooperation is absolutely essential to the success of the domestic cultivation market. Jean Giblette of High Falls Gardens feels the same way, and she and I have been working for years as volunteers to support this type of cooperative endeavor. Feel free to join us— collectively we can proceed together through http://www.localherbs.org. As Jean says, "Historically farmers, suffering the vagaries of the marketplace, have been forced to compete against each other in a spiral of diminishing returns. Little incentive for quality

and other values exists in the global commodity system."[15] Organized professional growers cooperating to offer an array of top quality medicinal plant products has the potency of a project that will truly prosper.

Customer Relations

There are a number of different markets besides wholesale and retail segments—progressive herbal pharmacies, OM practitioners with whole herb and different compounding products they make, Western herbalists and their products, and the nutriceutical and supplement markets and cosmetic trade. Each of these markets operates within a different scale. Local retail herb stores tend to buy just a pound or so of any one herb, while wholesale herb tea buyers may only want herbs in hundred-pound lots—and they want it cut and sifted to specification. There are also even larger markets, but this is not the place to start.

When you've made the commitment to supply a buyer, it becomes extra important to calculate how much you need to plant to meet the obligation. Plant more than is contracted or needed; contract fulfillment is an important component for continued success in grower/buyer relations. If the crop produces more than a fresh order, great—dry it for later sale. Suffice it to say that buyers do not love to hear the words "crop failure." Review the Planting section in chapter 3 for tips on how to decide how much to plant so you'll have some built-in "crop insurance."

GOOD AGRICULTURAL PRACTICES

No description of marketing agricultural crops in the twenty-first century would be complete without a discussion of Good Agricultural Practices (GAPs),

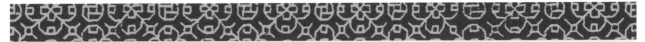

NOTES FROM THE CHINESE MEDICINAL HERB FARM   BY DANIEL MCQUILLEN

A Small but Growing Community

Being a medicinal herb farmer is not the lonely profession it once might have been. Many farms across the United States have joined together into a group called the Medicinal Herb Consortium (MHC), a nonprofit group where US medicinal herb growers work together to service market demand and build connections with practitioners.

Herb farm owner Jean Giblette serves as the MHC's coordinator while running High Falls Gardens in Philmont, New York. She explains how the consortium is trying to organize growers and markets so that a complete system can sprout, grow, and flourish. This is why Giblette and others formed the MHC: to get information to the farmers, assess the results of their efforts, and offer contracts with guaranteed prices. A farmer that wants to grow jié gěng may know a lot about balloon flower plants, but is her farm the right place to grow *Platycodon*

grandiflorus to produce medicinally effective jié gěng? Ultimately, OM practitioners are the best judge of the quality of the final product. The MHC makes that practitioner knowledge available to the farmers. "So the farmer grows a little jié gěng, gets the nod and the contract, then grows a lot more with less risk," she explains. "The farmers and the practitioners have to go through a process together to get what they want. We're beginning that process right now." (The group has a Website at http://www.localherbs.org.)

The MHC is working to help herb farmers like Peg Schafer—who cofounded the group with Giblette—organize, collaborate, and exchange information and techniques. But in the end there is still a big requirement of ingenuity and a trust in nature. "How do I know what to do?" asks Schafer. "Nature is guiding me. It makes me feel good about what I do."

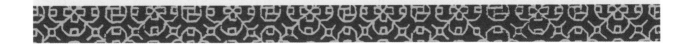

which are guidelines for growers covering everything from planting stock and methods of cultivation to harvesting and storage of crops. Currently there are no mandated regulations—only recommendations, and several organizations have created their own albeit competing guidelines. These collections of principles will have more impact as time progresses and protocols are organized and enacted. In a nutshell, GAPs address safety through proper botanical identity, cleanliness, quality assurance, environmental stewardship, farm systems, and economic and social issues. Although I have always been careful about ensuring the identity of the herbs we sell, it is medicine after all; we are even more careful now, and I am working on a herbarium of each herb accession we grow out for future identification and verification. I also offer to e-mail this scanned material, and invite buyers to the farm to see the crops while they are growing. The United States Department of Agriculture (USDA), the Food and Drug Administration, and the Food and Agriculture Organization of the United Nations all have guidelines. More directly applicable to the herb industry are the guidelines crafted by the American Herbal Products Association in cooperation with the American Herbal Pharmacopoeia.[16] Another resource is the World Health Organization Guidelines on Good Agricultural and Collection Practices (GACP) for Medicinal Plants.[17] (These guidelines are not to be mistaken for the Good Manufacturing Practices [GMPs], which are legally enforceable and apply to manufacturing processes—including value-added products.)

MAKE ALLIANCES

There are so many Chinese herbs to grow—literally hundreds—that it makes good sense to form alliances with other growers and work cooperatively. Besides the fact that cultivation of some herbs is more regionally appropriate for some areas than others, it is good to have help growing different varieties and sharing orders to satisfy market demand, troubleshooting problems from germination to drying, and locally sharing such things as equipment and harvest help. Alliances with buyers and buyer groups also make sense; the Sonoma County Herb Exchange (http://www.sonomaherbs.org) is but one example of this type of community-minded entrepreneurial relationship. I am proud to be a founding member of this organization offering many helpful services to growers and buyers alike. Several of the benefits are an herb brokering system and a group organic certification, so the expenses are lower than for an individual grower going it alone. Local connections between growers, practitioners, medicine makers, and product manufacturers can be synergistically powerful. Going beyond the local geographical region to a national enterprise focusing predominantly on Asian herbs, we have the all-volunteer MHC coordinating growers and buyers. Both of these organizations are a win-win proposition for growers and buyers interested in quality herbal material.

CHAPTER FIVE

Conservation and Global Trade in Medicinal Plants

We were a small group of Chinese licensed acupuncturists, Chinese herb students, and one lone Chinese herb farmer who came to China to see Chinese herbs growing in their native habitats. I was thrilled—we walked up a mountain almost every day. Robert Newman L.Ac., a Chinese herbalist who introduced the growing of Asian herbs to the United States, had generously given in to the many requests—and here we were on our first day in China. The mountain of the day—Bai Wang Shan Forest Park, near our entry point of Beijing. It was cloudy when we arrived at the park, but we started in an orderly fashion ascending the mountain pathways looking at the multitude of herbs and the beautiful scenery. I paused ever so briefly to take a picture. Then it started to rain—really hard—and after I took my photo I turned to see that everyone had dispersed. Five separate groups, of one to three people each, made their way back down the mountain through the deluge. We learned that if we wanted to see the herbs we had to have a

plan and know where we were going—and that we had to make contingency plans as well. Luckily for us it was only rain, but you never know what environmental or political event might separate herbalists from their herbs.

CURRENT STATUS: FACTORS AND REASONS FOR CONCERN

India and China share the distinction of being the world's largest medicinal plant consumers. More than 90 percent of the traded medicinal plants in India are wild-collected, most of them unsustainably. As a result, at least 300 species are assessed as threatened.[18] In reference to Chinese herbs, in 2007 the United States was the third top importer, at $147 million worth, of Chinese traditional medicines.[19]

China has approximately 30,000 endemic plant species—about twice the number native to North America. Of the more than 4,000 of these species used in Asian medicine, roughly 600 to 800 are in common use. The majority of those (75–80 percent) are wild-harvested. However, the remaining 20–25 percent are cultivated, and these represent the bulk of the most commonly used herbs, accounting for 70 percent of the total volume of Chinese medicinal plant production.[20]

Fueled by strong market demand, the worldwide trade for Eastern medicinal plants is expanding at an annual rate of 10 percent. The traditional medicine and pharmaceutical industry markets are increasing, within China as well as internationally, placing unrelenting pressure on Asia's already depleted wild reserves. This has resulted in 15–35 percent of all Asian medicinal plants currently considered to

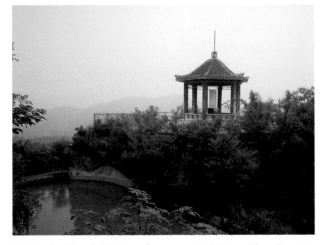

This is the "fateful" photo from atop Bai Wang Shan Forest Park, China.

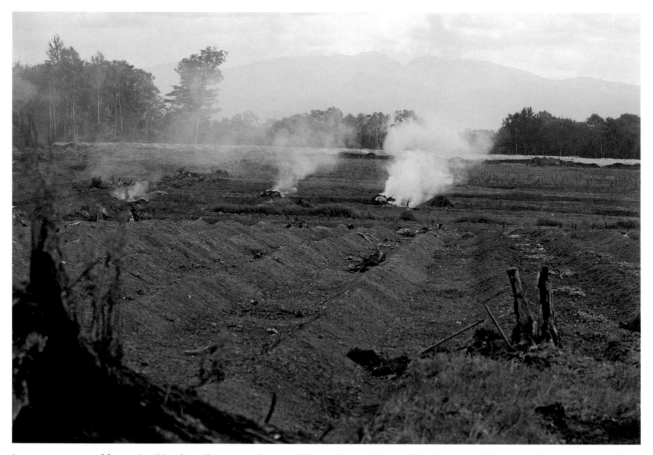

Large expanses of forest in China have been cut down and burned to make way for ginseng cultivation. Photo courtesy of Paul W. Meyer, Morris Arboretum of the University of Pennsylvania.

be in endangered status.[21] The *China Plant Red Data Book: Rare and Endangered Plants*, the latest volume of which was published in 1992, indicates that there were 168 species of endangered medicinal plants, which amounted to over 42 percent of the total number of endangered plants in China.[22] If this trend has continued for the nearly twenty years since this data was published, the situation of endangerment now is almost assuredly more critical.

A new middle class in China is becoming ever more active in consuming wild herbal material. Other Asian countries and many populations in the West are also increasingly utilizing these wild resources. As health care costs increase, especially in the United States, medicinal plants will be further explored and the market niches will expand. This pressure has already placed a heavy burden on the environment as a result of overcollecting practices and is currently exceeding the carrying capacity of China *and* its neighboring countries. If these botanical reserves are not protected, and regulations are not enforced, we will all be without these valuable resources.

WHO NEEDS PROTECTION?

Wild-harvesting (combined with the even larger issue of climate change), along with loss of habitat due to urban expansion (and the consequent agricultural expansion), soil erosion, disruptive mining, and other extractive technologies—all contribute to sharp declines in wild medicinal plant resources. While some of the more opportunistic botanicals maintain healthy populations, others are becoming increasingly rare and some are on the brink of extinction.[23]

The species most at risk are those from

fragile or unique ecosystems, of limited or fragmented geographic distribution, and those that are either slow-growing or slow to reproduce. In terms of climate change, high-altitude mountainous and polar regions are the most vulnerable. Severe weather events, as well as longer-term shifts in weather patterns, adversely impact plants. If at-risk plants are to survive, they have to either adapt to the changes or they (and their pollinators) must move. A tall order when plants are polar or already endemic to high altitudes! Ironically, it may be that the biochemical mechanisms these plants have evolved to thrive in such ecosystems are what make them valuable as medicinal herbs: "Plants that grow in such extreme climates often produce chemical compounds to protect themselves against the cold and UV radiation."[24] As we know, these chemicals are the medicine.

PROTECTIVE MEASURES

Two fundamental ways to protect threatened plants are to conserve existing populations and to regulate collection practices.

For conservation purposes it is always easier to preserve what already exists than to try to recreate intact viable populations and the biodiversity in which all is interwoven. In-situ and ex-situ conservation of plants in ecological preserves, parks, and botanic gardens—as well as other areas designated as important plant areas—will serve an increasingly important function as genetic reservoirs.

Currently there are a plethora of Chinese policies on the books for the protection of endangered plants. Unfortunately that is where they stay—on paper. These policies are not well known to the people at the starting point of the supply chain for some of these increasingly rare plants. Rural harvesters and herb middlemen do know that medicinal plants are increasingly difficult to find, but economic pressures force them to continue what most likely are unsustainable harvesting practices. Unfortunately, in other Asian countries besides India, there are very few regulations for either ascertaining at-risk status or for the protection of endangered plants. Currently, the most important tool for regulating trade in endangered plants is the international trade control treaties such as the Convention on International Trade in Endangered Species of Wild Fauna and Flora (CITES) and the Convention on Biological Diversity (CBD) (a significant agreement, but focused more on conserving ecological systems than individual species). Both CITES and CBD are legally binding but solely between signatory countries. Among the largest and most active conservation groups are the International Union for the Conservation of Nature (IUCN) and the World Wildlife Fund (WWF), which also have a joint program—TRAFFIC—to monitor the trade of endangered plants and animals. Another is the German Federation Agency for Nature Conservation (BfN). All of these groups have dynamic programs and projects aimed at protecting biodiversity and indigenous peoples.

The *International Standard for Sustainable Wild Collection of Medicinal and Aromatic Plants* (ISSC-MAP), prepared and published in 2007 by the Medicinal Plant Specialist Group of the Species Survival Commission and IUCN serves as the accepted global guideline and was created to improve industry and management practices.

HOW EFFECTIVE ARE THE PROTECTIVE STRATEGIES?

The work of these organizations is commendable, but how effective are they? Conservation and legal protective strategies are based on research data that is limited, fragmented, and incomplete—due, in part, to the vastness of the project and extensive rural geography. And even in those instances where particular species of medicinal plants have been reviewed, established as threatened, and integrated into trade control policies, the protocols have been largely ineffective in protecting those plants. According to a study released in 2008 by the IUCN, "Reviews of the status, wild collection and trade of a number of CITES-listed medicinal plant species found that implementation of collection and trade control was generally low, and in some cases non-existent."[25]

Table 5-1. CITES-Listed Asian Herbs			
Botanical Name	CITES Appendix	Pinyin Medicinal or Plant Name	Common Trade Name
Aquilaria spp.	II	chén xiāng	Agarwood
Cibotium barometz, (L) J. Sm.	II	gǒu jǐ	Chain Fern
Cistanche deserticola, Y.C.Ma	II	ròu cōng róng	Broomrape
Dioscorea deltoidea, Wall ex Griseb	II	sān jiǎo yè shǔ yù	No common name
Nardostachys jatamansi (D. Don) DC.	II	gān sōng	Indian Valerian, Nard
Synonym: *Nardostachys grandiflora*, DC.			
Orchidaceae spp. including:			
Bletilla striata (Thunb.) Rchb.f.	II	bái jí	Hardy Ground Orchid
Cremastra appendiculata (D.Don) Makino	II	shān cí gū	No common name
Dendrobium spp.	II	shí hú	No common name
Pleione bulbocodioides (Franch.) Rolfe	II	shān cí gū	No common name
Pleione yunnanensis (Rolfe) Rolfe	II	shān cí gū	No common name
Panax ginseng, C.A. Mey. (Russian Federation populations only.)	II	rén shēn	Asian Ginseng
Panax quinquefolius, L.	II	xī yáng shēn	American Ginseng
Picrorhiza kurrooa, Royle	II	hú huáng lián	Kutki
Podophyllum hexandrum, Royle	II	guǐ jiù	Himalayan Mayapple
Synonyms: *P. emodi* var. *chinense*, Sprague			
Sinopodophyllum hexandrum (Royle) T.S.Ying			
Sinopodophyllum emodi (Wall.ex Royle) T.S.Ying			
Pterocarpus santalinus, L.f.	II	zǐ tán	Red Sanders
Rauvolfia serpentina, (L.) Benth. ex Kurz	II	yìn dù luó fú mù	Serpentine Root
Saussurea costus (Falc.) Lipsch.	I	mù xiāng	Costus
Synonyms: *Saussurea lappa* (Decne.) Sch.Bip.			
Auklandia lappa, Decne.			
Taxus wallichiana, Zucc.	II	xǐ mǎ lā yǎ hóng dòu shān	Himalayan Yew
© 2011 Peg Schafer and Steven Foster			

CITES-listed plants are classified in three appendices. Appendix I includes species threatened with extinction; trade in these species is permitted only in exceptional circumstances. Appendix II includes species not necessarily threatened with extinction, but for whom trade must be controlled in order to avoid utilization incompatible with their survival. Appendix III contains species that are protected in at least one country that has asked other CITES member countries for assistance in controlling traffic. To complicate matters, the taxonomic nomenclature is rather fluid, with numerous botanical synonyms. It should also be noted that wild-collecting practices frequently include mixed species. All wild-harvested CITES-listed plants sold internationally require supporting paperwork.

A comprehensive list of endangered wild medicinal herb plants does not exist. CITES Listed Asian Herbs, see table 5-1, is a condensed version for Asian medicinal plants; please note that there are parts and derivative exceptions for all listed herbs and that extract products, from these or other plants, are not included at all in the convention. This list is for all herb users to be aware of which herbs to avoid purchasing. Currently all, or almost all, of these plants are wild-collected and of Asian export. Unfortunately, any CITES-listed plant can be found in any herb shop in any major US city—and yes, it is completely illegal. This list will also indicate to growers highly valuable medicinal plants; cultivation conditions will need to be developed, but they are in much demand.

CULTIVATE TO CONSERVE

The circumstances for medicinal plants to come under cultivation include (1) a demand for herbs that are coveted enough and have had enough pressure in the wild to create a shortage and thus drive up the market value, (2) where control over a modified or more standardized base product is desired, such as in the pharmaceutical trade, or (3) perhaps a circumstance where local or rural enterprises are encouraged. These conditions are beginning to emerge, and the cultivation of many botanicals will be necessary to satisfy demand.

To bring wild species under cultivation will require time and support. It is costly and will take years of evaluation. Support from governments, agricultural institutions, and industry stakeholders is necessary. In the United States the land grant colleges used to take the role of crop introduction, but unfortunately those schools are now heavily financed by large corporations to conduct research on proprietary products that are often genetically modified or patented. As a result, it is community-based, small-scale, entrepreneurial agricultural operations—such as the MHC and the Sonoma County Herb Association—that are taking the lead, often in conjunction with innovative medicinal plant product businesses.

As wild medicinal crops become scarcer, the efforts expended to collect them will start to fall more in line with the increased efforts and costs of farming inputs. The 2008 study from the IUCN notes that "Cultivation is routinely promoted as the preferred (and sometimes the only) solution to the problem of dwindling supplies and overcollection of wild medicinal plant populations. Given the interest in cultivation it might be expected that

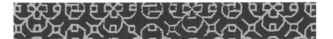

Supporting Sustainable Wild-Collection

Rural populations, often landless and with few options for generating income, should be included as stakeholders in policies concerning sustainable wild-collection practices. To ignore their need to maintain their living through collection of wild herbs is not only unconscionable, but applies undue financial pressure, potentially forcing the wild-collection market underground in regions notoriously difficult to effectively patrol. Regulatory programs such as organic certification and the various ecological labeling organizations (Fairtrade, FairWild, Rainforest Alliance, Ecocert) provide frameworks, albeit far-ranging and with competing ideals, for farmers and wild-crafters. Those affiliations are designed to raise product, environmental, and often social justice standards and thus command a higher price for their members. However, it is difficult to monitor and verify the complex label claims from distant and convoluted supply chains.[26]

Wild-harvesting of some Asian medicinal plants occurs in areas of the world outside Asia. As much as 25 percent of the traditional Chinese plants used medicinally are endemic to other regions. Some of them are native to more than one continent, such as *Prunella vulgaris* (heal all, xià kū cǎo); others, like *Siegesbeckia pubescens* (xī xiān cǎo), are simply invasive.

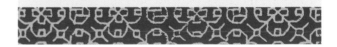

information on the scale of cultivation of medicinal plant species would be more readily accessible."[27] At least some CITES-listed medicinal plants, among them *Cistanche deserticola* (ròu cōng róng) have been the focus of preliminary cultivation trials, many with promising results and all with at least some success.[28] The first of many challenges will be finding germplasm, though occasionally seeds or plants are listed in the nursery trade. One of the more important herb plants that we are lacking germplasm for in the United States is *Panax notoginseng* (sān qī)—so if you obtain seed give me a call!

For a win-win situation where growers and consumers support each other and the environment, the cultivated herbs will have to be efficacious and available in sufficient quantities—and the buyers have to pay the cost of producing them. The alternative is that no one wins. The default would be large industrial monotypic agricultural systems that do not support ecological diversity and do not generally grow efficacious medicine. These types of operations are increasingly common for food and medicinal plants—in the United States and in China—and are more about the bottom line than they are about healthful food and medicine. Choose your medicine wisely.

HOW TO BE PART OF THE SOLUTION

As herb users, the first solution is to avoid purchasing endangered or threatened wild-harvested species. Unfortunately, origins are often difficult to determine. Transparency and accountability are key components; be vigilant and inquire of suppliers. Is the product labeled with the origin? Are the genus and species listed? When were they harvested? Remember that you as the consumer are the motivating factor in commerce—voices will be heard when customers vote with their money. As groups representing sustainable wild-crafters and growers become better organized, this may be a way to support responsible efforts.

Another option is to buy domestically grown medicinal plants and their products. The shorter supply chain, with fewer middlemen, experiences fewer quality failures. Shorter travel distances coupled with smaller businesses, and a culture of openness and accountability, usually mean fresher products. Domestic products require fewer travel miles from field or farm to customer, which benefits the environment and delivers the botanicals to the end user more quickly. Supporting domestic medicinal plant production also defends access to herbs, thereby ensuring practitioners access to the tools of their profession.

Botanical medicine is on the rise worldwide. As the global herbal community faces the challenges of worldwide climate change and ecological uncertainties, as well as unsustainable levels of wild-collection, it is more imperative than ever that everyone takes a conscientious role in the conservation of these treasured medicinal plants. Every stakeholder—the people who originally identified and still work with the medicinal plants, cultivators everywhere, the people who engage in trade, the medicine makers, the manufacturing companies, herbal practitioners, and consumers—all need to come together to responsibly address sustainable resource management and long-term species survival. Time is of the essence. It is clear that a combination of cultivation as well as collection of wild medicinal plants will be necessary to satisfy global market needs. We can engage in conservation and meet the demand for Asian medicinal plants with applied agro-ecological cultivation, sustainable wild-collection practices, and responsible trade. The future of Asian botanical medicine, and consequently the health of the people who utilize it, are depending on it.

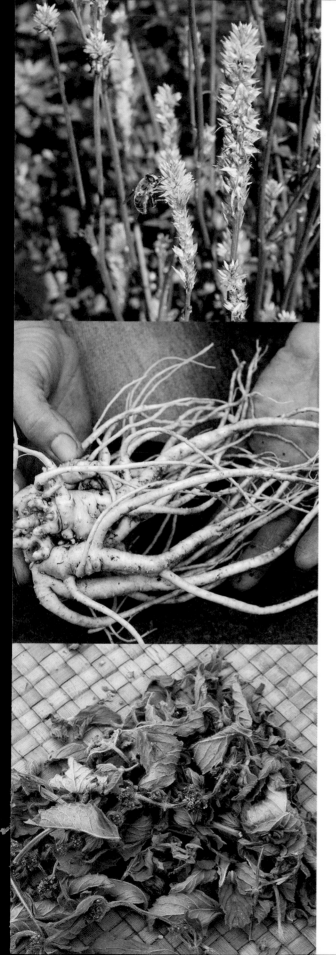

PART TWO

MEDICINAL HERB PROFILES

Medicinal Herb Profile Introduction

The following 79 cultivation profiles represent some very promising medicinal herbs for domestic cultivation. Starting with a list of over 250 different Asian herbs, I narrowed the field through repeated trials at the Chinese Medicinal Herb Farm. This book is a pioneering effort and there are many worthy plants that do not grow in my region, thus I have less data for them. Or perhaps they grow too well—*Leonurus heterophyllos* (Chinese motherwort, yì mǔ cǎo/chōng wèi zǐ) is invasive here but grows in New York without exhibiting invasive qualities, as reported by grower Jean Giblette.

For clarity the profiles are organized alphabetically by botanical name. If you don't know the botanical name of an herb you'd like to read about, refer to the quick cross-reference name tables at the back of the book. One table lists plants alphabetically by common name and another by pinyin name, thus allowing you to quickly find a plant and ascertain its botanical name.

Some of the plant profiles have *botanical synonym* designations directly under the botanical name; these are plants that (unfortunately) have more than one botanical name in use. The authority utilized for the most accepted species was http://www.theplantlist.org.

Another designation listed is *medicinal synonym*. Plants listed as such are (usually) a different species from the specific profile but they share the same function and medicinal pinyin name. They usually share similar cultivation preferences as well. These are listed as standard species used in the book *Chinese Herbal Medicine: Materia Medica* (3rd ed., comp. and trans. Dan Bensky, Steven Clavey, Erich Stöger with Andrew Gamble [Seattle: Eastland Press, 2004]).

An example of a medicinal synonym is *Lilium lancifolium* and *Lilium brownii*—two different lilies, but both are used as bǎi hé.

Finally there are a few profiles designated as *alternate species*; these are different plants from the specific profile, but they share the same function and medicinal pinyin name. This differs from a medicinal synonym in that they are listed as nonstandard but accepted alternate species in *Chinese Herbal Medicine: Materia Medica*.

I've used standard botanical terminology in the Plant Description section of the profiles because it is precise and space efficient. If your botanical vocabulary is rusty, look to the glossary at the back of the book for definitions of terms such as *pinnate* and *lanceolate*. The glossary also includes a separate listing of terminology used by OM practitioners. If you're not a practitioner, you may find these definitions helpful when reading the Medicinal Uses feature of a profile.

In the Propagation section, I've included information aimed not only at farmers and gardeners, but also for commercial nursery use. It's my hope that people will specialize, as I have discovered that it is indeed a long row to hoe and then return from the field to propagate nursery starts. Gardeners looking for ornamental use of plant material will find additional useful information in the Garden and Polyculture Planting section.

Due to the amazing amount of climate variability in North America the lists of Suitable Companions are meant as guidelines only and are best bets—they will work in most, but probably not all, situations. As noted in chapter 3, some medicinal herbs have invasive tendencies in certain regions or habitats. Among the herb profiles, I've chosen to include five herbs known to have overly persistent tendencies because they are already commonly available in North America. These plants are:

Arctium lappa, burdock, niú bàng zǐ
Artemisia annua, sweet annie, qīng hāo
Dioscorea opposita, Chinese yam, shān yào
Fallopia multiflora, fo ti, shǒu wū/yè jīao
  téng
Glycyrrhiza uralensis, Chinese licorice,
  gān cǎo

I have not included these plants in any of the Suitable Companions lists because they are not very suitable companions for other herbs! If you choose to grow these plants, please do so responsibly—take measures to ensure they do not escape cultivation.

All information on crop yield and ratio of fresh weight to dry weight of harvested material is based on actual harvest data from the Chinese Medicinal Herb Farm. I encourage you to keep your own harvest data because the yield of any particular herb will vary by climate, cultural, and management conditions.

Writing these herb profiles has been a goal for me for over ten years; I am happy to finally be able to share this information with you. Experiment and have fun growing these valuable medicinal plants. Welcome to our collective journey!

Acanthopanax gracilistylus (W.W.Smith)

Botanical Synonym: *Eleutherococcus gracilistylus* (W.W.Sm.) S.Y.Hu
Common Name: None
Pinyin: Wŭ jiā pí
Family: Araliaceae
Part Used: Root bark

Plant Description

Acanthopanax's plant family is the source of many medicinals worldwide. Growing as a large woody shrub, this important Chinese medicinal can form a ten-foot-high thicket. Its stiff branches bear fierce, backward-facing thorns and glossy trifoliate or palmate leaves, at the junction of which arise small green flowers in umbels in summer. The blueberry-flavored black fruits mature late in the fall, just before the plants go dormant.

Flora of China states that *Acanthopanax gracilistylus* grows in "forest margins, scrub fields, mountain slopes, valleys, stream banks, roadsides; below 1000 m[eters] in the E[ast] and 3000 m[eters] in W[estern] part of range."[29] Because of this wide range of adaptation—from 3,000 feet high inland to 9,000 feet high closer to the coast— *Acanthopanax gracilistylus* may grow well in many areas of USDA hardiness zones 5–10.

Propagation

Fresh seed, cleaned of its fleshy black fruit when harvested in the fall, is best. Sow immediately or the following spring. Germination from fall-sown seed is variable, starting at three weeks, and is temperature dependent. Stratification may be needed if the seed is older than one year. Hardwood cuttings taken in late fall yield well if given bottom heat. Layering naturally occurs when stems have good soil contact. Plants hold well in pots and make dependable transplants for nursery sale.

Garden and Polyculture Planting

Grow in full sun to part shade in well-drained soil. Place it deep within or at the back of the border or hedgerow, and leave a respectful amount of space around it. Due to its long, arching branches and unfriendly thorns, *Acanthopanax gracilistylus* is best in a large-scale garden or arboretum. For long-term placement, space ten feet apart. Watering needs are average, but *Acanthopanax* is not drought tolerant.

Suitable Companions

Allium macrostemon, xiè bái
Allium tuberosum, Garlic Chives, jiǔ cài zǐ

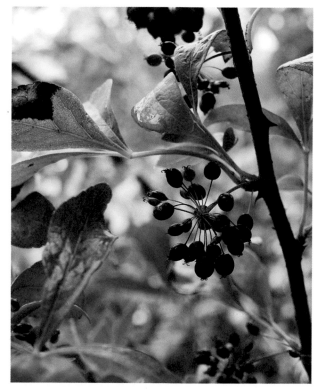

Acanthopanax **fruit ripening in autumn.**

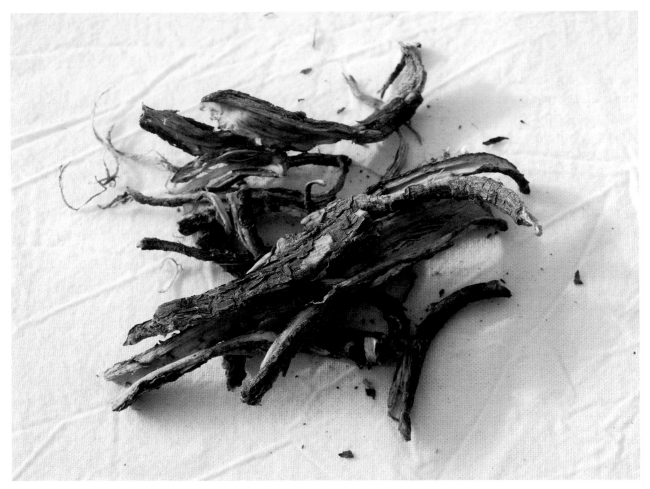

Dry *Acanthopanax* root bark (wǔ jiā pí).

Anemarrhena asphodeloides, zhī mǔ
Belamcanda chinensis, Blackberry Lily, shè gān
Clerodendrum trichotomum, Glorybower, chòu wú tóng
Cornus officinalis, Dogwood, shān zhū yú
Crataegus pinnatifida, Chinese Hawthorn, shān zhā
Eriobotrya japonica, Loquat, pí pá yè
Eucommia ulmoides, Hardy Rubber Tree, dù zhòng
Ginkgo biloba, Ginkgo, bái guǒ
Ligusticum jeholense, Chinese Lovage, gǎo běn
Lilium lancifolium, *L. brownii*, Lily, bǎi hé
Magnolia denudata, xīn yí huā
Platycodon grandiflorus, Balloon Flower, jié gěng
Salvia miltiorrhiza, *S. przewalskii*, *S. bowleyana*, Red Sage, dān shēn
Saposhnikovia divaricata, Siler, fáng fēng
Scutellaria baicalensis, Baikal Skullcap, huáng qín

Field Production

For production purposes one-year-old nursery-grown plants can be set on three-foot centers (as opposed to garden specimens, which need more space and are more horizontal in habit than many other members of this plant family). Plant in full sun except in hot summer areas (there, plant in part shade and give moderate amounts of water). Prune while the plant is winter dormant to keep in bounds and away from pathways. Try planting *Acanthopanax* down the center of a four-foot bed, with smaller root herbs placed at the sides for harvest at the same time or a season before. Due to the thorny nature of *Acanthopanax*, avoid planting leaf or seed crops nearby.

Pests and Diseases

Gophers occasionally consume the roots (but it is not their first choice) and deer browse the flowers and leaves. Prolonged wet winters may cause roots to rot. Ripe fruit is desirable to birds.

Harvest and Yield

Harvest root bark in the summer or fall after a minimum of four years' growth. To avoid the thorns, prune back branches to the crown before harvesting roots; roots are not especially deep or difficult to remove. For whole root cut crosswise; for root bark use a knife to pry bark off the woody interior and thorns, which pierce the bark. The best final product is thick without inner wood. Four-year-old plants yield five pounds of fresh whole root per plant or three pounds of fresh root bark. Ratio of fresh to dry for whole root and root bark is 2:1.

Notes

Most often this herb is sold as whole, crosswise-cut roots; however, it is the root bark that is traditionally used. Check with your market or buyer before embarking—or debarking—because this process takes a lot of time.

Medicinal Uses of Wǔ jiā pí

Wǔ jiā pí is the root bark of *Acanthopanax gracilistylus*. Warm, acrid, and bitter, it dispels wind damp cold, addresses bi (painful obstruction) syndrome, nourishes the kidney and liver, and strengthens the tendons and bones. It has secondary functions of draining dampness to address fluid retention. It is used to address issues such as arthritic pain and muscle pain (particularly when the pain is worsened by damp and cold), pain due to trauma, weakness of the lower back and knees, and delayed development in children. In recent times it has come to be considered an important adaptogenic herb (increasing the body's ability to adapt to stress), and its use has been expanded to include strengthening the immune system, decreasing inflammation, and supporting cardiovascular health.

Wǔ jiā pí is used both alone and in combination with other herbs. Common methods of administration include alcohol extracts, decoctions, powders, concentrated granules, tablets, and pills.

Achyranthes bidentata (Blume).
Common Name: Oxknee
Pinyin: Huái niú xī
Family: Amaranthaceae
Part Used: Root

Plant Description
This perennial reaches an overall size of three by three feet in its first season of growth. It has simple, opposite, pubescent green leaves. At leaf nodes the stem produces swollen joints resembling an ox's knee (thus the common name). The plant crowns slowly expand in successive seasons and go dormant in winter. Inconspicuous flowers bloom in dense spikes on the stem terminals in the fall. The green flowers then turn to brown and yield light brown seed.

Humidity and heat are prevalent in southern China and other climes where oxknee is indigenous, but the crop also does well in the arid western United States. Plants are reported to self-sow in the southeast United States, so always monitor for invasive tendencies. Oxknee is hardy to ten to fifteen degrees, making it suitable for USDA hardiness zone 8.

Propagation
The seed remains viable and germinates well for at least five years. Compliant in the nursery, oxknee germinates at five days with bottom heat and fourteen days in cool soil conditions. Sow in spring and do not allow to become pot-bound or the roots will always retain the shape of the pot.

Garden and Polyculture Planting
Oxknee is not necessarily considered an ornamental, but its informal habit fills in the midborder well in a mixed planting. Quite undemanding, it does best in full sun in well-drained soil, with moderate soil fertility and average to low irrigation needs. It adapts well to a range of growing conditions, generally thrives even when neglected, and is companionable with many other plants.

Suitable Companions
Agastache rugosa, Korean Mint, tǔ huò xiāng
Angelica dahurica, bái zhǐ
Angelica pubescens, dú huó
Artemisia annua, Sweet Annie, qīng hāo
Aster tataricus, Tartar Aster, zǐ wǎn

One-year-old *Achyranthes bidentata*.

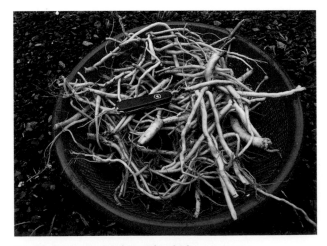
Freshly harvested *Achyranthes bidentata* roots.

Belamcanda chinensis, Blackberry Lily, shè gān
Carthamus tinctorius, Safflower, hóng huā
Chrysanthemum morifolium, Mum, jú huā
Cyathula officinalis, Hookweed, chuān niú xī
Dolichos lablab, Hyacinth Bean, bái biăn dòu
Lilium lancifolium, L. brownii, Lily, băi hé
Lonicera japonica, Honeysuckle, jīn yín huā
Momordica charantia, Bitter Melon, kŭ guā
Prunella vulgaris, Heal All, xià kū căo
Rheum palmatum, Chinese Rhubarb, dà huáng
Salvia miltiorrhiza, S. przewalskii, S. bowleyana,
    Red Sage, dān shēn
Saposhnikovia divaricata, Siler, fáng fēng
Scutellaria baicalensis, Baikal Skullcap, huáng qín
Withania somnifera, Ashwagandha

Field Production

Set out transplants on two-foot spacing in full sun. Pruning stems in midsummer encourages root production; if left unpruned the top portions will be quite large compared to the root mass come harvest time. Moderate amounts of fertilizer are beneficial; yields are poor in lean soils. For best results keep moderately weeded and irrigated.

Pests and Diseases

Gophers occasionally consume the roots and deer occasionally browse the foliage. Prolonged wet conditions may result in root rot.

Harvest and Yield

Collect or dig two-year or older roots from late fall to early spring, when the plants are dormant. Roots are white to yellow in color and should be straight with a larger main root and smaller side roots. Following traditional Chinese processing methods I first grade the crop by cutting off the root crown and pruning off and composting the small rootlets prior to cleaning. Wash the roots with a power washer, being careful not to damage the root bark. Then the roots are sliced lengthwise from the top down before drying. To facilitate even drying, take care to make cuts of

Medicinal Uses of Huái niú xī

Huái niú xī is the root of *Achyranthes bidentata*. Bitter, sour, and neutral, it activates the blood circulation, dispels blood stagnation, tonifies the kidney and liver, and strengthens the tendons and bones. It has secondary functions of promoting urination and directing fire and blood downward. It is one of the herbs most commonly used to address issues such as chronic and acute joint pain in the lower body as well as pain due to external injury. It is commonly used in gynecology to address menstrual pain, irregular menstruation, and amenorrhea (lack of a period). Less common uses include treating painful urination, toothache, and mouth ulcers.

Huái niú xī is usually used in combination with other herbs. Common methods of administration include decoctions, powders, concentrated granules, alcohol extracts, tablets, and pills. It is in formulas such as Zuo Gui Wan (Restore the Left Kidney Pill), Si Miao San (Four Marvels Powder), and Zhen Gan Xi Feng Tang (Sedate the Liver and Extinguish Wind Decoction).

equal thickness. Two-year-old roots yield an average of a quarter pound per plant when fresh. Ratio of fresh to dry herb is 2:1.

Notes

Achyranthes aspera is a rather uncommon plant here in the United States. It has the same cultural needs as oxknee (*A. bidentata*) and I have found yields are basically the same. In China this variety of huái niú xī is both cultivated and wild-collected.

Agastache rugosa (Fisch. & C.A.Mey.) Kuntze

Common Name: Korean Mint
Pinyin: Tŭ huò xiāng
Family: Lamiaceae
Part Used: Herb

Plant Description

Agastache rugosa bears purple-blue flowers three to four inches high atop five-foot-tall anise-scented stems in midsummer. The flowers attract various species of butterflies as well as honeybees and native bees. Green cordate leaves are lightly serrate and show purple hues in response to cooler temperatures. This east Asia native is a long-lived deciduous perennial and a close relative of anise hyssop (*Agastache foeniculum*). It is winter hardy down to at least zero degrees, so it is suitable for USDA hardiness zones 5–11.

Propagation

Unlike other mints, Korean mint does not produce runners. The main way to propagate it is to sow seed in spring or fall; germination occurs in from six to fourteen days. Transplant into a permanent planting area in spring or early summer. Sowing seeds in the fall in a greenhouse will produce higher yields the following summer than spring-sown seed. This is especially helpful if the crop is being grown in cold-winter regions where it is treated as an annual.

Garden and Polyculturel Planting

A worthy and ornamental garden addition, Korean mint communes well with other plants and fits in nicely in the midborder. It is columnar in habit; plant it in groupings to optimize the harvest as well as its visual appeal. Easy to grow in full shade to part shade, it makes a good cut flower that holds well in the vase.

Suitable Companions

Achyranthes bidentata, Oxknee, huái niú xī
Allium tuberosum, Garlic Chives, jiŭ cài zĭ
Anemarrhena asphodeloides, zhī mŭ
Angelica dahurica, bái zhĭ
Aster tataricus, Tartar Aster, zĭ wăn
Belamcanda chinensis, Blackberry Lily, shè gān
Carthamus tinctorius, Safflower, hóng huā
Celosia argentea, qīng xiāng zĭ
Celosia cristata, Cockscomb, jī guān huā
Chrysanthemum morifolium, Mum, jú huā
Codonopsis pilosula, Poor Man's Ginseng, dǎng shēn
Coix lacryma-jobi, Job's Tears, yì yĭ rén
Cornus officinalis, Dogwood, shān zhū yú
Dianthus superbus, Fringed Pink, qú mài
Eriobotrya japonica, Loquat, pí pá yè
Lilium lancifolium, *L. brownii*, Lily, bǎi hé
Magnolia denudata, xīn yí huā

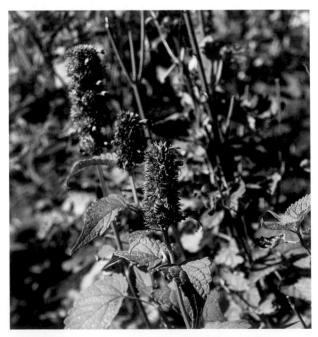

Agastache rugosa flowers are popular with honeybees.

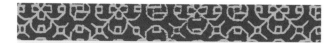

Korean Mint Recipes

The young leaves of Korean mint are most often used in tea, but you can also chop them to add to marinades for fish and chicken. Or combine Korean mint with basil in a simple syrup to serve over fresh fruit.

For tea: Pour boiling water over dried or fresh whole leaves and steep for two to three minutes. Use a larger quantity of fresh leaves to dried, but adjust the amount to your taste. If desired, stir a teaspoon of honey into each individual cup. Chilled, the tea makes a refreshing hot-weather drink.

For marinade: Combine 1 cup dried leaves, a ½ cup olive oil, 3 tablespoons soy sauce, and 2 mashed cloves of garlic. Whisk to incorporate the ingredients. Use as a marinade for chicken, fish, or shellfish.

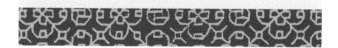

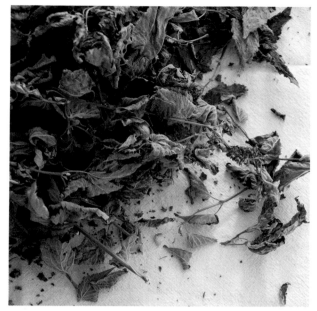

Freshly dried tǔ huò xiāng.

Ocimum sanctum, Sacred Basil, Tulsi
Platycodon grandiflorus, Balloon Flower, jié gěng
Prunella vulgaris, Heal All, xià kū cǎo
Salvia miltiorrhiza, S. przewalskii, S. bowleyana, Red Sage, dān shēn
Saposhnikovia divaricata, Siler, fáng fēng
Schizonepeta tenuifolia, Japanese Catnip, jīng jiè
Scutellaria baicalensis, Baikal Skullcap, huáng qín

Field Production

In spring, set out starts at least ten weeks old; plant two feet on center. Korean mint prefers full sun, a moderate amount of summer water, and an average loam—but it will tolerate wet winters and heavy soils. Provide average soil fertility; offering more increases production but yields an inferior product and leaves plants subject to insect predation. Plants tolerate some drought pressure. Drip irrigation is better than overhead; the leaves stay dry. Weed to avoid resource competition. I have noticed a decrease in production after three years.

Pests and Diseases

Gophers only occasionally eat Korean mint, and deer do not browse it. Insect pests include Diabrotica, the cucumber beetle, which chew holes in the leaves. Cucumber beetles can be hand picked when temperatures are cool and they are slow, but I have found that it is not a cost effective measure and tend to let the damage occur. Mites can cause light leaf damage.

Harvest and Yield

Harvest the leaves, young flowers, and stems in June through August of the first and subsequent seasons when the plants are growing vigorously and the weather is warm or hot (the volatile oils will not be as concentrated if you harvest during the cooler months). The best quality herb has an intense fragrance. The Western tea trade prefers leaf while Chinese medicine utilizes leaf as well as stem material.

Two good harvests are possible per season. I use a gas hedge trimmer to make quick work cutting Korean mint for the hang-to-dry method. When dry, gently roll the plant material on a four-inch mesh screen to riddle the leaves and flowers off the stems.

If you want fresh herb, harvest by hand instead; remove the terminal five inches of stems, but pick lower leaves individually. They wilt easily, so harvest early in the day and cool them down soon after picking. Harvesting early will also avoid bee activity and the possibility of stings. The best quality product consists of whole leaves and young flowers. The yield is one pound per plant per season (fresh). Ratio of fresh to dry herb is 6:1.

Notes

- Alone or mixed with other tea ingredients, Korean mint makes a fragrant and pleasant tea. If you are growing Korean mint in quantity, try marketing to Western tea companies as well as the Chinese herb market to diversify sales.
- Korean mint is cultivated throughout China, Japan, and in North America for medicinal use as well as a source of essential oil. Tŭ huò xiāng has been utilized in Asian medicine for over 1,500 years and was recorded in *Miscellaneous Records of Famous Physicians* in 510 CE.
- Due to its ornamental qualities, Korean mint has been extensively hybridized. If you're growing it for medicinal use, make sure to choose the species or unselected (unhybridized) seed—or medicinal properties may not be present.
- The cut flowers hold well and dry successfully.

Medicinal Uses of Tŭ huò xiāng

Tŭ huò xiāng, also referred to as huò xiāng, is the aerial part or herb portion of *Agastache rugosa*. Slightly warm, acrid, and aromatic, it transforms dampness, releases the exterior, relieves summer-dampness, and addresses nausea and vomiting. Tŭ huò xiāng is most commonly used for its ability to gently but effectively transform dampness, harmonize the stomach, and treat nausea and vomiting. It is used to alleviate morning sickness, stomach flu, and chronic digestive weakness leading to nausea. It is also an important herb in combinations used to address upper respiratory tract infections that appear in the summertime. Topically, it is used to address fungal infections of the hands and feet.

Tŭ huò xiāng is usually used in combination with other herbs. Other methods of administration include pills, tablets, powders, decoctions, and concentrated granules. Tŭ huò xiāng is one of the key ingredients in the popular Traditional Chinese Medicine (TCM) patent remedy "Pill Curing" that is used for a variety of digestive disorders and is a major component of the well-known formula Huo Xiang Zheng Qi San (*Agastache* Rectify the Qi Powder).

Albizia julibrissin (Durazz.)

Common Name: Mimosa
Pinyin: Hé huān pí/huā
Family: Fabaceae
Part Used: Flower, bark

Plant Description

Albizia is a popular, long-blooming landscape tree, but the attractive pink flowers with dense stamens that look like puffballs only last a day. Quick-growing to thirty-five feet tall and spreading to forty feet wide, it is winter deciduous. Its feathery, light-green leaves are twice divided; bark is smooth and greyish-brown. *Albizia* has been widely planted—some would say overplanted—in part because it tolerates problem soils where other trees will not thrive. In some regions *Albizia* tends to reseed; in the southeast United States it is considered invasive. USDA hardiness zones 8–10.

Propagation

The leguminous seeds have a hard coat that needs scarification; alternatively, plant into a nursery bed or large flat in the fall and let the winter weather and the soil's biological activity naturally break down the testa. Nursery-grown plants are readily available; remember to avoid stock that has been bred for ornamental qualities (named varieties). Mimosa is fast growing; keep young plants in containers no longer than two years before planting out.

Garden and Polyculture Planting

Adaptable to heat as well as cool coastal conditions, this rather flat-topped tree is quite suitable for the ornamental or function-designed landscape. Roots are shallow but are compatible with ground covers and some shade-loving plants. Hummingbirds are frequent visitors. Mimosa can be a nice specimen tree, but it's best to site it away from decks and entries due to its habit of dropping leaf and twig litter. Otherwise it is quite low maintenance.

Suitable Companions

Agastache rugosa, Korean Mint, tǔ huò xiāng
Andrographis paniculata, Kalmegh, chuān xīn lián
Angelica pubescens, dú huó
Coix lacryma-jobi, Job's Tears, yì yǐ rén
Eclipta prostrata, Eclipta, mò hàn lián

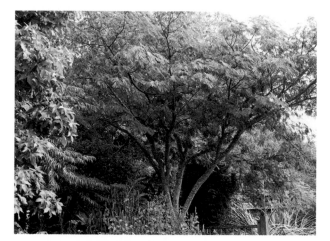

Fifteen-year-old *Albizia julibrissin* tree.

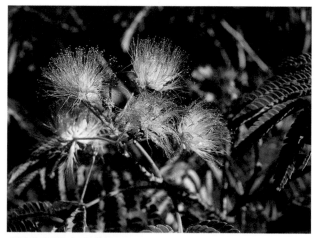

***Albizia julibrissin* flowers.**

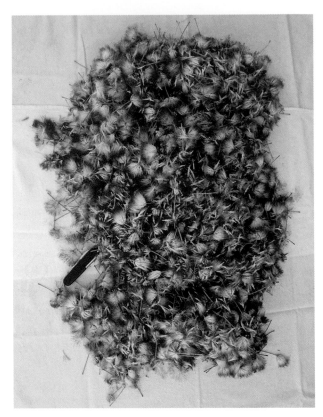

Fresh harvest of *Albizia julibrissin* flowers.

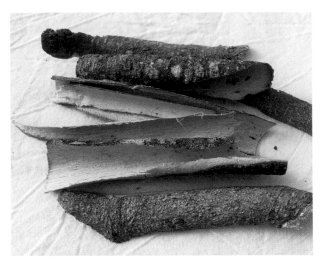

Dried bark of *Albizia julibrissin* (hé huān pí/huā).

Houttuynia cordata, yú xīng cǎo
Lonicera japonica, Honeysuckle, jīn yín huā
Mentha haplocalyx, Field Mint, bò hé
Ophiopogon japonicus, Lilyturf, mài mén dōng
Schisandra chinensis, Five Flavored Fruit, wǔ wèi zǐ

Field Production

Plant trees that are a minimum of one year old on fifteen-foot spacing in spring. Mimosa is drought tolerant; however, regular watering produces better specimens and higher herb yields without sacrificing quality. Plant in full sun to part shade. Even in drought-prone areas trees will begin to produce flowers in three or four years with some irrigation. Bark is best when taken from trees that are at least five years old. The trees grow rapidly enough and I grow sufficient quantities so that I can harvest bark by either chainsawing down five- or ten-year-old whole trees or large limbs at least every other year. Alternately trees can be coppiced (a process of cutting the trees down and then allowing the stumps to regenerate for

a few years before harvesting); this will keep flowers within OSHA harvesting regulation height (a safety measure), but they will not produce every year—making multiyear staggered harvesting necessary for yearly flower production. In addition, coppicing results in an inferior bark product, because the limbs you remove will be young and will not yield thick bark.

Pests and Diseases

None.

Harvest and Yield

Harvest in the morning after the dew has evaporated and the day's new flowers are open, but before the heat of the day arrives. For maximum harvest efficiency, avoid the temptation to pick when a tree first begins to bloom. Instead wait and pluck clustered flowers when they are in full bloom in summer. Overall yields are lower, but pounds per hour increase when you can harvest more than one flower with each movement. Use an orchard ladder and carry a basket slung over your shoulders or around your waist. Harvest every other day and collect no more than one pound at a time before transferring to the refrigerator; the flowers are fragile and crush easily as well as heat up rapidly. Cool down immediately by refrigerating in baskets or thin layers until the day's harvest is complete and they can be either sold fresh

Medicinal Uses of Hé huān pí/huā

Hé huān pí is the bark and hé huān huā is the flower of *Albizia julibrissin*. Sweet and neutral, hé huān pí calms the shen, relieves constrained qi, invigorates the blood, and reduces swelling. Hé huān huā calms the shen, regulates the qi, and harmonizes the liver and stomach. Some sources say that hé huān huā also nourishes the blood and benefits the spleen. Hé huān huā is a key herb for addressing insomnia due to liver qi stagnation.

Both hé huān pí and hé huān huā are traditionally used to address insomnia, irritability, anxiety, emotional tension, and pain and swelling due to trauma. Hé huān pí is also used for swellings and abscesses, while hé huān huā is also used for pain and tightness in the limbs, tightness in the abdomen and stomach pain, or digestive issues due to emotional tension.

Both hé huān pí and hé huān huā are most commonly used in combination with other herbs as well as individually (typically for milder situations). Common methods of administration include as a form of tea, decoctions, powders, alcohol extracts, concentrated granules, and in tablet and pill form.

Hé huān can be translated as "Collective Happiness," making a literal rendition of hé huān huā "Flower of Collective Happiness" and hé huān pí "Bark of Collective Happiness."

or put into the drying shed. Expect about twenty pounds per each ten- to fifteen-year-old tree. Cull out any old dry flowers (after chilling) that may have been accidentally picked with the harvest; best quality is intact flowers with a strong, aromatic fragrance.[30] Ratio of fresh to dry flowers is 5:1. Drying the flowers takes only a few days; the best quality retains the pink color.

Harvest bark from trees at least five years old, and only when they are dormant. I power wash or scrub the tree trunks or limbs with water and a brush, then use a chainsaw to cut down trunks or large limbs. With a draw knife or similar tool, peel off the bark in thick slabs down to the cambium layer. The best herbal material is "dry, tender pieces of bark with distinct lenticels and without cork layers."[31] On average a ten-year-old tree yields ten to fifteen pounds of fresh bark. Bark dries easily; ratio of fresh to dry weight is 2:1.

Notes

- Commercial hé huān huā from China does not include the small flower stems, but the stems are difficult to remove. Inform potential buyers if you leave the stems attached.
- Magnolia coco is an adulterant frequently sold as hé huān huā.

Alisma plantago-aquatica, subsp. orientale (Sam.)

Botanical Synonym: *Alisma orientale* (Sam.) Juz.
Common Name: Water Plantain
Pinyin: Zé xiè
Family: Alismataceae
Part Used: Root

Plant Description

Alisma is a perennial aquatic herb that grows in shallow water or mud along lake margins, marshes, and ponds in sun to part shade. Submerged and rooted in mud, the broad, spoon-shaped, basal rosette of rubbery leaves rises 1½ feet above water on long, thick petioles. Small white flowers arranged in umbels bring the total height to 2 feet. *Alisma* is widely distributed in China from the extreme northeast through Mongolia and far into the south; it is not found in the more arid western region. USDA hardiness zones 4–10.[32]

Propagation

In late fall, the seeds mature into tan whorls comprised of flattened seeds. Surface-sow seeds in spring into mud (saturated field soil) in pots without drainage. Germination is ongoing starting at two weeks. The plants containerize well—even on a permanent basis

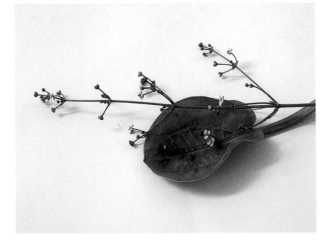

Leaf and flower of *Alisma plantago-aquatica* subsp. *orientale*.

if the vessel is large enough. Although these are suitable potted plants, do not offer them for standard commercial sale due to potential invasiveness and the possibility of escape into the environment via people planting them into natural bodies of water.

Garden and Polyculture Planting

A good location is a water garden that is isolated from natural bodies of water. There are some nice-looking water troughs on the market that can be repurposed, and even old bathtubs are serviceable. Plant eight inches to one foot apart, into mud, in conditions from muddy-wet to water from six to ten inches deep. (When water plaintain is grown in soil that is merely muddy, there will be more weed pressure.) No fertilizer is necessary.

Suitable Companions

For a muddy location rather than actual standing water, try these companions:

Bacopa monnieri, Brahmi
Houttuynia cordata, yú xīng cǎo
Plantago asiatica, Plantain, chē qián zǐ

Some Chinese herbs not covered in this book also make good companions for water plantain—including lotus, water lily, and duckweed, to name a few.

Field Production

Direct seed or transplant from eight inches to one foot apart into mud in a marsh or margin of a pond (make sure there is no outlet into streams or other natural bodies of water), or plant into a suitable

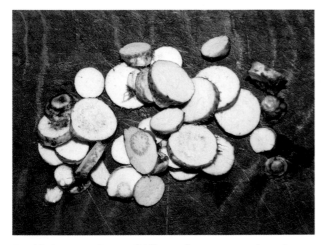

Freshly harvested root of *Alisma plantago-aquatica* subsp. *orientale* sliced and ready for drying.

artificial vessel. Any field soil is a suitable medium as long as it is waterlogged from six to ten inches deep. Plant in full sun to part shade exposure. No fertilizers are necessary, but do weed to keep resource competition low.

Pests and Diseases

None.

Harvest and Yield

Wait to harvest until plants are at least three years old. In the winter, remove foliage at the crown and cut off the hairy roots and leaf sheaths; the remaining volume will be very small compared to the initial mass of the plant. The desired herb is the white roundish rhizome—"good quality consists of large, heavy rhizomes with a solid texture."[33] Make eighth-inch parallel slices and dry; they dry to a light yellow-white color. Deadheading, or removing the flowering stalk, does not increase the size of the rhizome. The yield from a three-year-old plant is a quarter-pound per plant fresh. Ratio of fresh to dry herb is 3:1.

Medicinal Uses of Zé xiè

Zé xiè is the rhizome of *Alisma plantago-aquatica* subsp. *orientale*. Sweet, bland, and cold, it is one of the most important herbs for regulating fluid circulation and resolving dampness and has important functions of clearing empty heat that is rising from the kidneys. It is also used to moderate and prevent tonic herbs from overheating the body. It is used to address issues such as edema (water swelling), many types of urinary disorders, vertigo, dizziness, and ringing in the ears and to normalize the bowels. In modern China it is also being used to lower cholesterol and to help to regulate weight.

Zé xiè is most commonly used in combination with other herbs. Common methods of administration include decoctions, powders, concentrated granules, alcohol extracts, tablets, and pills. Well-known formulas that have zé xiè as an important ingredient include Liu Wei Di Huang Wan (Six Flavor *Rehmannia* Pills) and all of its derivatives, Wu Ling San (Five Ingredient Powder with *Poria*), and Zhu Ling San (*Polyporus* Powder).

Allium macrostemon (Bge.)

Medicinal Synonym: *Allium chinense* (G. Don)
Common Name: None
Pinyin: Xiè bái
Family: Alliaceae
Part Used: Bulb

Plant Description

Looking like the onions they are, both of these *Allium* species are more petite in bulb and leaf than the garden-variety bulbing onions, and their hollow greens are not as robust as scallion tops. *A. macrostemon* bulbs are globular to a half inch, and *A. chinense* bulbs have poorly defined necks from one quarter to one inch in diameter. *A. macrostemon* reaches a mere 1 foot tall whereas *A. chinense* can grow to 1½ feet tall. Both species are herbaceous and have many pale purple flowers arranged in umbels atop flowering stalks that rise above faceted foliage and very narrow, bladelike leaves. Both are clumping varieties with the typical onion odor when crushed. *A. macrostemon* grows in western China, Japan, Korea, Mongolia, and eastern Russia.[34] *A. chinense* grows on the Chinese eastern seaboard and is widely cultivated as a vegetable throughout southern China.[35] Uncommonly cultivated in the United States (and therefore extrapolating from the native extent), *A. macrostemon* would be suitable for USDA hardiness zones 5–9 and *A. chinense* for USDA hardiness zones 8–11.

Propagation

Sow the small black seeds in spring in average nursery media. Having said this, I must point out that the *A. chinense* we've planted at the Chinese Medicinal Herb Farm has never set seed—lots of pretty flowers, but no seed production. Another method to increase stock is to separate clumps and replant them. These species make excellent permanent potted plants.

Garden and Polyculture Planting

Of these sweet little cousins of the onions, *A. chinense* possesses more ornamental qualities than *A. macrostemon*. It is a carefree grower in average garden soil in a full sun site; water as you would regular onions.

Suitable Companions

Acanthopanax gracilistylus, wǔ jiā pí
Achyranthes bidentata, Oxknee, huái niú xī
Agastache rugosa, Korean Mint, tǔ huò xiāng
Allium tuberosum, Garlic Chives, jiǔ cài zǐ
Andrographis paniculata, Kalmegh, chuān xīn lián
Anemarrhena asphodeloides, zhī mǔ
Angelica dahurica, bái zhǐ

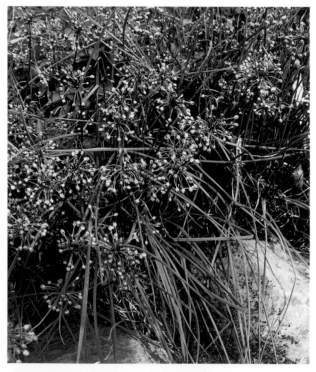

***Allium chinense* blooming in the garden.**

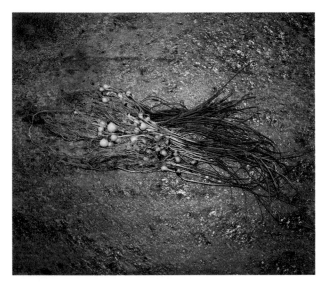

Freshly harvested *Allium macrostemon*.

Medicinal Uses of Xiè bái

Xiè bái is the bulb of *Allium macrostemon* (although it also comes from *Allium chinense*). Acrid, bitter, and warm, it opens the yang qi, moves the qi, and disperses stagnation. Its primary use is for painful obstruction bi of the chest, particularly when accompanied by phlegm. It is used to address issues such as angina characterized by pain and pressure in the chest, loud wheezing, shortness of breath, and stabbing pain in the chest. It is also used for certain types of diarrhea and dysentery.

Xiè bái is suitable as a culinary herb. Medicinally it is used in combination with other herbs. It is used both topically and internally. Internally, it is usually administered by decoction, powder, concentrated granule, or pill.

Angelica pubescens, dú huó
Aster tataricus, Tartar Aster, zǐ wǎn
Atractylodes macrocephala, Chinese Thistle Daisy, bái zhú
Belamcanda chinensis, Blackberry Lily, shè gān
Bupleurum chinense, Hare's Ear, chái hú
Carthamus tinctorius, Safflower, hóng huā
Celosia argentea, qīng xiāng zǐ
Celosia cristata, Cockscomb, jī guān huā
Chrysanthemum morifolium, Mum, jú huā
Clerodendrum trichotomum, Glorybower, chòu wú tóng
Cornus officinalis, Dogwood, shān zhū yú
Crataegus pinnatifida, Chinese Hawthorn, shān zhā
Cyathula officinalis, Hookweed, chuān niú xī
Dianthus superbus, Fringed Pink, qú mài
Dolichos lablab, Hyacinth Bean, bái biǎn dòu
Eriobotrya japonica, Loquat, pí pá yè
Eucommia ulmoides, Hardy Rubber Tree, dù zhòng
Ginkgo biloba, Ginkgo, bái guǒ
Ligusticum jeholense, Chinese Lovage, gǎo běn
Ligustrum lucidum, Chinese Privet, nǚ zhēn zǐ
Lilium lancifolium, *L. brownii*, Lily, bǎi hé
Momordica charantia, Bitter Melon, kǔ guā
Ocimum sanctum, Sacred Basil, Tulsi
Platycodon grandiflorus, Balloon Flower, jié gěng
Prunella vulgaris, Heal All, xià kū cǎo
Rehmannia glutinosa, Chinese Foxglove, dì huáng
Rheum palmatum, Chinese Rhubarb, dà huáng
Salvia miltiorrhiza, *S. przewalskii*, *S. bowleyana*, Red Sage, dān shēn
Saposhnikovia divaricata, Siler, fáng fēng
Schizonepeta tenuifolia, Japanese Catnip, jīng jiè
Scrophularia buergeriana, Figwort, běi xuán shēn
Scutellaria baicalensis, Baikal Skullcap, huáng qín
Trichosanthes kirilowii, Chinese Cucumber, guā lóu/tiān huā fěn
Withania somnifera, Ashwagandha

Field Production

Plant in average, well-drained soil on eight-inch to one-foot spacing in rows with one foot between rows. Grow each species for two to three seasons to obtain sizable bulbs. Cultivate to reduce competition, and mulch and irrigate in regions where there is little summer rain. Flowers are insect pollinated but do not cross outside of their species.

Pests and Diseases
None.

Harvest and Yield
Plants of both species mature for two to three years before bulbs start to bulk up. The traditional seasons of harvest are spring through fall. Simply dig up the shallow roots, cut the green leaves off the bulb, and wash (if not selling or using fresh, set to dry); good quality is "dry, large, full, heavy and solid, yellowish-white, translucent bulbs."[36] Harvest yield for *A. chinense* three-year stock is a half pound per six-inch clump. Ratio of fresh to dry is unknown. *A. macrostemon* yields smaller roots.

Notes
- Xiè bái is the bulb of *A. macrostemon* or *A. chinense*, more precisely named huá xiè bái (as with many traditional medicinal herbs, there is more than one botanical species used identically).

Allium tuberosum (Rottl. ex Spreng.)
Common Name: Garlic Chives
Pinyin: Jiǔ cài zǐ
Family: Alliaceae
Part Used: Seed

Plant Description
In Asia *Allium tuberosum* has a long history of both culinary and medicinal use. This herb is a long-lived herbaceous perennial with flat, narrow, arching leaves that are a half-inch wide and one foot long. Mounding one-foot-wide clumps produce white, starlike flowers in clusters on multiple two-foot-tall stiff stems. Summer flowers yield black-faceted seed in autumn. This *Allium* is native to southeast Asia. USDA hardiness zones 5–11.

Propagation
Reproduction is easy by seeds or plant division. The seed of many *Alliums* does not retain viability for more than a year or two, and garlic chives is no exception. For seed culture, sow in spring in a heated greenhouse or warm location; germination time is two weeks. Pot little clusters of seedlings in each container when they are a few inches tall. Division couldn't be easier—in spring simply cut vertically through the thick rhizomes to separate a clump into pieces, and replant. In very cold regions, dig whole plants in the fall to overwinter in a protected environment if desired. Obviously, though, the rate of return with this technique would not be economically viable on a large scale.

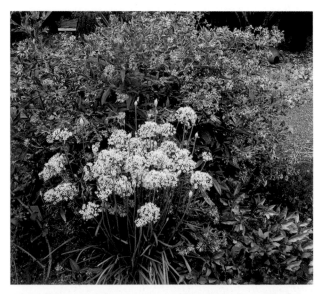

White-flowered *Allium tuberosum* in full bloom—with blue-flowered *Aster* sp., yellow-flowered *Bupleurum chinense*, and sunburned *Ardisia japonica*—in a plot near the nursery.

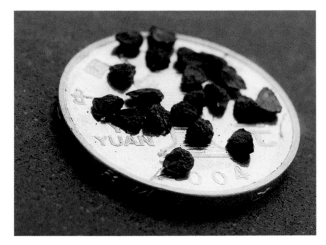

Jiŭ cài zĭ, **the dry seed of *Allium tuberosum*. Photo by Nina Zhito.**

Garden and Polyculture Planting

With its neat ornamental habit and pretty flowers, garlic chives is as easy to grow as it is aesthetically pleasing. Try planting it in the front of the border in groups of threes or fives. Garlic chives prefer a rich, moist, well-drained soil and tolerate short periods of drought. Transplant one foot apart or seed directly in a full sun to part shade position. Garlic chives occasionally reseed.

Suitable Companions

Acanthopanax gracilistylus, wŭ jiā pí
Achyranthes bidentata, Oxknee, huái niú xī
Agastache rugosa, Korean Mint, tŭ huò xiāng
Allium macrostemon, xiè bái
Anemarrhena asphodeloides, zhī mŭ
Angelica dahurica, bái zhĭ
Angelica pubescens, dú huó
Aster tataricus, Tartar Aster, zĭ wăn
Atractylodes macrocephala, Chinese Thistle Daisy, bái zhú
Belamcanda chinensis, Blackberry Lily, shè gān
Bupleurum chinense, Hare's Ear, chái hú
Carthamus tinctorius, Safflower, hóng huā
Celosia argentea, qīng xiāng zĭ
Celosia cristata, Cockscomb, jī guān huā
Chrysanthemum morifolium, Mum, jú huā
Clerodendrum trichotomum, Glorybower, chòu wú tóng

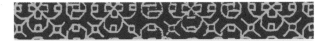

Garlic Chives Recipes

The white flowers and flat leaves are delicious chopped and added at the last minute to soups and stir-fry. Do not overcook as this deprives them of flavor and color and renders them stringy and sometimes bitter.

Scrambled Eggs with Chinese Chives

Chives and eggs are a traditional pairing, and the garlic chives, with their robust flavor, add more personality to a gentle scramble of eggs for a late breakfast or supper.

> 2 teaspoons canola oil
> 1 cup garlic chives, cut into 1-inch lengths
> Pinch of coarse sea salt
> Freshly ground pepper to taste
> 1 teaspoon soy sauce
> 4 eggs, lightly beaten

Serves 2

In a medium-size saucepan, heat the canola oil. When the oil is hot, stir in the chives and cook for two minutes. Add the salt, pepper, and soy sauce to the beaten eggs, stir, and pour into the saucepan. Lower heat and cook until eggs reach a soft curd, stirring continually. Serve immediately.

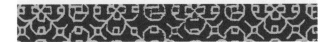

Codonopsis pilosula, Poor Man's Ginseng, dǎng shēn
Cornus officinalis, Dogwood, shān zhū yú
Crataegus pinnatifida, Chinese Hawthorn, shān zhā
Cyathula officinalis, Hookweed, chuān niú xī
Dianthus superbus, Fringed Pink, qú mài
Eriobotrya japonica, Loquat, pí pá yè

Eucommia ulmoides, Hardy Rubber Tree, dù zhòng
Ginkgo biloba, Ginkgo, bái guŏ
Ligusticum jeholense, Chinese Lovage, gǎo běn
Lilium lancifolium, *L. brownii*, Lily, bǎi hé
Magnolia denudata, xīn yí huā
Ocimum sanctum, Sacred Basil, Tulsi
Paeonia lactiflora, Chinese Peony, bái/chì sháo
Paeonia suffruticosa, Tree Peony, mǔ dān pí
Platycodon grandiflorus, Balloon Flower, jié gĕng
Prunella vulgaris, Heal All, xià kū cǎo
Rehmannia glutinosa, Chinese Foxglove, dì huáng
Rheum palmatum, Chinese Rhubarb, dà huáng
Salvia miltiorrhiza, *S. przewalskii*, *S. bowleyana*,
   Red Sage, dān shēn
Saposhnikovia divaricata, Siler, fáng fēng
Schizonepeta tenuifolia, Japanese Catnip, jīng jiè
Scrophularia buergeriana, Figwort, běi xuán shēn
Scutellaria baicalensis, Baikal Skullcap, huáng qín
Scutellaria barbata, Barbat Skullcap, bàn zhī lián
Sophora flavescens, kǔ shēn
Trichosanthes kirilowii, Chinese Cucumber, guā
   lóu/tiān huā fěn
Withania somnifera, Ashwagandha

Field Production

Place transplants on one-foot spacing or direct sow three to five seeds per foot or emitter. Plants tolerate a variety of soil types but need fertility and good drainage. Weed in the first season to reduce resource competition; in the following season the plants will be more robust, and spacing should exclude weeds. To keep production active, top dress, or mulch, with compost after the first season.

Medicinal Uses of Jiŭ cài zǐ

Jiŭ cài zǐ, also called jiŭ zǐ, is the seed of *Allium tuberosum*. Warm, acrid, and sweet, Jiŭ cài zǐ tonifies the liver and kidney, supplements the yang and consolidates the jing (essences), with secondary functions of warming and regulating the stomach. Its most common application is in the treatment of kidney yang deficiency and stomach cold patterns. It is used to address issues such as impotence, weakness, coldness, frequent urination, profuse clear vaginal discharge, soreness of the back and knees, nausea, vomiting, and hiccups due to cold.

Jiŭ cài zǐ is used individually and in combination with other herbs. Common methods of administration include powders, decoctions, concentrated granules, tablets, and pills.

Pests and Diseases

Slugs are often present but do little actual damage.

Harvest and Yield

Seed matures in fall over a period of time; plan for at least two harvests to avoid losing the seed crop to adverse weather. Collect seeds when the papery cover splits and they are almost dry. Dry further, and for best quality winnow off any extraneous material. Yield is one to two ounces per plant each season.

Andrographis paniculata (Burm. f.) Nees.

Botanical Synonym: *Justicia paniculata (Burm. f.)*
Common Name: Kalmegh
Pinyin: Chuān xīn lián
Family: Acanthaceae
Part Used: Herb

Plant Description

Good at colonizing and adapting to new environmental conditions, *Andrographis paniculata* reaches three feet tall when in its element. An upright tender perennial (commonly treated as an annual) with many branches, this plant has lanceolate leaves up to three inches long and three-quarters of an inch wide. Very floriferous, its white flowers are marked with red, pink, or dark purple and are borne in stiff terminal panicles. Flowers and seed occur at the same time, often with successful seed set. Long, ridged capsules form, and when seed is ripe and humidity is low, the tiny dark yellow seeds disperse by bursting forth and shooting far and wide. Kalmegh is a heat-loving plant of tropical or subtropical origins in southern India and Sri Lanka, growing in plains and forests and introduced throughout tropical Asia.[38] It is also found in moist areas near water, as well as fallow land.[39] Assigning hardiness zones is not that useful for kalmegh, because it is not cold hardiness that determines its success but a subtropical-like warm, humid summer. This would describe the Atlantic and Gulf Coast plains, from southeast Texas east and all through Florida and up the Atlantic seaboard into South Carolina. USDA hardiness zones 8–11.

Propagation

Sow seed in spring directly into warm soil or in average media in the nursery or indoors. In my experience, germination rates are low, with sporadic germination from two weeks onward. Keep well watered and warm. Kalmegh keeps well as a potted plant; it will reseed in the greenhouse from potted specimens.

Garden and Polyculture Planting

Plant near the front of the garden or border. Plants are adaptable, preferring to grow where summers are humid and warm; warm nights and ample moisture encourage kalmegh to thrive. Plants produce flowers and seed in cooler northern regions as well; however, the plants may not grow very tall—even with a very long season. Native bees and honeybees visit the nectar-rich flowers.

Suitable Companions

Bacopa monnieri, Brahmi
Celosia argentea, qīng xiāng zǐ
Celosia cristata, Cockscomb, jī guān huā
Centella asiatica, Gotu Kola, jī xuě cǎo
Coix lacryma-jobi, Job's Tears, yì yǐ rén
Eclipta prostrata, Eclipta, mò hàn lián
Gynostemma pentaphyllum, Sweet Tea Vine, jiǎo gǔ lán
Houttuynia cordata, yú xīng cǎo

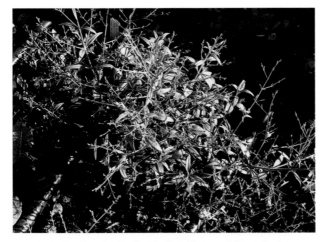

A young planting in the field of *Andrographis paniculata*.

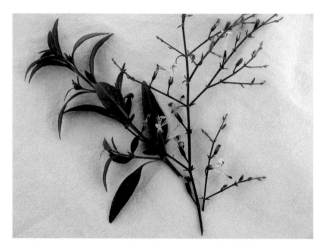

Fresh harvest sample of *Andrographis paniculata*.

Lonicera japonica, Honeysuckle, jīn yín huā
Momordica charantia, Bitter Melon, kǔ guā
Ocimum sanctum, Sacred Basil, Tulsi
Ophiopogon japonicus, Lilyturf, mài mén dōng
Pinellia ternata, bàn xià
Plantago asiatica, Plantain, chē qián zǐ
Platycodon grandiflorus, Balloon Flower, jié gěng
Prunella vulgaris, Heal All, xià kū cǎo
Schizonepeta tenuifolia, Japanese Catnip, jīng jiè
Scrophularia buergeriana, Figwort, běi xuán shēn
Scutellaria barbata, Barbat Skullcap, bàn zhī lián

Field Production

Plant one to two feet apart in sun or shade in a warm site and irrigate regularly. Kalmegh prefers soils that are well drained and of average fertility. In northern climes grow plants in a season extension hoophouse or high tunnel in the field if possible to even out temperatures and add humidity. The plants are not cold tolerant.

Pests and Diseases

None.

Harvest and Yield

Harvest kalmegh in the first season after 95–120 days, when the flower initiates start to develop. Wash plants a few days before harvest to rinse off dust and impurities. Cut aerial portions of the plants into three- to four-inch segments and dry. Drying is easy and should

Medicinal Uses of Chuān xīn lián

Chuān xīn lián is the herb or aerial part of *Andrographis paniculata*. Bitter and cold, chuān xīn lián, although a relatively recent addition to the official materia medica, has become one of the most important herbs in TCM to clear heat and eliminate toxins. It has secondary functions of clearing heat and drying dampness. It is used to address issues such as upper respiratory tract infections with sore throat, fever, and cough (including bronchitis and pneumonia); skin disorders characterized by redness and swelling; eczema; venomous bites; certain types of diarrhea; and urinary tract infections. Part of its popularity in modern China comes from its effectiveness in treating infection while simultaneously stimulating the immune system.

Chuān xīn lián is commonly used as a single herb as well as in combination with other herbs. It is used topically and internally. Common methods of administration are decoctions, powders, concentrated granules, tablets, pills, and capsules. It is the chief ingredient in the formula Chuan Xin Lian Pian.

be uneventful. The Chinese quality criterion for this herb specifies at least 35 percent leaves (plants tend to have a lot of stem material), a dark green color, and very bitter flavor.[40] Yield is one to three pounds per plant fresh. Ratio of fresh to dry is 3:1.

Notes

Occasionally Ayurvedic practitioners will also want roots to be included in the harvest, though no one has ever asked me for them.

Anemarrhena asphodeloides (Bge.)
Common Name: None
Pinyin: Zhī mǔ
Family: Anthericaceae
Part Used: Rhizome

Plant Description

Rare in cultivation, this herbaceous perennial has clumping basal leaves, to 1½ feet tall, and looks a lot like lawn grass, especially when young—maturing into looking more like mounding ornamental grass. Small white, pink, or lavender vase-shaped flowers are arranged in clusters on stiff racemes that rise above the foliage, making the total plant 4 feet tall. Laterally growing rhizomes have orangish exteriors and yellowish interiors. This Asian native occurs as far north as Mongolia and is considered cold hardy. USDA hardiness zones 3–9.

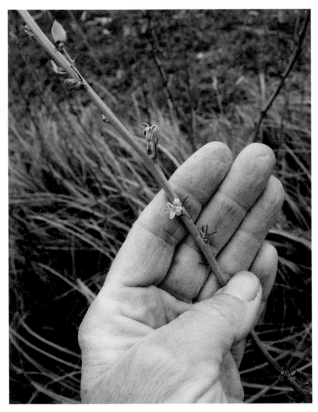

Anemarrhena asphodeloides–flower, seed pod, and leaf.

Propagation

Black-faceted seeds form in chambered tan capsules that should be separated before sowing (if seed was not received as such). Sow seeds in spring or fall. The seeds are somewhat fragile. Seedlings grow slowly, so plan to keep them in the nursery for a year or more before planting in the field. Do not allow to dry out. We have achieved 90 percent germination by spring-sowing seed in a heated greenhouse and also by sowing outdoors in the fall in wooden flats. Emergence takes place in one to two weeks, or in spring if fall sown. Seed stored at a constant temperature remains viable for more than four years. But the plants grow faster to harvest size if propagated vegetatively; to do so, cut off the last 1½ inches of the growing tip of the harvested rhizome, along with two to three roots, and replant in the field. Keep in mind that propagating by root cuttings makes for a less genetically diverse—and thus more vulnerable to environmental pressures—stock offering less genetic complexity to the end user. This herb holds well in pots and makes dependable, albeit slow, transplants for containerized sale.

Garden and Polyculture Planting

Not particularly ornamental, this valuable medicinal is quite durable. Plants that are at least one year old are recommended for planting—try not to mistake it for grass and weed it out! Group these neat and tidy growers one to two feet apart in the front of the border to give them presence—otherwise these humble-looking plants might be visually lost.

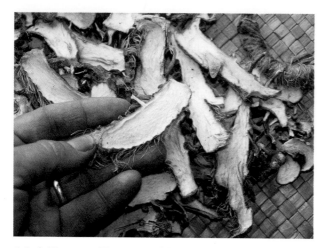

Dried rhizomes of four-year-old *Anemarrhena asphodeloides*, zhī mǔ.

Suitable Companions

Agastache rugosa, Korean Mint, tǔ huò xiāng
Allium macrostemon, xiè bái
Allium tuberosum, Garlic Chives, jiǔ cài zǐ
Angelica dahurica, bái zhǐ
Aster tataricus, Tartar Aster, zǐ wǎn
Belamcanda chinensis, Blackberry Lily, shè gān
Celosia argentea, qīng xiāng zǐ
Celosia cristata, Cockscomb, jī guān huā
Chrysanthemum morifolium, Mum, jú huā
Codonopsis pilosula, Poor Man's Ginseng,
    dǎng shēn
Coix lacryma-jobi, Job's Tears, yì yǐ rén
Cornus officinalis, Dogwood, shān zhū yú
Dianthus superbus, Fringed Pink, qú mài
Ligusticum jeholense, Chinese Lovage, gǎo běn
Magnolia denudata, xīn yí huā
Ocimum sanctum, Sacred Basil, Tulsi
Plantago asiatica, Plantain, chē qián zǐ
Platycodon grandiflorus, Balloon Flower, jié gěng
Prunella vulgaris, Heal All, xià kū cǎo
Saposhnikovia divaricata, Siler, fáng fēng
Scutellaria baicalensis, Baikal Skullcap, huáng qín
Scutellaria barbata, Barbat Skullcap, bàn zhī lián

Field Production

Cultivate this medicinally important, slow-growing herb in full sun to part shade with well-drained,

Medicinal Uses of Zhī mǔ

Zhī mǔ is the rhizome of *Anemarrhena asphodeloides*. Cold, bitter, and sweet, it is an important herb for clearing heat and fire with a strong secondary effect of nourishing the yin and supporting the fluids. It is used to clear excess heat and fire from the lung or stomach and deficient heat of the kidneys, and as an assistant in herbal formulas to prevent warming herbs from overheating the body. Zhī mǔ is commonly used to address problems related to menopause and is particularly well known for treating hot flashes and other menopausal symptoms when used in combination with the herb *Phellodendron chinense*, huáng bái. It is also used to address issues such as gastric reflux and stomatitis, inflammatory joint conditions, and lung conditions characterized by dryness and inflammation. In modern China it is an important component of many formulas that are used in the treatment of diabetes.

Zhī mǔ is usually used in combination with other herbs. Common methods of administration include decoctions, powders, concentrated granules, and tablets and tea pills. It is in formulas such as Zhi Bai Di Huang Wan (*Anemarrhena*, *Phellodendron*, and *Rehmannia* Pills) and Yu Nu Jian (Jade Woman Combination).

average soil; it tolerates clay soils well. Plant one-year-old starts into a cultivated bed with even spacing, one foot on center and one foot between rows. Regular irrigation is recommended; this is not a drought resistant plant. Keep weeded, especially when young, to avoid confusion with grassy weeds.

Pests and Diseases

Occasionally deer browse the flowers, and birds eat the maturing seed. Prolonged wet winters may cause roots to rot.

Harvest and Yield

The shallow thickened rhizomes of this herb look quite like iris rhizomes. Dig them while dormant in the fall or winter after three years or more of growth. To facilitate washing, remove the thickened roots close to the rhizome, and any persistent foliage—a power washer is helpful. Slice lengthwise in large, flat slabs and dry. Drying is quick and rhizomes do not tend to reabsorb moisture from the environment. "Good quality consists of large rhizomes, with a compact and soft texture. The cross section is yellowish white with a slightly greenish tinge."[41] Store zhī mǔ in an evenly cool, dry, dark location. Average yield at four years is a half pound per plant fresh. Ratio of fresh to dry herb is 3:1.

Angelica dahurica (Hoffm.) Benth.
Common Name: None
Pinyin: Baí zhǐ
Family: Apiaceae
Part Used: Root

Plant Description

This herbaceous biennial or short-lived perennial has thrice-divided, coarsely toothed, two- to three-foot leaves with long purple-blushed petioles. In the first season of vegetative growth, overall plant size is roughly three feet square. In the second (reproductive) season, the upright flower stalks give the plant the potential to reach seven feet tall. This species of

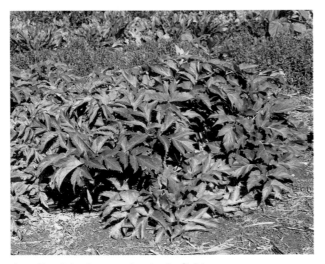

Angelica dahurica **growing in the field.**

Angelica is more columnar in shape than either the common western *Angelica archangelica* or the eastern *A. pubescens*, and is more robust than *A. sinensis*. The floral umbel can reach almost a foot across and consists of many tiny white flowers that attract pollinating insects. Each plant bears several flowering stalks, which are hollow and thick. Each plant produces hundreds of tan, flat, viable seeds. The richly fragrant one-foot-long light brown roots with white interiors are soft, round, and thick. *Angelica dahurica* is endemic to moist grasslands in north and central China and along China's northeast coast as well as in Siberia, Russia, and Taiwan[42]; USDA hardiness zones 4–9 or 10.

Propagation

Success is easy; this species does not exhibit delayed germination tactics. Surface-sow seeds outdoors in large flats in fall or early spring. Outdoor germination is variable and weather dependent. On our farm, seed stock remains viable for several years; however, there are reports of other landraces that are short-lived (this is not uncommon for the Apiaceae family).

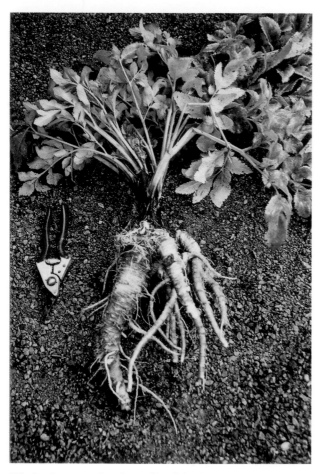

Whole plant sample of *Angelica dahurica*.

Pot up seedlings in average media to keep these fast growers from becoming either too crowded or pot-bound. This herb is not a good candidate for long-term pot culture.

Garden and Polyculture Planting

Angelica dahurica is a very companionable and undemanding plant in the garden, and large and bold enough for the hedgerow. Transplant two to three months after sowing. Plant in full sun to part shade three feet apart, in average but friable, well-drained soil. For best results irrigate when drought threatens.

Suitable Companions

Agastache rugosa, Korean Mint, tǔ huò xiāng
Allium tuberosum, Garlic Chives, jiǔ cài zǐ
Anemarrhena asphodeloides, zhī mǔ

Medicinal Uses of Bái zhǐ

Bái zhǐ is the root of *Angelica dahurica*. Warm and acrid, bái zhǐ releases the exterior, dispels wind, and is one of the most important herbs for opening the "upper orifices" (specifically the nose and sinuses). It also has primary functions of warming and relieving pain, particularly in the upper part of the stomach channel along the face and head. It is less commonly used for transforming dampness to address diarrhea, and eliminating toxins and reducing pus and swellings. It is most often used for opening the sinuses and is in both traditional and modern combinations that address sinus conditions ranging from sinusitis and allergic rhinitis to the common cold. Due to its regional effect on the face and head, it is also one of the most widely used herbs for addressing headaches from a variety of causes.

Bái zhǐ is usually used in combination with other herbs. Common methods of administration include powders, decoctions, concentrated granules, and tablets and tea pills. Most formulas that are well known for addressing allergies or sinus congestion contain bái zhǐ, including Cang Er Zi San (*Xanthium* Seed Powder) and Xin Yi San (Magnolia Flower Powder). It is also in the widely used formulas Huo Xiang Zheng Qi San (*Agastache* Rectify the Qi Powder), Xiao Feng San (Eliminate Wind Powder), and Chuan Xiong Cha Tiao San (*Ligusticum* Powder to Be Taken with Green Tea).

Asparagus cochinchinensis, tiān mén dōng
Aster tataricus, Tartar Aster, zǐ wǎn
Belamcanda chinensis, Blackberry Lily, shè gān
Chrysanthemum morifolium, Mum, jú huā

Eucommia ulmoides, Hardy Rubber Tree, dù zhòng
Forsythia suspensa, lián qiào
Ligustrum lucidum, Chinese Privet, nǚ zhēn zǐ
Lilium lancifolium, *L. brownii*, Lily, bǎi hé
Lonicera japonica, Honeysuckle, jīn yín huā
Paeonia lactiflora, Chinese Peony, bái/chì sháo
Paeonia suffruticosa, Tree Peony, mǔ dān pí
Platycodon grandiflorus, Balloon Flower, jié gěng
Prunella vulgaris, Heal All, xià kū cǎo
Rehmannia glutinosa, Chinese Foxglove, dì huáng
Rheum palmatum, Chinese Rhubarb, dà huáng
Salvia miltiorrhiza, *S. przewalskii*, *S. bowleyana*,
   Red Sage, dān shēn
Saposhnikovia divaricata, Siler, fáng fēng
Schizonepeta tenuifolia, Japanese Catnip, jīng jiè
Scrophularia buergeriana, Figwort, běi xuán shēn
Scutellaria baicalensis, Baikal Skullcap, huáng qín
Scutellaria barbata, Barbat Skullcap, bàn zhī lián
Sophora flavescens, kǔ shēn
Trichosanthes kirilowii, Chinese Cucumber, guā
   lóu/tiān huā fěn

Field Production

Plant in full sun or part shade where summers are hot. Soil should be well drained but moist and of average fertility. Though this may not be true of all *Angelica dahurica* landraces, the stock grown at the Chinese Medicinal Herb Farm has all been strictly biennial in nature and thus must be treated as an annual and harvested in the first season. If you delay harvest until the second spring, the emerging flower stalk will shoot up and the plant's energy will go to support flower production—and the root (and medicine) will be wasted. In mild winter regions plant early in the season (January through February) for the largest roots possible. For cold winter areas sow in fall or in the cold greenhouse.

Pests and Diseases

None except the occasional spring aphid on nursery stock.

Harvest and Yield

The perfumed thin-barked roots are a joy to harvest; they should be large, thick, and ropy—not hairy. After digging the roots, I saw off the crowns; wash and cut in parallel slices from the crown downward in quarter-inch slabs. It is interesting to note that there will be oil in the wash water if the herb is soaked for even a short amount of time. Drying is easy and uneventful. The traditional time for harvesting is noted as "summer or autumn when the leaves turn yellow,"[43] but if you harvest in summer the roots will not be very large, so I recommend harvesting in fall instead. Individual plants are highly variable in their root size and weight. In my experience, for the same stock grown out together, yields per plant have ranged from a ¼ pound to almost 2½ pounds. Average weight is 1¼ pounds per plant fresh. Ratio of fresh to dry weight is 4:1.

Angelica pubescens (Maxim.)

Botanical Synonym: *Angelica biserrata* (Shan & Yuan)
Common Name: None
Pinyin: Dú huó
Family: Apiaceae
Part Used: Root

Plant Description

What an appealing fragrance this *Angelica* root has—like good quality perfume. A member of a large and diverse family, the species is either a biennial or a short-lived perennial—only the plant's DNA knows for sure. It has dark green, three-foot-long, thrice-divided leaves wrapped around the stem in prominent purple sheaths. The individual leaflets are coarsely toothed and lightly fuzzy. In its first year, the plant forms a mound two to three feet tall by three feet wide. When in full bloom in the second or successive seasons, total height ranges from four to twelve feet tall, depending on how much sun is available. The white-flowered umbels are borne on terminal stalks; one naturalized part-shade-grown plant I saw at the University of California Berkeley Botanical Garden had an impressive central terminal flower fourteen inches wide. Flowers are insect pollinated and produce copious amounts of tan seed in fall. The roots are thick and cylindrical. *Angelica pubescens* grows in moist areas from 3,000 to 5,500 feet in elevation in four central and eastern Chinese provinces along the 30th parallel.[44] USDA hardiness zones 8–9.

Propagation

Sow seed in autumn in large deep flats, letting the winter have its vernalizing ways, and in spring seedlings will appear. If seedlings fail to appear, apologize to the cook, and put the whole flat in the refrigerator for two to three weeks. Don't delay too long before transplanting, or plant roots will kink and not recover.

Garden and Polyculture Planting

Uncommon but an asset to the ornamental garden as well as the hedgerow, *Angelica pubescens* can be placed toward the middle or back of the border in full sun to part shade. Soils should be somewhat fertile, and moist but well drained. Space three feet apart. Because of its large stature, place it away from diminutive plants.

Suitable Companions

Agastache rugosa, Korean Mint, tǔ huò xiāng
Allium tuberosum, Garlic Chives, jiǔ cài zǐ
Anemarrhena asphodeloides, zhī mǔ

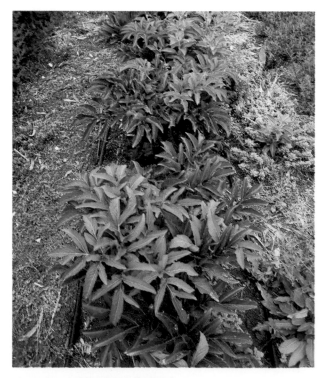

First-season *Angelica pubescens*.

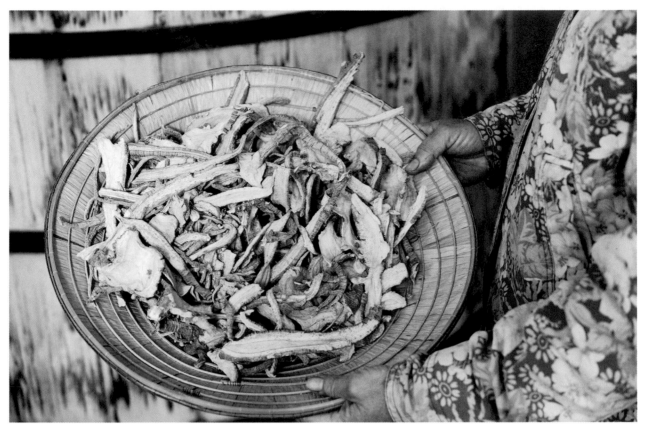

Dried *Angelica pubescens*, dú huó. Photo by Nina Zhito.

Asparagus cochinchinensis, tiān mén dōng

Aster tataricus, Tartar Aster, zǐ wǎn

Belamcanda chinensis, Blackberry Lily, shè gān

Chrysanthemum morifolium, Mum, jú huā

Clerodendrum trichotomum, Glorybower, chòu wú tóng

Codonopsis pilosula, Poor Man's Ginseng, dǎng shēn

Coix lacryma-jobi, Job's Tears, yì yǐ rén

Cornus officinalis, Dogwood, shān zhū yú

Crataegus pinnatifida, Chinese Hawthorn, shān zhā

Eclipta prostrata, Eclipta, mò hàn lián

Eucommia ulmoides, Hardy Rubber Tree, dù zhòng

Forsythia suspensa, lián qiào

Gentiana scabra, lóng dǎn cǎo

Gentiana straminea, qín jiāo

Ginkgo biloba, Ginkgo, bái guǒ

Gynostemma pentaphyllum, Sweet Tea Vine, jiǎo gǔ lán

Houttuynia cordata, yú xīng cǎo

Lilium lancifolium, *L. brownii*, Lily, bǎi hé

Lonicera japonica, Honeysuckle, jīn yín huā

Ophiopogon japonicus, Lilyturf, mài mén dōng

Paeonia lactiflora, Chinese Peony, bái/chì sháo

Paeonia suffruticosa, Tree Peony, mǔ dān pí

Plantago asiatica, Plantain, chē qián zǐ

Platycodon grandiflorus, Balloon Flower, jié gěng

Prunella vulgaris, Heal All, xià kū cǎo

Rheum palmatum, Chinese Rhubarb, dà huáng

Salvia miltiorrhiza, *S. przewalskii*, *S. bowleyana*, Red Sage, dān shēn

Saposhnikovia divaricata, Siler, fáng fēng

Schisandra chinensis, Five Flavored Fruit, wǔ wèi zǐ

Schizonepeta tenuifolia, Japanese Catnip, jīng jiè

Scrophularia buergeriana, Figwort, běi xuán shēn

Scutellaria baicalensis, Baikal Skullcap, huáng qín

Scutellaria barbata, Barbat Skullcap, bàn zhī lián

Sophora flavescens, kǔ shēn

Trichosanthes kirilowii, Chinese Cucumber, guā lóu/tiān huā fěn

Field Production

Plant *Angelica pubescens* on three-foot spacing in full sun to part sun with well-draining average to fertile soil. It sometimes self-sows (particularly in a lightly forested area) but is not considered invasive, though it is very adaptable. Overhead or drip irrigation is necessary in regions where there are no summer rains. If cultivated when young to remove competition, the plant will fill in and crowd out unwanted weeds.

In an effort to obtain larger roots, some growers remove the emerging flower stalks, but I wasted hundreds of plants into oblivion trying that technique. Perhaps it's a function of the original landrace genetics, but my plants exhibited a strong desire to reproduce—every other week I had to remove new floral stalks. Ultimately, the plants succumbed and died—and *all* of that root shriveled. Shall we call it flower power?

If you plan to collect seed for this herb, be aware that if other species of *Angelica* are in bloom nearby, cross-pollination may occur. This must be avoided; if there is any risk, remove all flowers except those of the species from which you want to save seed. Closely related species of *Heracleum* may serve as a pollen source, too; remove flowers from nearby *Heracleum* plants also.

Pests and Diseases

Gophers gladly eat the roots.

Harvest and Yield

Harvest in the late fall or early winter when cold has withered the leaves. After digging the roots, I saw off the crowns; wash and cut in parallel slices from the crown downward in quarter-inch slabs. Harvest before flowers initiate their show. I conducted trials with seed of different origins and found significant differences in time to sexual maturity—from one to four years, although most of the plants flowered in the second year. It is safest, and most convenient, to sow very early in the year and transplant as soon as the field is available so you can harvest roots that first fall. The roots should be very fragrant; larger is good. Yield for one-season-old root is 0.9 pounds per plant. Ratio of fresh to dry is 4:1.

Medicinal Uses of Dú huó

Dú huó is the root of *Angelica pubescens*. Warm, bitter, and acrid, it dispels wind and dampness, unblocks the channels to relieve pain, and has secondary functions of releasing the exterior. Dú huó is one of the most important herbs in TCM for addressing bi (painful obstruction) patterns; arthritic pain; acute or chronic muscle and joint pain, particularly of the lower body; and weakness of the knees and lower back. It also is used to address symptoms such as muscle aches, pain and headaches that accompany colds and flu, and for various types of headaches.

Dú huó is usually used combined with other herbs in formulas. Common methods of administration include decoctions, alcohol extracts, powders, concentrated granules, tablets, and pills. Many formulas that deal with arthritic pain (particularly when aggravated by cold and damp) contain dú huó as an important ingredient, including the well-known formula Du Huo Ji Sheng Tang (*Angelica pubescens* and *Loranthus* Decoction).

Angelica sinensis (Oliv.) Diels

Alternate Species: *Angelica acutiloba* (Siebold & Zucc.) *Kitag., Angelica polymorpha* var. *sinensis* (Oliv.)
Common Name: Dang Gui
Pinyin: Dāng guī
Family: Apiaceae
Part Used: Root

Plant Description

Perennial and herbaceous, *Angelica sinensis* grows up to four feet tall with the typical white- to green-flowering umbel in summer followed in fall with flattish, slightly furrowed brown seed. The round, many-branched, white roots are quite aromatic.

Overall the plants are much more delicate, brighter green, and less coarse than the western *Angelica archangelica* or the Asian *A. dahurica* and *A. pubescens.* Ten-inch-long leaves are divided into three leaflets (bipinnate) and are light green, sometimes with a blue-green hue but more often with purple overtones on the

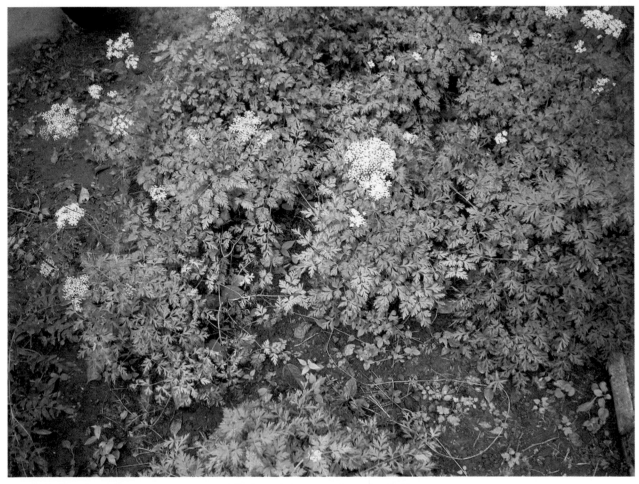

Angelica sinensis **in bloom at the Institute of Medicinal Plant Development, Beijing.**

petioles, and leaf margins are serrated or toothed. Not surprisingly, the whole plant smells like celery, which belongs to the same family. The *Flora of China* notes that *Angelica sinensis* is native to central China and grows "wild or cultivated in forests, shrubby thickets; 2500–3000 meters in Gansu, Hubei, Shaanxi, Sichuan, Yunnan."[45] USDA hardiness zones 6–9.

Propagation

Angelica sinensis can be challenging to grow. "The plants like a cool, moist environment with deep, rich, sandy soil, high in organic matter. It does best in very high and cold conditions in a shaded location."[46] Many varieties of seed in the Apiaceae family are considered short-lived, but I've had close to 100 percent germination several times with February-sown seed that was just over two years old. As with many in the *Angelica* genus, seeds are cool soil germinators; surface sow or cover only lightly and keep flats in a moist shaded location. For nursery-started plants sow fresh seed into deep wooden flats with a mixture of forest soil and nursery media. In a mountainous forest environment direct sowing is possible. *Angelica sinensis* is a slow growing plant.

Garden and Polyculture Planting

Place *Angelica sinensis* one to two feet apart in a shady ornamental or garden setting. Environs should be cool; avoid sunny sites where plants would suffer from too much heat. A forested situation with deep, moist soil and duff cover is ideal. Consistent rainfall is best, or provide it with irrigation. Do not crowd this coveted perennial; competition can overwhelm it. Mark the plant locations so as to avoid disturbing them while they are dormant.

Suitable Companions

Codonopsis pilosula, Poor Man's Ginseng, dǎng shēn
Cornus officinalis, Dogwood, shān zhū yú
Crataegus pinnatifida, Chinese Hawthorn, shān zhā
Eriobotrya japonica, Loquat, pí pá yè
Eucommia ulmoides, Hardy Rubber Tree, dù zhòng
Gentiana scabra, lóng dǎn cǎo

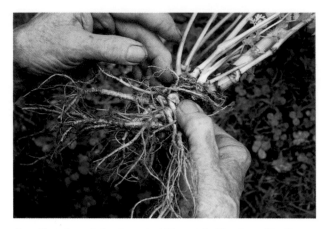

Angelica sinensis **fresh root at Mountain Gardens, North Carolina. Photo courtesy of Jean Giblette.**

Gentiana straminea, qín jiāo
Ginkgo biloba, Ginkgo, bái guǒ
Magnolia denudata, xīn yí huā
Schisandra chinensis, Five Flavored Fruit, wǔ wèi zǐ

Field Production

Evergreen forest is predominant in the Chinese provinces where dang gui is native,[47] and thus semiwild forest cultivation is superior to standard field production. Either direct sow fresh seed or use the nursery method described above. Grow plants on one- to two-foot centers in part shade. This species is not drought resistant. In arid regions or times of drought provide overhead irrigation, or perhaps use a nearby creek (with water rights) or a truck or ATV outfitted with a water tank. On a small scale in remote areas a water backpack used for fighting wildfires could be of service. Keep weeded and mulched, and try not to compact the soil surrounding the plants.

Pests and Diseases

On my farm, gophers devour all unprotected *Angelica polymorpha* var. *sinensis* specimens; however, they passed over, or should I say under, hundreds of *Angelica sinensis*. Prolonged excessively wet periods may cause roots to rot.

Harvest and Yield

Harvest in the fall after two or more years. In *Herbal Emissaries*, Foster notes that dang gui is harvested in

Medicinal Uses of Dāng guī

Dāng guī is the root of *Angelica sinensis*. It is one of the most widely used tonic herbs within TCM and has become one of the most well-known Chinese medicinal herbs throughout the world. Sweet, acrid, and warm, it tonifies the blood, invigorates the blood circulation, relieves pain, moistens the intestines, and stops cough. It is used to address a wide variety of conditions that involve the blood and is one of the primary herbs used to treat many gynecological problems, including scant menstruation, irregular menstrual cycle, menstrual cramping, and PMS. It is also used to address issues such as anemia, dry skin and hair, dizziness, palpitations, insomnia, traumatic injuries, numbness and pain, constipation, and certain types of coughs.

Dāng guī is traditionally used in dietary therapy as a nourishing food in soups, congees (porridges), and other dishes. Medicinally it is used alone, but also often in formulas combined with other herbs. Along with being used in TCM, it is now commonly used in western herbal medicine, naturopathic medicine, and as a dietary supplement (sold at health food markets and herb shops). Common methods of administration include decoctions, alcohol extracts, powders, concentrated granules, and in tablet and pill form. It is also used topically, usually as part of a plaster. Dāng guī is in many major formulas, including Si Wu Tang (Four Substances Decoction), Xiao Yao San (Free and Easy Wanderer Powder), Dang Gui Bu Xue Tang (*Angelica* Tonify the Blood Decoction), Gui Pi Tang (Restore the Spleen Decoction), and Xue Fu Zhu Yu Tang (Drive Out Stasis in the Mansion of Blood Decoction).

autumn after two or three years of growth and that one-year plants are not harvested as they yield inferior medicine. He also states that the best quality is very aromatic and the roots are plump and long. Roots are white when freshly dug and dry to a dark yellow color. In a Chinese study conducted in Gansu province, optimal and suitable habitat niches produced between 1,075 and 3,769 pounds per acre per year.[48]

Notes

- *Angelica sinensis* has specific site preferences; lucky is the grower with the correct conditions. With limited experience, I've found *Angelica polymorpha* var. *sinensis* and *A. acutiloba*, also plant sources of dāng guī, to be much easier to cultivate.
- This is a primary herb in the materia medica and much in demand; efforts should be widely made to grow this important crop.

Arctium lappa (L.)
Common Name: Burdock
Pinyin: Niú bàng zǐ
Family: Asteraceae
Part Used: Seed, root

Plant Description

Although *Arctium lappa* is a rather weedy plant, I've included it due to its long-term naturalization and "common and useful" status. *Arctium lappa* has escaped cultivation in many areas of the United States and is considered invasive in many regions of both Canada and the United States. This large-scale, hardy, herbaceous biennial grows up to nine feet tall, with large, coarse, ovate- to heart-shaped leaves that are green on top and white pubescent on the underside. The purple flower is burrlike. A significant stout taproot can grow three feet deep and three inches across—in five to six months! Brown-skinned roots are white within and discolor rapidly when exposed to air, sometimes turning pink if not processed rapidly. USDA hardiness zones 4–10.

Propagation

Burdock's large, dark, gray-brown seeds are easy to sow directly on the soil surface. Seedlings are large and grow fast, so all is effectively done in situ. Nursery sowing is also easy. Germination is quick, and it's important to transplant seedlings without delay. I recommend waiting until summer to plant burdock; otherwise the root can become very large and hard to dig—smaller is easier.

Garden and Polyculture Planting

Place burdock in the rear of the border, allowing a planting site at least four feet across. Direct sow in full sun in soil of average fertility that is sandy and well drained. Several varieties of butterflies enjoy the flower nectar. If you plant burdock in a hedgerow, don't forget to remove either the flower or young seedhead to prevent reseeding.

Suitable Companions

Achyranthes bidentata, Oxknee, huái niú xī
Agastache rugosa, Korean Mint, tǔ huò xiāng
Angelica dahurica, bái zhǐ
Angelica pubescens, dú huó
Aster tataricus, Tartar Aster, zǐ wǎn
Belamcanda chinensis, Blackberry Lily, shè gān
Carthamus tinctorius, Safflower, hóng huā
Celosia argentea, qīng xiāng zǐ
Celosia cristata, Cockscomb, jī guān huā
Chrysanthemum morifolium, Mum, jú huā
Clerodendrum trichotomum, Glorybower, chòu wú tóng
Cyathula officinalis, Hookweed, chuān niú xī
Dolichos lablab, Hyacinth Bean, bái biǎn dòu
Eriobotrya japonica, Loquat, pí pá yè
Eucommia ulmoides, Hardy Rubber Tree, dù zhòng

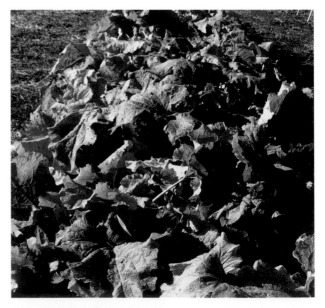

Row of *Arctium lappa*, first season.

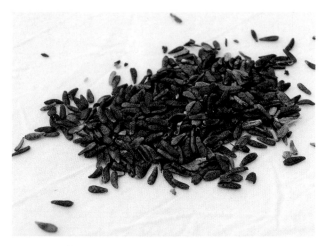

Dry seed of *Arctium lappa*, niú bàng zǐ.

Ligustrum lucidum, Chinese Privet, nǚ zhēn zǐ
Lilium lancifolium, L. brownii, Lily, bǎi hé
Lonicera japonica, Honeysuckle, jīn yín huā
Lycium chinense, Chinese Wolfberry, gǒu qǐ zǐ/dì gǔ pí
Magnolia denudata, xīn yí huā
Momordica charantia, Bitter Melon, kǔ guā
Prunella vulgaris, Heal All, xià kū cǎo
Rheum palmatum, Chinese Rhubarb, dà huáng
Salvia miltiorrhiza, S. przewalskii, S. bowleyana, Red Sage, dān shēn
Scutellaria baicalensis, Baikal Skullcap, huáng qín
Sophora flavescens, kǔ shēn
Trichosanthes kirilowii, Chinese Cucumber, guā lóu/tiān huā fěn

Field Production

Burdock can manage in heavy clay, but sandy soil makes more attractive roots and easier harvesting. Heavy clay makes them difficult to dig and so large as to be hollow cored; when this happens root quality suffers. For a root crop, sow burdock in spring for fall harvest or in fall for spring harvest. Spring- to summer-sown root crops are ready in as little as two months. For seed crops, sow in spring to summer so the root can obtain enough strength to throw flowers the following year. Place burdock on two-foot spacing in the row. Provide water if drought threatens. There are many varieties on the market to choose from. If sown early enough, some varieties in some locations may set seed in the first fall.

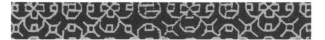

Burdock Cooking Tips

Small burdock roots can be lightly scrubbed, sliced thinly like carrots, and added to stir-fry. They are delicious oven roasted in combination with other root vegetables such as carrots and potatoes, tossed with olive oil, lightly salted, and topped with toasted sesame seeds.

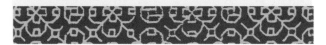

Pests and Diseases

Gophers eat the roots; on occasion, insects consume the seed.

Harvest and Yield

Roots are dug in the fall of the first season, and seed is usually not available until the second. It's physically impossible to harvest both roots and seed from the same plant. After digging roots, wash and (if they are to be dried) cut them crosswise in one-inch rounds. Cut open to check for doneness during the drying process. Good quality roots have a fresh smell and are dense and not pithy.

Seed harvest is trickier. There are tiny hooks in the seedhead that get loose and embed themselves in skin, lungs, eyes, and so on—the itch can be terrible. The hooks bother dogs and probably other mammals as well. Carefully harvest just the mature flower heads. If you don't plan to sell them fresh, put them aside to gently dry for a few days, whereupon the seed will come loose from the receptacle more easily. The processing setup is all about protection: wear a raincoat with the hood up, rain pants, goggles, rubber gloves, and boots. You'll also need a clean chipper/shredder, clean tarp, several fans, and a winnowing basket or vessel. Place the chipper outside on the tarp with the fans behind you. Don your getup and, with the fans on, run the flower heads through the chipper.

Be sure the hooks and nonseed material will blow away from you, not toward you. When all is done and the seed is in a pile below the machine, move the chipper away and winnow the chaff from the seed. The chaff is light and will blow further onto the tarp (compost the chaff later). Only a few winnowings are needed and the crop of seed is clean and ready to dry. (I have found that this setup is only time and cost effective if you are processing more than roughly twenty-five plants.) After the seed has dried, put it in the refrigerator or it will become rancid in just a few month's time. Good quality seed is plump and has a different—but also a fresh (not rancid)—smell.

Yield for spring-sown root crops for the variety 'Watanabe' is 2½ pounds per plant; the variety 'Gobo' is ¾ pound per plant. Ratio of fresh to dry is 4:1. The fresh yield for seed is up to ¼ pound per plant. Ratio of fresh to dry is 1.5:1.

Notes

- With dual Eastern and Western markets and heavy-yielding production, burdock is an attractive crop. It has the added advantage of opening up and improving the structure of heavy soils.
- Burdock root is a popular food in Asia and is used in Western herbalism. In the Chinese herbal tradition the seed is also employed.

Medicinal Uses of Niú bàng zǐ

Niú bàng zǐ is the fruit of *Arctium lappa*. Acrid, bitter, and cold, it dispels wind, clears heat, eliminates toxins, vents rashes, and clears toxic heat from the throat. It is used to address issues such as sore throat, swollen tonsils, headache, fever, cough and phlegm (usually yellow), and many chronic and acute dermatological disorders that involve itching, rashes, and swelling.

Niú bàng zǐ is usually used in combination with other herbs. Common methods of administration include powders, decoctions, concentrated granules, tablets, and pills. It is in formulas such as Yin Qiao San (*Forsythia* and *Lonicera* Powder), Xiao Feng San (Eliminate Wind Powder), and Pu Ji Xiao Du Yin (Universal Benefit Decoction to Eliminate Toxins).

Artemisia annua (L.)

Common Name: Sweet Annie
Pinyin: Qīng hāo
Family: Asteraceae
Part Used: Herb

Plant Description

An annual, *Artemisia annua* has insignificant yellow flowers borne in a profusion of panicles. Leaves are green, deeply divided, and four inches long on many-branched eight-foot-tall-by-four-foot-wide plants. It has an upright, open form and a vigorous habit. *Artemisia annua*, native to Asia and eastern Europe, is quite aromatic and has been widely cultivated for many years as foliage for the floral industry, for aromatic oil, and increasingly for its medicinal properties. Due to its tendency to naturalize it is widely distributed in the United States and Canada. USDA hardiness zones 4–9.

Propagation

Direct seed in the spring after the last frost or start seeds in the nursery or indoors; emergence occurs in about one week. The seed is very small, almost dustlike; barely cover with soil and water gently. Use bottom heat or keep seed flats in a heated greenhouse to encourage faster seedling growth. This *Artemisia* is a fast grower and does not hold well in pots.

Garden and Polyculture Planting

A carefree grower, sweet annie is an attractive, large-scale herb suitable for the back of the border in sunny, hot locations—or try planting it as a summer hedge or as short term screening. Set plants five feet apart. To use as cut foliage, harvest before the flowers open. Even though pollen production is very high, bees do not seem particularly drawn to the plants.

Suitable Companions

Agastache rugosa, Korean Mint, tǔ huò xiāng
Allium tuberosum, Garlic Chives, jiǔ cài zǐ
Angelica dahurica, baí zhǐ
Angelica pubescens, dú huó
Aster tataricus, Tartar Aster, zǐ wǎn
Belamcanda chinensis, Blackberry Lily, shè gān
Carthamus tinctorius, Safflower, hóng huā
Chrysanthemum morifolium, Mum, jú huā
Cornus officinalis, Dogwood, shān zhū yú
Crataegus pinnatifida, Chinese Hawthorn, shān zhā
Cyathula officinalis, Hookweed, chuān niú xī
Eucommia ulmoides, Hardy Rubber Tree, dù zhòng
Ligustrum lucidum, Chinese Privet, nǚ zhēn zǐ
Lilium lancifolium, L. brownii, Lily, bǎi hé
Lonicera japonica, Honeysuckle, jīn yín huā
Magnolia denudata, xīn yí huā
Momordica charantia, Bitter Melon, kǔ guā
Prunella vulgaris, Heal All, xià kū cǎo
Rheum palmatum, Chinese Rhubarb, dà huáng

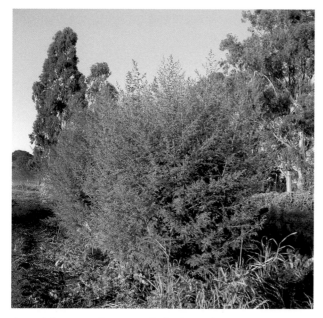
***Artemisia annua* almost ready for harvest.**

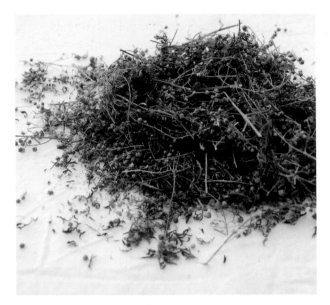

Dry *Artemisia annua*, qīng hāo.

Salvia miltiorrhiza, S. przewalskii, S. bowleyana
    Red Sage, dān shēn
Scutellaria baicalensis, Baikal Skullcap, huáng qín
Sophora flavescens, kǔ shēn
Withania somnifera, Ashwagandha

Field Production

Sweet annie grows well in full sun in well-drained, moderately fertile soils. For production it needs ninety-five frost-free days. Space plants four feet apart in the row. It has average water needs and is easy to grow, not being particular about soil conditions. High winds may break branches.

Pests and Diseases

None.

Harvest and Yield

As usual, in preparation for harvest, wash standing plants with potable water a day or two before collection. Collect leafy stems just before or as they are coming into flower in late summer to fall. If harvesting for fresh sale, collect only the nonwoody flowering tops with tips up to eight inches long. For dry herb sales, whole plants that are cut down can be hooked via branch stubs and hung to dry—or smaller branches can be bundled and rubber-banded together

Medicinal Uses of Qīng hāo

Qīng hāo is the herb or aerial portion of *Artemisia annua*. Bitter, acrid, and cold, qīng hāo clears heat and treats malaria; clears yin; deficient heat, summer heat and liver heat; and cools the blood. It is widely recognized, both traditionally and pharmacologically, for its ability to treat malaria and is now also being used in the treatment of Lyme disease. Traditionally, it is used to address tidal fever (fever that comes up in the night), absence of perspiration, "five center heat" (heat in the palms, soles, and center of the chest), eye disorders, and certain types of jaundice.

Qīng hāo is commonly used as a single herb as well as in combination with other herbs. To treat malaria it is often administered as a juice or as a large amount of the fresh herb in a quick decoction. It is also generally administered in decoctions (added in near the end of the cooking time), concentrated powders, alcohol extracts, tablets, and pills.

The modern pharmaceutical group of drugs called artemisinins originally came from *Artemisia annua*. In combination with other drugs, they are now standard treatment throughout the world for malaria.

and hung or placed on drying racks. Riddle the dry bundles on a four-inch mesh screen to remove the leaf from the stem material. Good quality dry herb should be very highly aromatic and have bright green leaf pieces and stem, not powder. The best quality in Chinese medicine is noted to be harvested before flowering and have yellow-green stems and dark green leaves.[49] The yield for *Artemisia annua* is 2½ pounds per plant when fresh. Flowering tops ratio of fresh to dry is 6:1; destemmed material 4:1.

Notes

• Occasionally Chinese herbal practitioners specify a preference for which part of the plant they would like, such as leaf and no stem, or stem and no leaf, or flowering tops only. As always it is best to inquire at the onset of contract negotiations. *Artemisia annua* has Eastern and Western herbal marketing potential.

• Plants can be invasive by seed, especially in areas with summer rain.

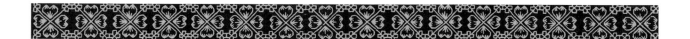

Asparagus cochinchinensis ([Lour.] Merr.)
Common Name: None
Pinyin: Tiān mén dōng
Family: Asparagaceae
Part Used: Root

Plant Description

This important herb is no garden variety asparagus. First off, the emerging shoots aren't nearly big enough to bother eating—the translucent, tuberous, two- to three-inch-long roots are where the action is. There are several important medicinal *Asparagus* species; this perennial herbaceous species can be identified by its very fine three-quarter-inch linear leaves that grow in whorls all along the spurred six-foot stems. Plants are dioecious (either male or female); for seed production both sexes must be present. Flowers are small, and female plants produce small, round, green berries, containing one or two seeds, distributed along the climbing stems. In China *Asparagus cochinchinensis* grows below the fortieth parallel on sparsely forested slopes at elevations from 5,000 feet to sea level over a range from Tibet to the eastern coast of China (as well as growing in other Asian countries). USDA hardiness zones 5–10.[50]

Propagation

Sown in spring, *Asparagus cochinchinensis* is a multicycle germinator and can take up to two years to germinate; be patient and keep the seed box moist. When the time is right a mass of seedlings appear that look very much like miniature garden asparagus. It is best to sow seed in large, deep, wooden flats—so they don't dry out—and leave them exposed to seasonal weather. Alternately, stratifying the seed by cycling it in and out of the

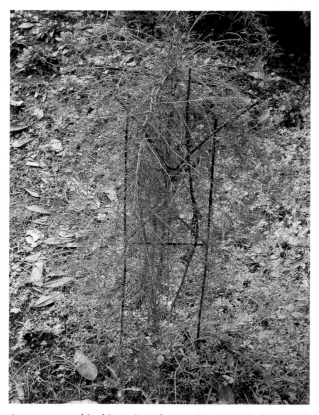

Asparagus cochinchinensis **at the Nanjing Botanical Garden.**

refrigerator should also aid germination. Since they are a longer term nursery item don't forget to protect them from drying out and from cats. Cat visits can be a problem—use upside-down black nursery flats to cover boxes; this aids in moisture retention as well. The seed coat is hard; in my experience, nicking the seed coat hasn't made a difference in germination rates or timeliness, nor has exposure to light or cleaning the seed coat (or not). Once the seedlings finally do come up, though, they hold well in nursery pots and make excellent permanent containerized plants.

Garden and Polyculture Planting

Asparagus cochinchinensis is ornamental and makes a welcome addition to the garden or hedgerow. Provide a light trellis for support and to keep the branches off the ground. Plant in full sun (or part shade in hot locations) on 1½-foot spacing. Soil should be well drained and fertile; water needs are average. If seed collecting is on the agenda keep in mind that members of the *Asparagus* genus outcross and must be separated from each other as far as a bee can fly in a day (roughly two miles). One way to prevent cross-pollination is to cover this plant with a cage covered with fine screening to exclude insects. Every other day, switch the cage to cover your other *Asparagus* varieties.

Suitable Companions

Acanthopanax gracilistylus, wǔ jiā pí
Achyranthes bidentata, Oxknee, huái niú xī
Agastache rugosa, Korean Mint, tǔ huò xiāng
Allium macrostemon, xiè bái
Allium tuberosum, Garlic Chives, jiǔ cài zǐ
Anemarrhena asphodeloides, zhī mǔ
Angelica dahurica, baí zhǐ
Angelica pubescens, dú huó
Aster tataricus, Tartar Aster, zǐ wǎn
Belamcanda chinensis, Blackberry Lily, shè gān
Bupleurum chinense, Hare's Ear, chái hú
Carthamus tinctorius, Safflower, hóng huā
Chrysanthemum morifolium, Mum, jú huā
Cornus officinalis, Dogwood, shān zhū yú

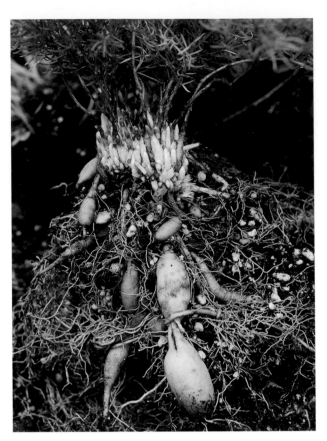

Sample of *Asparagus cochinchinensis* whole plant, four years old. Photo by Nina Zhito.

Crataegus pinnatifida, Chinese Hawthorn, shān zhā
Cyathula officinalis, Hookweed, chuān niú xī
Dianthus superbus, Fringed Pink, qú mài
Eucommia ulmoides, Hardy Rubber Tree, dù zhòng
Ginkgo biloba, Ginkgo, bái guǒ
Ligusticum jeholense, Chinese Lovage, gǎo běn
Lilium lancifolium, *L. brownii*, Lily, bǎi hé
Paeonia lactiflora, Chinese Peony, bái/chì sháo
Paeonia suffruticosa, Tree Peony, mǔ dān pí
Platycodon grandiflorus, Balloon Flower, jié gěng
Prunella vulgaris, Heal All, xià kū cǎo
Rehmannia glutinosa, Chinese Foxglove, dì huáng
Rheum palmatum, Chinese Rhubarb, dà huáng
Salvia miltiorrhiza, *S. przewalskii*, *S. bowleyana*,
    Red Sage, dān shēn
Saposhnikovia divaricata, Siler, fáng fēng
Scrophularia buergeriana, Figwort, běi xuán shēn
Scutellaria baicalensis, Baikal Skullcap, huáng qín
Scutellaria barbata, Barbat Skullcap, bàn zhī lián

Field Production

Transplant in spring on two-foot centers after at least one year of growth. Choose a site with fertile, friable, well-drained soil in full sun. Where summers are hot, part shade is appropriate. The crown shoots increase annually; provide support with stakes or a light six-foot trellis. Cultivate shallowly to keep weed competition low.

Pests and Diseases

None.

Harvest and Yield

Asparagus cochinchinensis is grown a minimum of four years before the swollen roots are harvested. It's traditional to harvest while the plants are winter dormant; the best "quality consists of thick, full, compact, yellowish white, and translucent roots."[51] It is possible to utilize the plants as an ongoing source by digging near the base of the plant and cutting off only a few of the shallow roots at any one time. Roots are easy to wash; cut them lengthwise to dry. Average yield is 0.4 pounds per plant. Ratio of fresh to dry is 3:1.

Medicinal Uses of Tiān mén dōng

Tiān mén dōng is the root of *Asparagus cochinchinensis*. Sweet, bitter, and very cold, it moistens dryness, nourishes the yin of the kidney and lung, and clears lung heat. It is used to address chronic and acute lung conditions that are characterized by dryness—such as dry cough, or cough with scant, sticky phlegm and dry mouth—as well as for clearing externally contracted dryness that has injured the lungs. It is also used to address issues such as constipation with dry stool, "wasting and thirsting disorders" (which often correspond to diabetes), and chronic and acute sore throat. In modern China its strong cooling and clearing properties have made it an important herb in addressing conditions such as tuberculosis, diabetes mellitus, and certain types of cancers.

Tiān mén dōng is usually used in combination with other herbs. Common methods of administration include decoctions, powders, concentrated granules, alcohol extracts, tablets, and pills. It is in formulas such as Tian Wang Bu Xin Dan (Emperor of Heaven's Special Pill to Tonify the Heart) and Zhen Gan Xi Feng Tang (Sedate the Liver and Extinguish Wind Decoction).

Aster tataricus (L.f.)
Common Name: Tartar Aster
Pinyin: Zǐ wǎn
Family: Asteraceae
Part Used: Root

Plant Description
A beautiful and potentially invasive plant in regions with summer rains, *Aster tataricus* gains traction by underground runners. This herbaceous perennial grows five to seven feet tall. Its stem-clasping, toothed leaves may be pointed or spatulate to obovate; up to two feet long; and covered with fine scratchy bristles. The leaf petiole is prominent and lighter green than the leaves. Early fall flowers are daisylike and typical of the Asteraceae family. Many flowers adorn the corymb or loose floral arrangement; each flower is 1½ inches wide. Disk flowers are yellow and the ray flower petals light purple. Roots are shaped like downward-facing stubby fingers. Native to southern Siberia, *Aster tataricus* has been available in the horticultural trade for many years. USDA hardiness zones 2–9 or 10.

Propagation
Sow seeds close to the surface of the soil in spring or fall. Spring-sown seed requires no additional heat and germinates in two to three weeks. If you plan to incorporate tartar aster into your nursery line, keep in mind that they need frequent dividing or potting up.

Garden and Polyculture Planting
Durable and pretty is a winning combination in this gardenworthy perennial. Overall the form is upright; flowers are bold and showy, attracting bees and other nectar-feeding insects. Plant tartar aster in full sun to part shade in average, well-drained soils. A good site might be a midborder planting—and it is vigorous enough to hold its own in a hedgerow. Plants are not considered drought tolerant and will not expand beyond the irrigated zone.

Suitable Companions
Acanthopanax gracilistylus, wǔ jiā pí
Achyranthes bidentata, Oxknee, huái niú xī
Agastache rugosa, Korean Mint, tǔ huò xiāng
Allium macrostemon, xiè bái
Allium tuberosum, Garlic Chives, jiǔ cài zǐ
Anemarrhena asphodeloides, zhī mǔ
Angelica dahurica, bái zhǐ
Angelica pubescens, dú huó
Belamcanda chinensis, Blackberry Lily, shè gān
Bupleurum chinense, Hare's Ear, chái hú
Carthamus tinctorius, Safflower, hóng huā
Celosia argentea, qīng xiāng zǐ
Celosia cristata, Cockscomb, jī guān huā
Chrysanthemum morifolium, Mum, jú huā
Clerodendrum trichotomum, Glorybower, chòu
    wú tóng
Cornus officinalis, Dogwood, shān zhū yú
Crataegus pinnatifida, Chinese Hawthorn, shān zhā
Cyathula officinalis, Hookweed, chuān niú xī
Dianthus superbus, Fringed Pink, qú mài

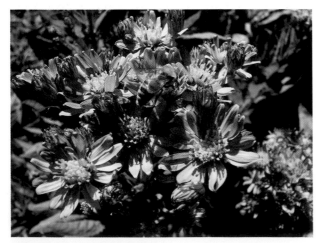
Aster tataricus with honeybee.

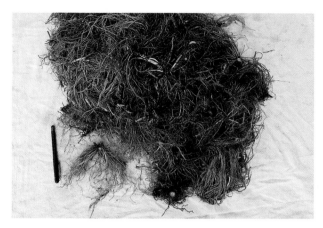

Freshly harvested *Aster tataricus* roots.

Eriobotrya japonica, Loquat, pí pá yè
Eucommia ulmoides, Hardy Rubber Tree, dù zhòng
Ginkgo biloba, Ginkgo, bái guǒ
Ligusticum jeholense, Chinese Lovage, gǎo běn
Ligustrum lucidum, Chinese Privet, nǔ zhēn zǐ
Lilium lancifolium, L. brownii, Lily, bǎi hé
Lonicera japonica, Honeysuckle, jīn yín huā
Lycium chinense, Chinese Wolfberry, gǒu qǐ zǐ/dì gǔ pí
Magnolia denudata, xīn yí huā
Momordica charantia, Bitter Melon, kǔ guā
Ocimum sanctum, Sacred Basil, Tulsi
Plantago asiatica, Plantain, chē qián zǐ
Platycodon grandiflorus, Balloon Flower, jié gěng
Prunella vulgaris, Heal All, xià kū cǎo
Rehmannia glutinosa, Chinese Foxglove, dì huáng
Rheum palmatum, Chinese Rhubarb, dà huáng
Salvia miltiorrhiza, S. przewalskii, S. bowleyana, Red Sage, dān shēn
Saposhnikovia divaricata, Siler, fáng fēng
Schizonepeta tenuifolia, Japanese Catnip, jīng jiè
Scrophularia buergeriana, Figwort, běi xuán shēn
Scutellaria baicalensis, Baikal Skullcap, huáng qín
Scutellaria barbata, Barbat Skullcap, bàn zhī lián
Sophora flavescens, kǔ shēn
Trichosanthes kirilowii, Chinese Cucumber, guā lóu/tiān huā fěn

Field Production

Transplant tartar aster on one-foot spacing. Use drip irrigation rather than overhead to keep powdery mildew

Medicinal Uses of Zǐ wǎn

Zǐ wǎn is the root of *Aster tataricus*. Bitter, sweet, and slightly warm, it has the preliminary application of addressing coughs and dissolving phlegm. It is an important ingredient in many formulas that treat coughing due to a variety of causes (including cough due to exterior influences, interior imbalances, and empty or full conditions).

Zǐ wǎn is used individually and in combination with other herbs. Common methods of administration are decoctions, powders, concentrated granules, tablets, and pills. It is in formulas such as Zhi Sou San (Stop Cough Powder), Zi Wan Tang (*Aster* Decoction), and Bu Fei Tang (Tonify the Lungs Decoction).

away. Soils with average fertility are best (actively avoid rich soils). Staking is not necessary as stems are rigid and strong. This aster manages weed pressure well.

Pests and Diseases

Powdery mildew occasionally presents itself; to prevent it, plant in areas that have good air movement.

Harvest and Yield

Dig roots in the second or successive years in late fall or early spring when the plants are dormant; both the rhizomatous and finer red roots are used. Remove persistent foliage at the crown of the plant and wash. I find that cleaning the roots to rid them of clinging soil takes more time than it does to dig them! Drying is easy and uneventful. Good quality is said to "consist of long, purplish red, pliable, and tough roots."[52] Average yield for three-year-old plant is 0.8 pounds per plant. Ratio of fresh to dry is 6:1.

Astragalus membranaceus (Bge.)
Common Name: Milk Vetch
Pinyin: Huáng qí
Family: Fabaceae
Part Used: Root

Plant Description

This important long-term crop resembles other members of the pea family, growing three to five feet tall with somewhat sprawling stems. *Astragalus membranaceus* is a deciduous perennial with pinnately compound light green leaflets on oppositely arranged leaves. Blossoms form out of leaf axils and develop into racemes with pealike yellow flowers in the fall, maturing into papery one- to two-inch-long seedpods. Naturally occurring as far north as Mongolia,[53] *Astragalus membranaceus* can generally be considered hardy, doing well in USDA hardiness zones 4–10.

Propagation

Sow these small tan seeds, which look like the little legumes that they are, in spring or fall. Because they have a hard seed coat it is common practice to scarify by rubbing with sandpaper or nicking

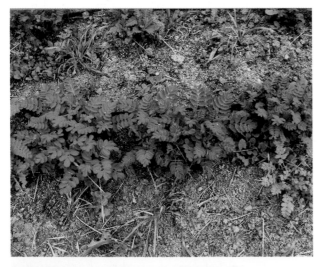

Spring emergence of three-year-old *Astragalus membranaceus*.

with a sharp knife or nail clippers. Soaking the seed overnight is another method to aid germination, as is using an inoculant indicated for vetches. At the Chinese Medicinal Herb Farm we have accomplished good germination without bothering to scarify the seeds; germination usually takes place in six to twenty days with bottom heat. In the nursery, twelve weeks from spring sowing to four-inch transplant or containerized sale is standard. Plants are drought tolerant in pots and field, and the nursery media should be extra well draining. Do not overwater; it is the most frequent reason for the loss of milk vetch.

Garden and Polyculture Planting

Because milk vetch needs very good drainage, it does not fit in well with herbs that need regular watering. Try placing it at the margins of areas where your sprinklers or soaker hoses reach. Space plants one to two feet apart in beds that are not well amended. Fertilizers and compost are not recommended. Milk vetch is such an important herb that its medicinal value may trump its lackluster ornamental value, but it does make an ideal rock garden plant.

Suitable Companions

Belamcanda chinensis, Blackberry Lily, shè gān
Carthamus tinctorius, Safflower, hóng huā
Ephedra sinica, Ephedra, má huáng/gēn
Lilium lancifolium, L. brownii, Lily, bǎi hé
Lycium chinense, Chinese Wolfberry, gǒu qǐ zǐ/dì gǔ pí
Withania somnifera, Ashwagandha
Ziziphus jujuba, Chinese Date, dà zǎo
Ziziphus jujuba var. *spinosa*, suān zǎo rén

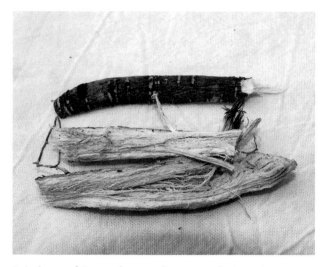

Dried root of *Astragalus membranaceus*, huáng qí.

Field Production

Grow drought-tolerant milk vetch in full sun and sandy soils that are very well drained (consider planting into raised beds if soil does not drain freely).

Plants in the Fabaceae family do not need much fertility, especially nitrogen; amendment inputs are low. Plant or sow one foot apart within the row and two feet between rows. Late spring direct seeding has worked well on our farm. Seed emergence is variable and takes place from two to four weeks. Transplants can be field planted at fourteen weeks.

Pests and Diseases

Gophers are a major pest—trap to control them. Thankfully, milk vetch is very capable of resprouting if the crown is left intact, but it makes for a smaller, less desirable finished crop. Deer occasionally browse the flowering tops.

Harvest and Yield

Roots are dug while dormant in the fall or spring after four years' growth. The long whitish-yellow tap roots grow three to four feet straight down, making

Medicinal Uses of Huáng qí

Huáng qí is the root of *Astragalus membranaceus*. It is one of the primary tonic herbs and is one of the most well-known Chinese medicinal herbs throughout the world. Sweet and slightly warm, it tonifies the spleen and lung qi, raises the yang, consolidates the exterior, and regulates the fluid circulation. It has less widely used, but important, functions of relieving pain and numbness, generating flesh, promoting the discharge of pus, and addressing wasting and thirsting (Xiao Ke) syndrome. It is used to address issues such as frequent colds and flu, fatigue, spontaneous sweating, loose stools, edema, and for postpartum recovery. It is probably best known for its use in enhancing energy and supporting the immune system. In modern China its ability to strengthen the body and enhance the healthy functioning of the immune system has made it an important herb in cancer treatment.

Huáng qí is often used in dietary therapy as a nourishing food in soups, congees (porridges), and other dishes. Huáng qí is also utilized in formulas combined with other herbs, as well as being used as a single herb. Along with being used in TCM, it is now commonly used in Western herbal medicine, naturopathic medicine, and as a dietary supplement. Common methods of administration include soups and congees, decoctions, powders, concentrated granules, alcohol extracts, tablets, capsules, and pills. Huáng qí is in many major tonic formulas, such as Yu Ping Feng San (Jade Windscreen Powder), Bu Zhong Yi Qi Tang (Tonify the Center and Benefit Qi Decoction), Dang Gui Bu Xue Tang (*Angelica* Tonify the Blood Decoction), and Gui Pi Tang (Restore the Spleen Decoction).

Pests and Diseases

Gophers occasionally eat the roots.

Harvest and Yield

This unusual but important medicinal needs to grow for one to two years before harvesting. The rhizome has a white interior and a tan to very dark thin-skinned root bark. Lift the rhizome in late fall or in winter (the latter is considered to be better).[56] Washing is easy, as the rhizomes are neither large nor convoluted; be sure to remove the small roots from the rhizome. In following Chinese tradition, slice roots from the crown downward. We've found that the average harvest weight per plant was the same for one- and two-year-old plants. The yield is low—0.2 pounds per plant fresh. Ratio of fresh to dry herb is 3:1.

Notes

- Rare in cultivation in North America, Chinese thistle daisy is one of two important Chinese botanical herbs in the genus *Atractylodes*, the other being *A. lancea* (cāng zhú).

- Despite its common name of Chinese thistle daisy, this herb is not known to be invasive.

Medicinal Uses of Bái zhú

Bái zhú is the rhizome of *Atractylodes macrocephala*. Sweet, bitter, and warm, bái zhú tonifies the qi, strengthens the spleen and stomach, transforms dampness, and stabilizes the exterior. It is also traditionally used to stabilize pregnancy and treat a restless fetus. It is one of the most commonly used Chinese medicinal herbs to address fatigue and weakness, poor digestive assimilation with loose stools or diarrhea, and lack of appetite. It is also used for edema, chronic phlegm, frequent colds and flu, and spontaneous perspiration. In certain cases it is used in combination with other herbs to help prevent miscarriage.

Bái zhú is usually used combined with other herbs in both traditional and modern formulas. Common methods of administration include decoctions, powders, concentrated granules, alcohol extracts, tablets, and pills. It is an important qi tonic that is included in most traditional formulas that treat qi deficiency, particularly spleen qi deficiency. This includes such fundamental formulas as Si Junzi Tang (Four Gentlemen Decoction) and all of its variations, Yu Ping Feng San (Jade Windscreen Powder), Shen Ling Bai Zhu San (Ginseng, *Poria*, and *Atractylodes* Powder) and Gui Pi Tang (Restore the Spleen Decoction).

Bacopa monnieri ([L.] Pennell)
Common Name: Brahmi
Hindi: Brahmi
Family: Scrophulariaceae
Part Used: Herb

Plant Description

Bacopa monnieri is an important herb in the ancient Indian Ayurvedic medical tradition; it is a semi-aquatic, creeping, tender perennial groundcover up to four inches tall. Succulent leaves and stems form a thick, spreading mat; stems root at leaf nodes. The leaves are a half inch or more long and a half inch wide, bright green, and spoon-shaped. Five-petaled flowers are white to pale blue and measure a half inch across. Originally from the tropics, the distribution of *Bacopa monnieri* is in wet muddy areas of India and South China, as well as in the southeast United States from Virginia to Florida and west into Texas.[57] *Bacopa monnieri* can withstand temperatures down to roughly twenty degrees. USDA hardiness zones 9–11.

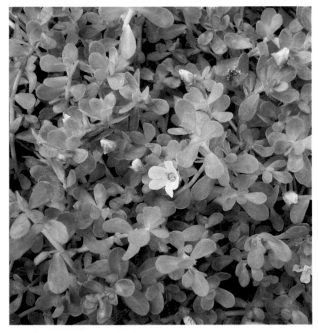

Bacopa monnieri, Brahmi.

Propagation

The easiest way to propagate brahmi is by division. Cuttings are also easy; clip stems with leaves and put the cut end in water to encourage roots to form. If you choose to sow seeds, do so in spring, using bottom heat for successful germination. With warm temperatures, plants grow quickly and do not keep long in small nursery pots; however, larger pots are suitable for permanent plantings. Keep well watered in part shade.

Garden and Polyculture Planting

Do you have a wet area in need of an herbal groundcover? Try brahmi. Plant it at the front of the border in partial shade or on muddy or watery edges of self-contained ponds. Or you can create an artificial bog out of a horse trough or an old bathtub and plant brahmi and several of its suitable companions there. Fertilizer needs are low, but brahmi is decidedly not drought tolerant. Where winters are cold, grow brahmi as a summer annual; before cold weather sets in, plant plugs back into the greenhouse or a more protected area to winter over.

Suitable Companions

Alisma plantago-aquatica subsp. *orientale*, Water Plantain, zé xiè
Centella asiatica, Gotu Kola, jī xuě cǎo
Coix lacryma-jobi, Job's Tears, yì yǐ rén
Eclipta prostrata, Eclipta, mò hàn lián
Gynostemma pentaphyllum, Sweet Tea Vine, jiǎo gǔ lán
Houttuynia cordata, yú xīng cǎo
Mentha haplocalyx, Field Mint, bò hé
Ophiopogon japonicus, Lilyturf, mài mén dōng
Plantago asiatica, Plantain, chē qián zǐ

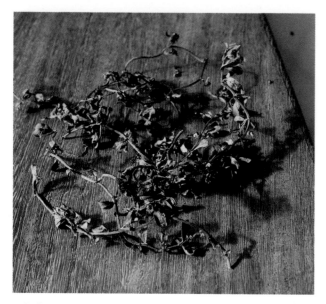

Dried *Bacopa monnieri*, Brahmi. Photo by Nina Zhito.

Field Production

Where winters are frost free, grow brahmi as a perennial crop. In temperate climates treat this tender perennial as an annual. Plant in partial shade on one-foot spacing, in soils of average fertility, and provide ample water to maintain a moist to wet environment. Ideally brahmi would love to grow in the tropics; a warm location yields vigorous growth. Row crop covers can add humidity and provide shade in an open field.

Pests and Diseases

None.

Harvest and Yield

Plan for three harvests a season (or possibly more in warm regions). The first harvest is in summer; subsequent harvests develop at four-week intervals. Cut stems and foliage with flowers, leaving a thick mat of rooted stems to produce future harvests or to divide to create next season's planting stock. Rinse the harvest and, if not selling fresh, put to dry. Drying is easy and quick, just a day or two. Expect yields of

Medicinal Uses of Brahmi

Brahmi is the whole herb (leaf, stem, and sometimes root) of *Bacopa monnieri*. It is an important Ayurvedic herb that, according to Ayurvedic classification, is light and cold, astringent, bitter, and sweet post-digestive and pacifies the kapha and pitta humor. It is particularly well known for its effect on enhancing mental functioning and is used to address issues such as difficulty focusing, poor memory, anxiety, skin disorders, anemia, certain types of cough, fever, asthma, and bronchitis and to promote lactation.

Brahmi is used as a single herb and in combination with other herbs. Common methods of administration include powders, oils, juices, decoctions, ghee mixtures, concentrated granules, tablets, and pills.

three-quarters of a pound per plant for the season. Fresh to dry ratio is 6:1.

Notes

- The common name brahmi is sometimes erroneously applied to *Centella asiatica*, and thus you need to be careful when buying plants to ensure that you are really getting *Bacopa* and not *Centella*—which is also readily available.
- *Bacopa monnieri* is known to bioaccumulate mercury, lead, chromium, and cadmium[58]—a reminder that it is always good to know your herb source.

Belamcanda chinensis ([L.] DC.)
Common Name: Blackberry Lily
Pinyin: Shè gān
Family: Iridaceae
Part Used: Rhizome

Plant Description

The sword-shaped, light green leaves grow up to three feet tall and are one inch wide in a fan-shaped arrangement. The plant is perennial and herbaceous and throws deep orange flowers on rigid branching stems rising to four feet tall. Each six-petaled flower is two to three inches across and maroon spotted; they bloom in late summer, and each one lasts just a day. Afterward the fertilized ovaries develop into green inflated seedpods that open up as they dry to reveal black shiny seeds that resemble blackberries.

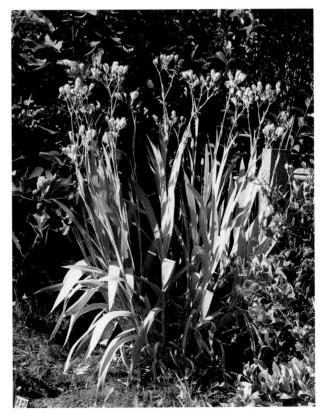

Fall seed pods on three-foot-tall *Belamcanda chinensis* plants.

Belamcanda chinensis is very hardy and has a wide native geographic distribution across the length and breadth of China, except the arid west.[59] USDA hardiness zones 4–9 or 10.

Propagation

Propagate blackberry lily by rhizome division or by seed. If dividing rhizomes, as you would with an iris, expose the cut ends to air for a day or so before replanting. This lessens the opportunity for pathogen entry into the wounded area. Seeds are easy—spring germination takes two to three weeks with the aid of heat. For saleable nursery stock, sow seeds the year before any projected sale. Blackberry lily holds very well in pots.

Garden and Polyculture Planting

Blackberry lily is durable; this is one survivor of gardens with challenging conditions. It is very ornamental, but happily it is not invasive; it spreads its basal clump of rhizomes in a neat and orderly manner. For the best display, plant in groups in the midborder of the garden or hedgerow in full sun to part shade. Plants topple over when growing in too much shade, but they still flower.

Suitable Companions

Achyranthes bidentata, Oxknee, huái niú xī
Agastache rugosa, Korean Mint, tǔ huò xiāng
Allium macrostemon, xiè bái
Allium tuberosum, Garlic Chives, jiǔ cài zǐ
Angelica dahurica, bái zhǐ
Angelica pubescens, dú huó
Aster tataricus, Tartar Aster, zǐ wǎn
Bupleurum chinense, Hare's Ear, chái hú

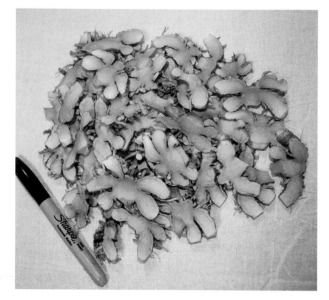

Freshly harvested *Belamcanda chinensis* rhizomes.

Carthamus tinctorius, Safflower, hóng huā
Celosia argentea, qīng xiāng zǐ
Celosia cristata, Cockscomb, jī guān huā
Chrysanthemum morifolium, Mum, jú huā
Clerodendrum trichotomum, Glorybower, chòu wú tóng
Cornus officinalis, Dogwood, shān zhū yú
Crataegus pinnatifida, Chinese Hawthorn, shān zhā
Cyathula officinalis, Hookweed, chuān niú xī
Dianthus superbus, Fringed Pink, qú mài
Dolichos lablab, Hyacinth Bean, bái biǎn dòu
Ginkgo biloba, Ginkgo, bái guǒ
Lilium lancifolium, *L. brownii*, Lily, bǎi hé
Lonicera japonica, Honeysuckle, jīn yín huā
Mentha haplocalyx, Field Mint, bò hé
Momordica charantia, Bitter Melon, kǔ guā
Ocimum sanctum, Sacred Basil, Tulsi
Paeonia lactiflora, Chinese Peony, bái/chì sháo
Paeonia suffruticosa, Tree Peony, mǔ dān pí
Platycodon grandiflorus, Balloon Flower, jié gěng
Prunella vulgaris, Heal All, xià kū cǎo
Rehmannia glutinosa, Chinese Foxglove, dì huáng
Rheum palmatum, Chinese Rhubarb, dà huáng
Salvia miltiorrhiza, *S. przewalskii*, *S. bowleyana*, Red Sage, dān shēn
Saposhnikovia divaricata, Siler, fáng fēng
Schizonepeta tenuifolia, Japanese Catnip, jīng jiè

Medicinal Uses of Shè gān

Shè gān is the rhizome of *Belamcanda chinensis*. Bitter and cold, shè gān clears heat and eliminates toxins, dispels phlegm, and stops wheezing that is due to an accumulation of heat or phlegm in the lungs. It is used to address cough and wheezing with profuse mucus and to address acute sore throats.

It is usually used in combination with other herbs. Common methods of administration include decoctions, powders, concentrated granules, tablets, and pills. It is in formulas such as Yin Qiao Ma Bo San (*Lonicera*, *Forsythia*, and Puff Ball Powder) and Gan Lu Xiao Du Dan (Sweet Dew Eliminate Toxin Special Pill).

Scutellaria baicalensis, Baikal Skullcap, huáng qín
Sophora flavescens, kǔ shēn
Trichosanthes kirilowii, Chinese Cucumber, guā lóu/tiān huā fěn

Field Production
Transplant blackberry lily on one-foot spacing in full sun. Loamy soils that are moderately fertile and freely draining are preferred; regular even watering is suitable, so irrigate in times of summer drought. Organic mulch or compost is helpful to conserve nutrients for this long-term crop.

Pests and Diseases
Gophers occasionally eat the rhizomes.

Harvest and Yield
Harvest rhizomes from plantings that are at least three years old, in late fall or early spring when the plant is dormant. Rhizomes grow horizontally and shallowly; dig, remove foliage at the crown and rootlets

from the rhizomes, and wash. Cut the rootlets close to the rhizome, as the rhizomes will be easier to wash and rootlets are not traditionally included in shè gān; a power washer makes for quick work. Before drying, slice the rhizomes in eighth-inch slabs. The best quality is said to be "dry, full rhizomes with a hard texture and without fibrous roots or soil on the surface. The cross section is yellow."[60] Yield for four-year root is 1½ pounds per plant fresh. Ratio of fresh to dry is 3:1.

Bupleurum chinense (DC.)

Alternate Species: *Bupleurum scorzonerifolium* (Willd.)
Common Name: Hare's Ear
Pinyin: Chái hú
Family: Apiaceae
Part Used: Root

Plant Description

Bupleurum chinense is a hardy, herbaceous perennial that has simple linear basal foliage. Plants grow to about three feet tall with stiff-stemmed, terminal-blooming yellow flower umbels that are rather airy in form. *Bupleurum chinense* is native to sunny exposures at elevation ranges from 300 feet to almost 9,000 feet, and from the central coast of China inland as far north as Mongolia, growing on grasslands, sunny slopes, and roadsides.[61] USDA hardiness zones 2–10.

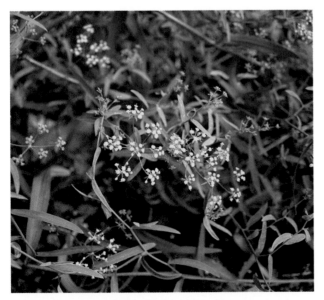

Yellow-flowered umbels of *Bupleurum chinense*.

Propagation

Fresh seed is a must for timely germination. If the seed is freshly dried a spring sowing can yield 100 percent germination rates. If not sown when freshly dried the seeds enter a protective dormant phase and may emerge in successive years, as long as they are kept watered. You can sow in the late fall and leave them outside to weather; the seed will naturally stratify—but again, do not allow them to dry out. Depending on how cold the weather is, they will emerge in four weeks to several months. It's also possible to cold/damp stratify the seeds in the refrigerator. Start checking them at four weeks for signs of germination. Hare's ear is a multicycle germinator: the seed requires a sequence of different (usually cold and warm) treatments to allow the seed to sprout. It responds well to containerization, though that may put a kink in the taproot.

Garden and Polyculture Planting

Hare's ear will thrive in a sunny ornamental herb garden if planted in an area that has good drainage and isn't watered much. However, I have seen it growing in areas that have very good drainage where overhead irrigation has been successful. Planted singly it is unimpressive, but a grouping of ten or more plants produces attractive masses of tiny flowers in fall.

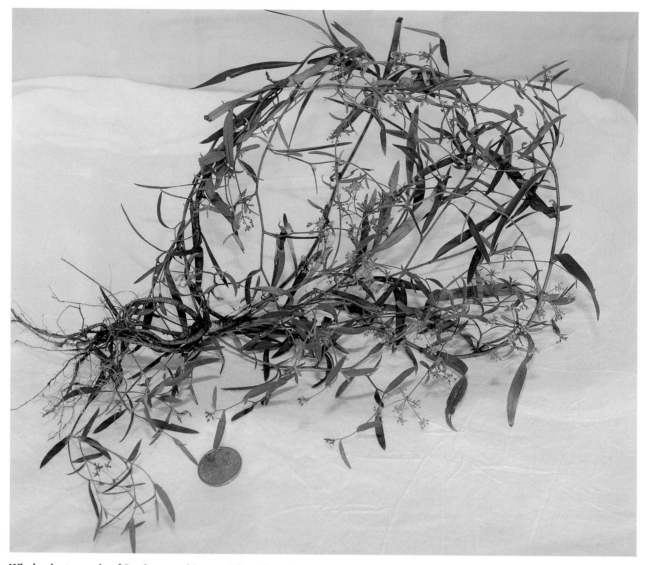

Whole plant sample of *Bupleurum chinense*. Photo by Nina Zhito.

Suitable Companions

Aster tataricus, Tartar Aster, zǐ wǎn

Astragalus membranaceus, Milk Vetch, huáng qí

Atractylodes macrocephala, Chinese Thistle Daisy, bái zhú

Belamcanda chinensis, Blackberry Lily, shè gān

Carthamus tinctorius, Safflower, hóng huā

Ephedra sinica, Ephedra, má huáng/gēn

Ligusticum jeholense, Chinese Lovage, gǎo běn

Lilium lancifolium, L. brownii, Lily, bǎi hé

Salvia miltiorrhiza, S. przewalskii, S. bowleyana, Red Sage, dān shēn

Withania somnifera, Ashwagandha

Field Production

This herb is sometimes challenging to cultivate; I continue to trial it under differing conditions with the modest goal of in-ground plant survival (at four or more years) and reasonable root size. Try planting it in full sun to part shade in somewhat dry, sandy, well-drained soils. Transplant out nursery starts when they are at least six months old, on one-foot centers; water needs are low. In terms of seed collection, the flowers are long lasting; flower and seed maturation take place at the same time—in summer through fall. It takes four or more months for the seed to mature (when they finally turn from green

Medicinal Uses of Chái hú

Chái hú is the root of *Bupleurum chinense*. It is one of the most commonly used Chinese medicinal herbs, particularly in North America and Japan. Bitter, acrid, and cool, it harmonizes the interior and exterior and spreads the liver qi to address liver qi stagnation. It has the important secondary function of lifting the yang qi in order to guide the effects of an herbal formula to the upper body. In combination with other medicinal herbs it addresses a wide range of health issues, including conditions such as premenstrual syndrome and other gynecological disorders, digestive disorders, allergies, malarial-type conditions, lingering cold and flu symptoms, chronic stress, and emotional tension.

Chái hú is occasionally used culinarily and primarily in combination with other herbs. Common methods of administration include decoctions, powders, concentrated granules, alcohol extracts, tablets, and pills. It is the chief herb in many important formulas such as Xiao Yao San (Free and Easy Wanderer) and its derivatives, all of the Chai Hu Tang (Bupleurum Decoction) variations (Xiao Chai Hu Tang, Chai Hu Jia Long Mu Tang, etc.), Si Ni San (Frigid Extremities Powder), and Chai Hu Shu Gan Tang (Bupleurum Spread the Liver Decoction).

to a dry brown-tan color). Be watchful, and collect seed as soon as it matures; otherwise the seed heads will shatter.

Pests and Diseases
Wet soils result in root rot.

Harvest and Yield
Harvest the oftentimes branched, tan, woody taproot in the fall or the spring after at least three seasons.

Expect roots to be small, about six inches long and three-quarters of an inch thick: "The best quality has a dry and long main root, no sprouts, and only a few hairy lateral roots."[62] Yield for three-year-old plants is a quarter-pound per plant fresh. Ratio of fresh to dry herb is 2:1.

Notes
Hare's ear is a very important Chinese botanical that needs to be brought into domestic production.

Carthamus tinctorius (L.)
Common Name: Safflower
Pinyin: Hóng huā
Family: Asteraceae
Part Used: Florets

Plant Description

Carthamus tinctorius is a quick-growing annual in warm weather. It is grown for its flowers, for oil pressed from the seed, or as a dye plant. The plants are stiff, many-branched, and grow 3–5 feet tall and 1½ feet wide. One-inch terminal flower heads with spiny or smooth rounded bracts are constricted below the yellow or orange inflorescences. Several varieties are available. The yellow spiny variety has random spines along the leaf edge while the more orange variety has soft rounded lobes on the leaf margins. Both develop into the orange-red characteristic of hóng huā. The leaves are variations on ovate, obovate, and lanceolate—all with nontoothed margins. *Carthamus tinctorius* is native to Eurasia and is reported to have escaped cultivation in Arizona, California, Colorado, Idaho, Illinois, Iowa, Kansas, Massachusetts, Montana, Nebraska, New Mexico, North Dakota, Ohio, Oregon, Utah, Washington, Europe, and British Colombia.[63]

Propagation

To grow this warm-season, undemanding annual, sow the quarter-inch white-faceted seed in late spring either directly in the garden or in the nursery/indoors with the aid of heat. A quick grower, it does not hold in pots very long. Under ideal conditions germination takes four to six days, and it takes four weeks from sowing to either four-inch transplant or sale. Media of average quality is sufficient.

Garden and Polyculture Planting

Ornamental as it is useful and easygoing in the garden, safflower is also bold enough for the hedgerow. Plant one to two feet apart in the middle of the border, and mass for the best ornamental value. Safflower prefers full sun and average, friable, well-drained soils—but it is drought tolerant and can manage in dry or moist, heavy soils.

Suitable Companions

Achyranthes bidentata, Oxknee, huái niú xī
Agastache rugosa, Korean Mint, tǔ huò xiāng
Allium macrostemon, xiè bái
Allium tuberosum, Garlic Chives, jiǔ cài zǐ
Angelica dahurica, bái zhǐ
Angelica pubescens, dú huó
Aster tataricus, Tartar Aster, zǐ wǎn
Astragalus membranaceus, Milk Vetch, huáng qí
Atractylodes macrocephala, Chinese Thistle Daisy, bái zhú
Belamcanda chinensis, Blackberry Lily, shè gān

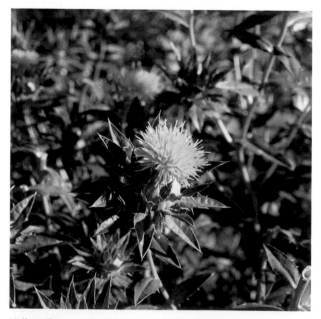
Yellow-flowered spiny variety of *Carthamus tinctorius*.

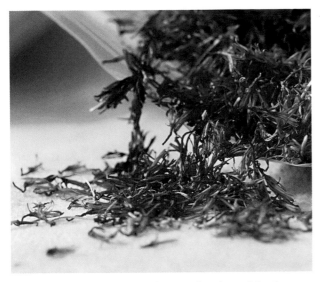

Dried flowers of the orange-flowered variety of *Carthamus tinctorius*. Photo by Nina Zhito.

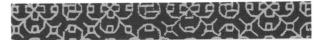

Safflower Recipes

The dried, bright orange flower petals add a yellow color to dishes, much like saffron, but with only a slight flavor. Use them sprinkled at the last minute over salads to add a dash of color or add one tablespoon to a pot of cooking rice to turn the grains a soft golden yellow.

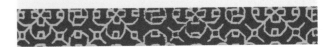

Bupleurum chinense, Hare's Ear, chái hú

Celosia argentea, qīng xiāng zǐ

Celosia cristata, Cockscomb, jī guān huā

Chrysanthemum morifolium, Mum, jú huā

Clerodendrum trichotomum, Glorybower, chòu wú tóng

Cyathula officinalis, Hookweed, chuān niú xī

Dianthus superbus, Fringed Pink, qú mài

Dioscorea opposita, Chinese Yam, shān yào

Dolichos lablab, Hyacinth Bean, bái biǎn dòu

Eucommia ulmoides, Hardy Rubber Tree, dù zhòng

Ginkgo biloba, Ginkgo, bái guǒ

Ligusticum jeholense, Chinese Lovage, gǎo běn

Lilium lancifolium, *L. brownii*, Lily, bǎi hé

Lonicera japonica, Honeysuckle, jīn yín huā

Lycium chinense, Chinese Wolfberry, gǒu qǐ zǐ/dì gǔ pí

Magnolia denudata, xīn yí huā

Ocimum sanctum, Sacred Basil, Tulsi

Platycodon grandiflorus, Balloon Flower, jié gěng

Prunella vulgaris, Heal All, xià kū cǎo

Rehmannia glutinosa, Chinese Foxglove, dì huáng

Rheum palmatum, Chinese Rhubarb, dà huáng

Salvia miltiorrhiza, *S. przewalskii*, *S. bowleyana*, Red Sage, dān shēn

Saposhnikovia divaricata, Siler, fáng fēng

Schizonepeta tenuifolia, Japanese Catnip, jīng jiè

Scutellaria baicalensis, Baikal Skullcap, huáng qín

Sophora flavescens, kǔ shēn

Trichosanthes kirilowii, Chinese Cucumber, guā lóu/tiān huā fěn

Withania somnifera, Ashwagandha

Ziziphus jujuba, Chinese Date, dà zǎo

Ziziphus jujuba var. *spinosa*, suān zǎo rén

Field Production

Direct sow or transplant after threat of frost with two feet apart in and between rows in full sun into warm soil of average fertility. Safflower is commonly dry-farmed in California's Central Valley, but it's a good idea to provide irrigation in times of extended drought. Direct-sown plants tend not to lodge, or fall over in high wind; they grow taller than transplanted material as well. Plant copiously to garner enough herb; this is a low production herb in terms of pounds per plant. Each plant will produce many flowers, especially if continuously harvested. To collect seed in short-season or cool-summer regions, plant as early as the soil warms—or start in the greenhouse and transplant, to leave ample time for seed maturation. If it rains toward the end of the ripening phase, the crop may be lost to seed germination in the head while still on the plant.

Medicinal Uses of Hóng huā

Hóng huā is the flower of *Carthamus tinctorius*. Acrid and warm, it activates the blood circulation, dispels blood stagnation, and opens the channels. Hóng huā is one of the most commonly used herbs to address blood stagnation in TCM, particularly for gynecological issues. It is used for a wide range of gynecological disorders, including menstrual cramping, lack of a menstrual cycle (amenorrhea), and excessive clotting during menstruation. It is also used to address issues such as abdominal accumulations and pain, joint pain, chest pain, and for certain types of dermatological disorders.

Hóng huā is primarily used in combination with other herbs. Common methods of administration include decoctions, powders, concentrated granules, alcohol extracts, and in tablets and pill form. It is a significant ingredient in important formulas such as Tao Hong Si Wu Tang (Four Substance Decoction with *Persica* and *Carthamus*).

To some degree, the functions of hóng huā are dosage dependent. In small doses it regulates and nourishes the blood, while in larger doses it breaks blood stagnation (strongly moves the blood circulation).

Pests and Diseases
None.

Harvest and Yield
To avoid potential bee stings collect florets while in full bloom early in the day—when it is still cool, just after the night's dew has dried. To maximize harvest potential, collect every third day. Work fast with two hands at once and the florets will fill the harvest container quickly. Drying is quick and easy—one day maximum. When dry the smell should be rich and fragrant. Traditionally the florets alone are used in Chinese medicine as hóng huā. It is more cost effective, for growers and buyers, to deal in whole flower heads instead of the florets. When the Chinese Medicinal Herb Farm explored this concept with practitioners, many were open to the idea. If you want to harvest whole flower heads, be sure to do two things: clear this form with your contract buyers before you harvest, and harvest the whole heads just as they are coming into bloom (if harvest is delayed the seeds develop and become a more pronounced portion of the herb). Some buyers will certainly prefer the florets over the whole head. Average weight for whole head harvest is a quarter-pound per plant per season fresh. Also try knocking the florets off by rolling around a bag full of dry flower heads. On any given harvest day the floret-only harvested weight is 0.02 pounds per plant (though a seasonal output was not measured, plants produce many flowers per plant throughout the season). Ratio of fresh to dry weight for whole head is 3:1; floret ratio is 5:1.

Notes
Even though safflower has escaped cultivation it is not aggressively invasive.

Celosia argentea (L.)
Common Name: None
Pinyin: Qīng xiāng zǐ
Family: Amaranthaceae
Part Used: Seed

Plant Description

Celosia argentea is a popular warm-season annual, used worldwide mainly as a garden ornamental, but also for its medicinal qualities in China and India. Decidedly upright plants have a branching central green-to-reddish fleshy stem; the species or unselected form grows twelve to sixteen inches tall and five inches wide. The two-inch linear-lanceolate leaves are sparse and small compared to the showy flowers, and they will drop off in response to moisture stress. The flower spikes are cone shaped and in unselected specimens are in light whitish tones with pink tips (while introduced cultivars are bright shades of red, orange, and pink). The seed, the source of qīng xiāng zǐ, is a small, shiny, jet-black, flattened sphere. *Celosia argentea* often reseeds and can become weedy. A truly cosmopolitan annual, especially in the tropics, it grows the width and breadth of China and in many other southeast Asian countries as well.[64]

Propagation

Seeds sown into warm soils in situ (in the garden) or in the greenhouse in spring germinate in two weeks. For best results barely cover the seed and keep evenly moist. *Celosia argentea* makes an attractive potted plant.

Garden and Polyculture Planting

Sow or transplant in the front of the garden, border, or hedgerow. Even with its small stature it is durable and will survive even if left neglected in a hedgerow. Plant en masse for the best ornamental effect. Irrigate regularly as moist but well drained soils are preferred. *Celosia argentea* is very ornamental and makes an excellent cut flower.

Suitable Companions

Acanthopanax gracilistylus, wǔ jiā pí
Achyranthes bidentata, Oxknee, huái niú xī
Agastache rugosa, Korean Mint, tǔ huò xiāng
Albizia julibrissin, Mimosa, hé huān pí/huā
Allium macrostemon, xiè bái
Allium tuberosum, Garlic Chives, jiǔ cài zǐ
Andrographis paniculata, Kalmegh, chuān xīn lián
Anemarrhena asphodeloides, zhī mǔ
Angelica dahurica, bái zhǐ
Angelica pubescens, dú huó
Aster tataricus, Tartar Aster, zǐ wǎn
Belamcanda chinensis, Blackberry Lily, shè gān

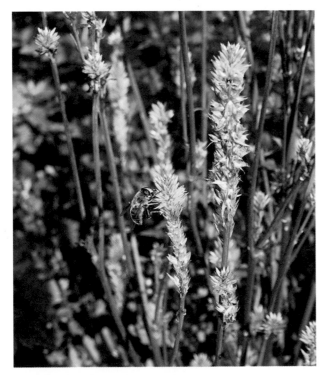

Honeybee visiting *Celosia argentea*.

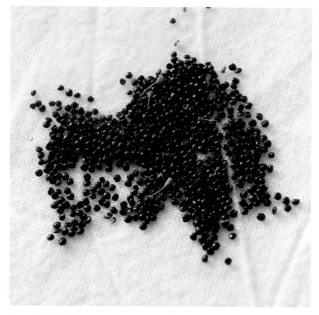

Seed of *Celosia argentea*, qīng xiāng zǐ.

Bupleurum chinense, Hare's Ear, chái hú
Carthamus tinctorius, Safflower, hóng huā
Celosia cristata, Cockscomb, jī guān huā
Chrysanthemum morifolium, Mum, jú huā
Clerodendrum trichotomum, Glorybower, chòu
  wú tóng
Cornus officinalis, Dogwood, shān zhū yú
Crataegus pinnatifida, Chinese Hawthorn, shān zhā
Cyathula officinalis, Hookweed, chuān niú xī
Dianthus superbus, Fringed Pink, qú mài
Dolichos lablab, Hyacinth Bean, bái biǎn dòu
Eriobotrya japonica, Loquat, pí pá yè
Eucommia ulmoides, Hardy Rubber Tree, dù zhòng
Forsythia suspensa, lián qiào
Ginkgo biloba, Ginkgo, bái guǒ
Houttuynia cordata, yú xīng cǎo
Ligustrum lucidum, Chinese Privet, nǔ zhēn zǐ
Lilium lancifolium, *L. brownii*, Lily, bǎi hé
Lonicera japonica, Honeysuckle, jīn yín huā
Magnolia denudata, xīn yí huā
Mentha haplocalyx, Field Mint, bò hé
Momordica charantia, Bitter Melon, kǔ guā
Ocimum sanctum, Sacred Basil, Tulsi
Plantago asiatica, Plantain, chē qián zǐ
Platycodon grandiflorus, Balloon Flower, jié gěng
Prunella vulgaris, Heal All, xià kū cǎo

Medicinal Uses of Qīng xiāng zǐ

Qīng xiāng zǐ is the seed of *Celosia argentea*. It is a less commonly used herb within TCM.

Bitter and cool, it clears liver fire—primarily when it is affecting the eyes or head or elevating the blood pressure. It is used to address eye disorders such as eye redness, swelling, and pain—as well as to address headaches and hypertension, often when these conditions are also present with the above-mentioned eye symptoms.

Qīng xiāng zǐ is usually used in combination with other herbs. Common methods of administration of formulas that contain it include decoctions, concentrated powders, tablets, and pills.

Rehmannia glutinosa, Chinese Foxglove, dì huáng
Rheum palmatum, Chinese Rhubarb, dà huáng
Salvia miltiorrhiza, *S. przewalskii*, *S. bowleyana*,
  Red Sage, dān shēn
Saposhnikovia divaricata, Siler, fáng fēng
Schizonepeta tenuifolia, Japanese Catnip, jīng jiè
Scrophularia buergeriana, Figwort, běi xuán shēn
Scutellaria baicalensis, Baikal Skullcap, huáng qín
Sophora flavescens, kǔ shēn
Trichosanthes kirilowii, Chinese Cucumber, guā
  lóu/tiān huā fěn

Field Production

Plant in a sunny, warm site with rich, moist soils on one-foot spacing. Drip irrigation is preferable to overhead sprinklers, to keep the flower heads dry. Impact sprinklers may knock the mature seed from the flowers. Seed ripens sequentially from the bottom on up the floral spike.

Pests and Diseases
None.

Harvest and Yield
Collect seed in the fall when it is ripe and readily falls from the floral bracts. The benchmark for quality is "full, black, and glossy seeds. Foreign matter should not exceed two percent of the content."[65] "Foreign matter" is most likely, in this case, chaff; winnow this off. Yield is 0.01 pounds per plant. Fresh and dry weights are almost equal.

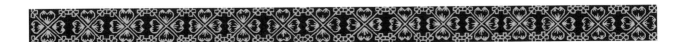

Celosia cristata (L.)
Botanical Synonym: *Celosia argentea* var. *cristata* ([L.] Kuntze)
Common Name: Cockscomb
Pinyin: Jī guān huā
Family: Amaranthaceae
Part Used: Flower

Plant Description
Celosia cristata is a much-recognized ornamental garden annual with a most curious-looking "cockscomb" flower. These convoluted, crested flowers come in shades of red, yellow, white, pink, and purple and bloom at the terminus of many branching upright stems. White or red colored flowers are traditionally used in Chinese medicine.[66] Leaves are elliptical and simple margined (no lobes or dentations) and sessile (directly attached to the stems). *Celosia cristata* blooms in late summer to fall. It was introduced long ago in the United States and now grows in disturbed areas in Alabama, Connecticut, Kansas, Louisiana, Missouri, North Carolina, Ohio, Rhode Island, Tennessee, Vermont, and Washington D.C.[67] *Celosia cristata* does best in warm regions.

Propagation
Sow directly or in the nursery/indoors into a warm medium; germination occurs in two weeks. For best results barely cover the seed and keep it evenly moist. In cool summer regions, sow in the nursery or indoors in early spring and transplant out to ensure that the crop has enough time to mature. It should be ten weeks from sowing to transplanting or sellable four-inch stock. Good in containers.

Garden and Polyculture Planting
Sow or transplant in the front or middle section of the garden or border in a warm location. Plant en

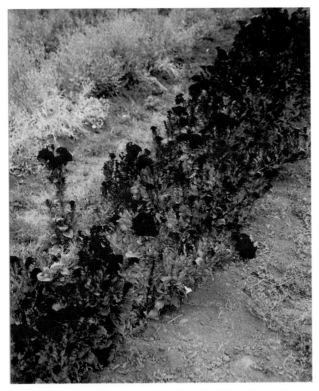

Field-grown *Celosia cristata*, ready to harvest.

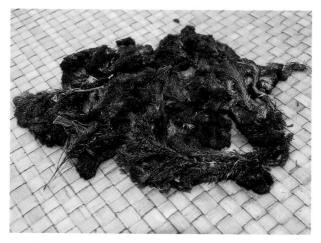

Dry flower heads of *Celosia cristata*, jī guān huā.

masse for best ornamental effects. Cockscomb prefers moist but well drained soils; be prepared to water it regularly. Cockscomb is very ornamental and makes an excellent cut flower.

Suitable Companions

Acanthopanax gracilistylus, wǔ jiā pí
Achyranthes bidentata, Oxknee, huái niú xī
Agastache rugosa, Korean Mint, tǔ huò xiāng
Albizia julibrissin, Mimosa, hé huān pí/huā
Allium macrostemon, xiè bái
Allium tuberosum, Garlic Chives, jiǔ cài zǐ
Andrographis paniculata, Kalmegh, chuān xīn lián
Anemarrhena asphodeloides, zhī mǔ
Angelica dahurica, bái zhǐ
Angelica pubescens, dú huó
Aster tataricus, Tartar Aster, zǐ wǎn
Belamcanda chinensis, Blackberry Lily, shè gān
Bupleurum chinense, Hare's Ear, chái hú
Carthamus tinctorius, Safflower, hóng huā
Celosia argentea, qīng xiāng zǐ
Chrysanthemum morifolium, Mum, jú huā
Clerodendrum trichotomum, Glorybower, chòu
    wú tóng
Cornus officinalis, Dogwood, shān zhū yú
Crataegus pinnatifida, Chinese Hawthorn, shān zhā
Cyathula officinalis, Hookweed, chuān niú xī
Dianthus superbus, Fringed Pink, qú mài
Dolichos lablab, Hyacinth Bean, bái biǎn dòu
Eriobotrya japonica, Loquat, pí pá yè

Medicinal Uses of Jī guān huā

Jī guān huā is the flower of *Celosia cristata*. It is a less commonly used herb within TCM.

Sweet and cool, it clears heat, cools the blood, stops bleeding, consolidates jing (essences), and stops diarrhea. Jī guān huā is used to stop bleeding, including intestinal and hemorrhoidal bleeding, abnormal uterine bleeding, and nosebleeds. It is also used to treat diarrhea and dysentery.

Jī guān huā is used by itself and in combination with other herbs. Common methods of administration include decoctions, powders, alcohol extracts, and concentrated granules.

Jī guān huā is charred to enhance its ability to stop bleeding and otherwise used unprocessed (dried).

Eucommia ulmoides, Hardy Rubber Tree, dù zhòng
Forsythia suspensa, lián qiào
Ginkgo biloba, Ginkgo, bái guǒ
Houttuynia cordata, yú xīng cǎo
Ligustrum lucidum, Chinese Privet, nǚ zhēn zǐ
Lilium lancifolium, *L. brownii*, Lily, bǎi hé
Lonicera japonica, Honeysuckle, jīn yín huā
Magnolia denudata, xīn yí huā
Mentha haplocalyx, Field Mint, bò hé
Momordica charantia, Bitter Melon, kǔ guā
Ocimum sanctum, Sacred Basil, Tulsi
Plantago asiatica, Plantain, chē qián zǐ
Platycodon grandiflorus, Balloon Flower, jié gěng
Prunella vulgaris, Heal All, xià kū cǎo
Rehmannia glutinosa, Chinese Foxglove, dì huáng
Rheum palmatum, Chinese Rhubarb, dà huáng
Salvia miltiorrhiza, *S. przewalskii*, *S. bowleyana*,
    Red Sage, dān shēn
Saposhnikovia divaricata, Siler, fáng fēng

Schizonepeta tenuifolia, Japanese Catnip, jīng jiè
Scrophularia buergeriana, Figwort, běi xuán shēn
Scutellaria baicalensis, Baikal Skullcap, huáng qín
Sophora flavescens, kǔ shēn
Trichosanthes kirilowii, Chinese Cucumber, guā lóu/tiān huā fěn

Field Production

Plant on one-foot spacing in full sun in a warm exposure. Preferred soils are somewhat fertile, moist, and well draining. I recommend drip irrigation, because overhead irrigation coupled with wind may blow down the top-heavy flowers.

Pests and Diseases

None.

Harvest and Yield

Harvest when the flowers are in full bloom at the end of the summer or in fall. Drying is easy and should be uneventful; when dry the flowers should retain their color. Yield is a quarter-pound per plant fresh. Ratio of fresh to dry is high at 8:1.

Notes

There are many introductions of this cultivar; stick with the most basic version you can find (the species). Many seed vendors offer this plant, but I prefer to obtain seed from herb seed sellers, because I trust that such seed was grown to retain the essential traits that contribute to the plant's medicinal effect and not selected for other traits such as flower color.

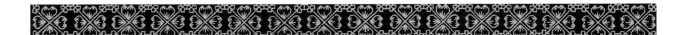

Centella asiatica ([L.] Urb.)

Botanical Synonym: *Hydrocotyle asiatica* (L.)
Common Name: Gotu Kola
Pinyin: Jī xuě cǎo
Family: Apiaceae
Part Used: Herb

Plant Description

The Indian Ayurvedic medical system brought us this popular and important herb. In very moist areas, *Centella asiatica* forms a thick spreading mat growing to one foot tall. There are a few forms; the larger one has a scalloped-edged, circular, three-inch, lightly pubescent leaf with a seven- to eight-inch petiole. The smaller cultivar has nearly heart shaped leaves that are totally fuzz-free and grow only to two inches wide. Both landraces are tender perennials. Insignificant white flowers produce seeds inside a rounded fruit a third of an inch wide. *Centella asiatica* is endemic to shady wet places in southern China and throughout many Asian tropical and subtropical countries.[68] USDA hardiness zones 7–11.

Propagation

Seed germination is difficult and slow; I surface sow thickly in spring in warm soil in a nursery flat, keep well watered, and expect low germination rates as sprouting occurs at four weeks. Vegetative propagation by plant division is easier and most of the time I divide plants—at any time of year. If the weather is not warm, use a heating mat to encourage new growth. It's convenient to divide plants when harvesting the crop, as described below.

Garden and Polyculture Planting

Gotu kola prefers warm, humid, and wet shady areas; plant on one-foot spacing. It is a low-growing groundcover, so place it near the front of the border or let it run around in a hedgerow planting, but keep

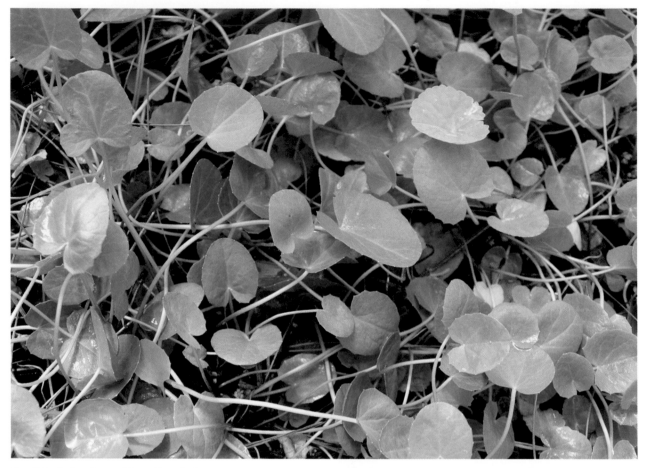

Small-leafed variety of *Centella asiatica*.

in mind that it is not drought tolerant. Alternately construct a bog from old bathtubs or other vessels. In cold winter regions, grow outdoors for the summer and plug into a deep flat in the nursery for the winter.

Suitable Companions

Alisma plantago-aquatica subsp. *orientale*, Water Plantain, zé xiè

Bacopa monnieri, Brahmi

Coix lacryma-jobi, Job's Tears, yì yǐ rén

Gynostemma pentaphyllum, Sweet Tea Vine, jiǎo gǔ lán

Houttuynia cordata, yú xīng cǎo

Pinellia ternata, bàn xià

Plantago asiatica, Plantain, chē qián zǐ

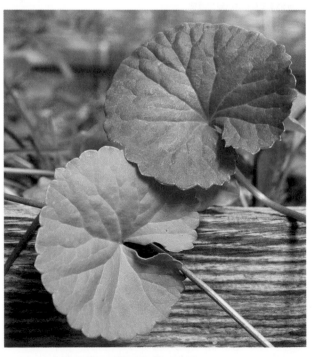

Large-leafed variety of *Centella asiatica*.

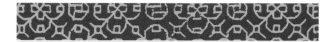

Gotu Kola Recipes

Add the young leaves to salads. Use the dried leaves to make a tonic tea, steeping longer if you prefer a stronger taste to this mild tea.

For tea: Pour boiling water over the dried or fresh whole leaves and steep for two to three minutes. Use a larger quantity of fresh leaves to dried, but adjust the amounts to your taste. Chilled, the tea makes a refreshing hot weather drink.

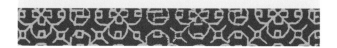

Field Production
Transplant onto one-foot spacing in a shady, fertile, well-irrigated location. Shade cloth or a row crop cover works well and also increases desired humidity.

Pests and Diseases
Gotu kola is subject to disfiguring virus attacks. When I have had this problem I have uprooted the plants and sent the virus to the landfill.

Harvest and Yield
Most often buyers want leaf only, but on rare occasions the whole herb with roots is requested. Whole plants weigh more, but washing is more laborious. Collect early in the day, wash immediately with ample water at washing stations or in large tubs with multiple rinses, and quickly refrigerate or dry as soon as possible. Harvesting is quick, but washing takes more time; especially for whole plants that have soil clinging to roots. If need be, hold harvested crop, of either leaf or whole plant, in large vessels of cold water. However, this should be done for only a few short hours or the crop will suffer. As with many water-loving crops, drying is quick and easy. Harvest the first season crop(s), then plug plantlets (crowns

Medicinal Uses of Jī xuě cǎo

Jī xuě cǎo, gotu kola, or Mandukaparni in Sanskrit, is the whole plant or herb of *Centella asiatica*. According to Ayurvedic principles, it is bitter and astringent, sweet post-digestive, and cold and alleviates all three doshas. It is used to enhance mental functioning, promote longevity, and address a wide range of issues—such as poor memory, senile dementia, skin problems, cough, asthma, hoarse voice, fever, insufficient lactation, seizures, agitation, and insomnia.

Gotu kola is usually used in combination with other herbs. It is used topically and internally. Common methods of administration include juices, infusions, cold infusions, pastes, and oils. It is sometimes eaten in salads. It is usually not decocted or cooked because its active ingredients are heat sensitive.

Gotu kola is sometimes also called brahmi, which is also the common name for *Bacopa monnieri*. Although there are similarities in application the two herbs are quite distinct.

with roots) into big deep flats in the greenhouse. The plantlets should establish well and will become the following year's crop. For leaf-only sales, at least two harvests a year are possible. Yield for fresh leaf and petiole is 0.5 pounds per plant per season; for whole fresh plant it is 1.2 pounds per plant. Ratio of fresh to dry is 6:1 for leaf and petiole.

Notes
This popular herb is not commonly used in Chinese herbal medicine; the market is Ayurvedic and Western.

Chrysanthemum morifolium (Ramat.)

Common Name: Mum
Pinyin: Jú huā
Family: Asteraceae
Part Used: Flower

Plant Description

This esteemed ornamental is a popular garden perennial and florist plant and has been cultivated in China for thousands of years. *Chrysanthemum morifolium* is thought to be a hybrid, with unknown origins.[69] In China varieties were selected for many years for slightly differing medicinal uses. However, nowadays most cultivated varieties offered for sale in the nursery trade are for ornamental rather than medicinal purposes. Choose species, medicinal cultivars, or unselected varieties found in the medicinal herb trade, or obtain cuttings or divisions grown for medicinal purposes. A bushy, herbaceous sub-shrub growing three to five feet tall, *Chrysanthemum morifolium* has leaves that are often deeply lobed and toothed. Flowers are variable in color, form, and size, from whites to yellows and reds, and singles to complete doubles. *Chrysanthemum morifolium* blooms in the fall and is generally considered hardy in USDA hardiness zones 6–9.

Propagation

Cuttings or plant division in spring or fall are good ways to propagate mums. Seed is not traditionally used to increase stock.

Garden and Polyculture Planting

Ornamental as a specimen or as a mass planting, mums are very useful in the garden and mixed plantings. Plant them one foot apart in the full sun in at least somewhat well-drained soils, or in a raised bed where soils are heavy or poorly drained. Vigorous and heavy yielding, just a few plants can provide enough flowers for a small household. As the flowers mature their weight pulls them earthward. Stake the plants to keep them looking attractive, for ease of harvest, and to ensure herb quality. Mums attract a host of beneficial insects, and they make excellent container specimens.

Suitable Companions

Acanthopanax gracilistylus, wǔ jiā pí
Achyranthes bidentata, Oxknee, huái niú xī
Agastache rugosa, Korean Mint, tǔ huò xiāng
Allium tuberosum, Garlic Chives, jiǔ cài zǐ
Anemarrhena asphodeloides, zhī mǔ

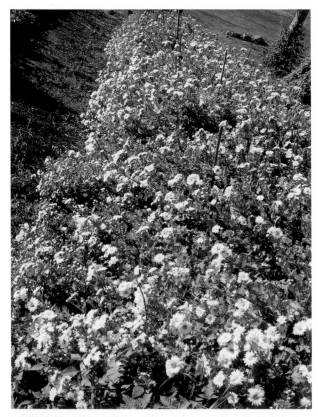

Medicinal cultivar of *Chrysanthemum morifolium* 'Bo Ju Hua.'

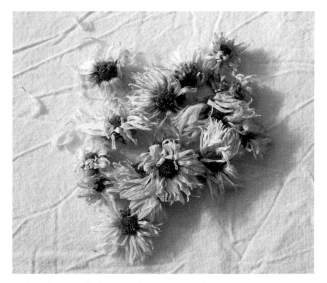

Dried flower of *Chrysanthemum morifolium* 'Bo Ju Hua.'

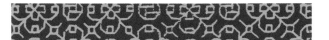

Mum Recipes

The lovely small flowers with yellow centers and white petals float beguilingly in a cup filled with boiling water. Add them with other tea ingredients if you wish. It is customary in Chinese cooking to add them to clear chicken broth.

For tea: Pour boiling water over dried or fresh whole flowers and steep for three to five minutes. Use a larger quantity of fresh flowers to dried, but adjust the amounts to your taste. Chilled, the tea makes a refreshing hot weather drink.

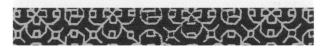

Angelica dahurica, bái zhǐ
Angelica pubescens, dú huó
Aster tataricus, Tartar Aster, zǐ wǎn
Belamcanda chinensis, Blackberry Lily, shè gān
Carthamus tinctorius, Safflower, hóng huā
Celosia argentea, qīng xiāng zǐ
Celosia cristata, Cockscomb, jī guān huā
Cornus officinalis, Dogwood, shān zhū yú
Crataegus pinnatifida, Chinese Hawthorn, shān zhā
Cyathula officinalis, Hookweed, chuān niú xī
Dianthus superbus, Fringed Pink, qú mài
Dolichos lablab, Hyacinth Bean, bái biǎn dòu
Eucommia ulmoides, Hardy Rubber Tree, dù zhòng
Forsythia suspensa, lián qiào
Ginkgo biloba, Ginkgo, bái guǒ
Ligusticum jeholense, Chinese Lovage, gǎo běn
Ligustrum lucidum, Chinese Privet, nǔ zhēn zǐ
Lilium lancifolium, L. brownii, Lily, bǎi hé
Lonicera japonica, Honeysuckle, jīn yín huā
Lycium chinense, Chinese Wolfberry, gǒu qǐ zǐ/dì gǔ pí
Magnolia denudata, xīn yí huā
Mentha haplocalyx, Field Mint, bò hé
Momordica charantia, Bitter Melon, kǔ guā
Ocimum sanctum, Sacred Basil, Tulsi
Platycodon grandiflorus, Balloon Flower, jié gěng
Prunella vulgaris, Heal All, xià kū cǎo
Rehmannia glutinosa, Chinese Foxglove, dì huáng

Rheum palmatum, Chinese Rhubarb, dà huáng
Salvia miltiorrhiza, S. przewalskii, S. bowleyana, Red Sage, dān shēn
Saposhnikovia divaricata, Siler, fáng fēng
Schizonepeta tenuifolia, Japanese Catnip, jīng jiè
Scutellaria baicalensis, Baikal Skullcap, huáng qín
Trichosanthes kirilowii, Chinese Cucumber, guā lóu/tiān huā fěn

Field Production

Mums enjoy a well-drained soil in a sunny position and have average water requirements. Use adequate fertilizer to maintain floral size and production. Plant on one-foot centers in early spring and they will fill in and achieve full production by fall. I use floral netting to prevent lodging and to make harvesting easier; it is available through farm suppliers. I use three horizontal layers, which I hold in place with fence T-posts. The flowers will grow though the grid support and be at a convenient height to pick. Use drip irrigation if possible because sprinkler irrigation weighs down the flower stems and can lead to fungal disease problems. I have found that the plants are vigorous enough that cutting back the terminal growth in late spring will not necessarily keep plants low enough to eliminate the task of staking, but it encourages branching—creating more terminal flowers. To reinvigorate your stock, divide it and replant in fresh ground every two or three seasons.

Pests and Diseases

I always freeze the dry flowers for twenty-four hours before placing the herb into storage to prevent insect infestation.

Harvest and Yield

Harvest flowers in the late fall when in full bloom. Pick the fully open young flowers just after the dew has dried, and hopefully before bee activity is high. The flowers produce internal heat when harvested, so cool them down or spread them out and put to dry as soon as feasible (or risk creating expensive compost). This herb requires repeat harvesting every few days to optimize quality and quantity. Dry the flowers with plenty of air movement and low heat; dehydrators produce the best quality. Do not overdry, as flower petals will fall off and produce an inferior product. Test for dryness by pressing the center of the flower with a thumbnail. Rain adversely affects the floral crop quality, so protect if possible with a temporary shelter (the ideal cultivation area would be a region with low rainfall in the autumn). The best quality dry material should smell and look like the fresh material (except a bit more yellow than white in color); flowers should be unbroken, fully open, and free from leaf matter. Yield varies from 0.75 to 1 pound per plant per season fresh, depending on what variety you grow and how often you repeat harvest. Yields for certain medicinal cultivars (named for their all-white flowers) are: 'Bo Ju Hua' (0.7 pounds per plant fresh), 'Gong Ju Hua' (0.4 pounds per plant fresh), and 'Chu

Medicinal Uses of Jú huā

Jú huā is the flower of *Chrysanthemum morifolium*. Acrid, sweet, bitter, and cool, jú huā dispels wind heat, clears liver heat, benefits the eyes, calms liver yang, and clears heat and toxins. It is used to address many kinds of headaches, fever, sore throat, red and painful eyes, blurred vision, near-sightedness, visual disturbances, dizziness, and hypertension. It is also used topically as a paste to address various dermatological conditions.

Jú huā is often used as a hot or cold steeped beverage. Medicinally it is used by itself as well or in combination with other herbs. Common methods of administration include decoctions, concentrated powders, tablets, pills, and infusions in hot water. Jú huā is used in formulas such as Sang Ju Yin (Mulberry and Chrysanthemum Decoction), Qi Ju Di Huang Wan (*Lycium*, Chrysanthemum, and *Rehmannia* Pills), and Ming Mu Di Huang Wan (Brighten the Eyes *Rehmannia* Pills).

Ju Hua' (0.4 pounds per plant fresh). Ratio of fresh to dry herb is 5:1.

Notes

'Bo Ju Hua' is a single-petaled flower that is the sweetest of the three mentioned above, and more sought after as a beverage tea. 'Gong Ju Hua' is a three-quarter-inch button mum and is the most bitter; 'Chu Ju Hua' is a fully double, rather tasty, but less vigorous cultivar.

Clerodendrum trichotomum (Thunb.)

Common Name: Glorybower
Pinyin: Chòu wú tóng
Family: Verbenaceae
Part Used: Leaf

Plant Description

Clerodendrum trichotomum is a deciduous multi-stemmed shrub or small single-trunked tree growing up to twenty feet tall with a spreading crown ten to fifteen feet wide. Softly pubescent, dark green, five-inch-long leaves are triangularly ovate with prominent venation, gentle serrate margins, and pointed tips. When leaves are damaged they emit an unpleasant odor. The showy fall-blooming flowers, on the other hand, emit a sweet, jasmine-scented fragrance. Emerging from hot pink calyxes are white, five-lobed, tubular flowers sporting long stamens. Fertilized flowers mature into round blue fruits surrounded by (still) hot pink calyxes in the fall. *Clerodendrum trichotomum* grows in the wild throughout China except in the arid west and far north and grows in India, Korea, and other southeast Asian countries as well.[70] Recommended USDA hardiness zones are 7–10 (it also grows in parts of USDA hardiness zones 5 and 6 but may freeze back to the ground in the winter).

Propagation

Planting seeds, taking cuttings, and rooting stem suckers work well for increasing stock. Sow seed in early spring in deep flats and leave outside to receive a short chilling period. Cuttings taken in summer from soft wood root easily and quickly in a warm bright area or heated greenhouse bench. Grow plants for a season before transplanting or selling (repot them to the next size up during that time to maintain vigorous growth). Fertilize twice a season if keeping containerized for more than a year.

Garden and Polyculture Planting

Glorybower is suitable for the back of the border or, better yet, the hedgerow or medicinal orchard; plants have a somewhat coarse appearance and show best at a short distance. They're not unattractive, just note: location, location, location! Later fall brings no coloration—glorybower blows it all on its summer and early fall display.

Suitable Companions

Acanthopanax gracilistylus, wǔ jiā pí
Achyranthes bidentata, Oxknee, huái niú xī
Agastache rugosa, Korean Mint, tǔ huò xiāng
Albizia julibrissin, Mimosa, hé huān pí/huā
Allium macrostemon, xiè bái
Allium tuberosum, Garlic Chives, jiǔ cài zǐ
Andrographis paniculata, Kalmegh, chuān xīn lián
Anemarrhena asphodeloides, zhī mǔ
Angelica dahurica, bái zhǐ
Angelica pubescens, dú huó

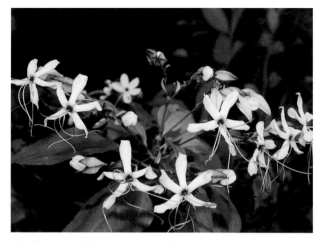

The flowers of *Clerodendrum trichotomum* are sweetly fragrant.

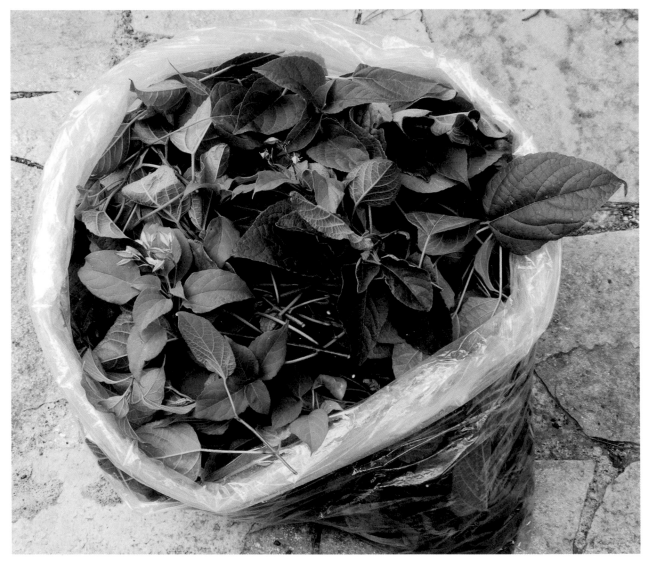

Fresh harvested *Clerodendrum trichotomum* leaves and stems.

Aster tataricus, Tartar Aster, zǐ wǎn

Atractylodes macrocephala, Chinese Thistle Daisy, bái zhú

Belamcanda chinensis, Blackberry Lily, shè gān

Bupleurum chinense, Hare's Ear, chái hú

Carthamus tinctorius, Safflower, hóng huā

Celosia argentea, qīng xiāng zǐ

Celosia cristata, Cockscomb, jī guān huā

Chrysanthemum morifolium, Mum, jú huā

Codonopsis pilosula, Poor Man's Ginseng, dǎng shēn

Cornus officinalis, Dogwood, shān zhū yú

Crataegus pinnatifida, Chinese Hawthorn, shān zhā

Cyathula officinalis, Hookweed, chuān niú xī

Dianthus superbus, Fringed Pink, qú mài

Dolichos lablab, Hyacinth Bean, bái biǎn dòu

Eriobotrya japonica, Loquat, pí pá yè

Eucommia ulmoides, Hardy Rubber Tree, dù zhòng

Forsythia suspensa, lián qiào

Ginkgo biloba, Ginkgo, bái guǒ

Ligusticum jeholense, Chinese Lovage, gǎo běn

Ligustrum lucidum, Chinese Privet, nǚ zhēn zǐ

Lilium lancifolium, *L. brownii*, Lily, bǎi hé

Lonicera japonica, Honeysuckle, jīn yín huā

Lycium chinense, Chinese Wolfberry, gǒu qǐ zǐ/dì gǔ pí

Medicinal Uses of Chòu wú tóng

Chòu wú tóng is the leaf of *Clerodendrum trichotomum*. Acrid, bitter, and cool, it dispels wind damp, addresses bi (painful obstruction) syndrome, lowers blood pressure, and (topically) is used to treat eczema and skin disorders characterized by itching and redness. It is used to treat musculoskeletal pain (particularly when characterized by heat and inflammation), numbness of the limbs, and paralysis. Its use in modern China has been expanded to include lowering high blood pressure.

Chòu wú tóng is used by itself and in combination with other herbs. Common methods of administration include decoctions, concentrated granules, as a wash (topical), and in tablet or pill form.

Magnolia denudata, xīn yí huā
Mentha haplocalyx, Field Mint, bò hé
Momordica charantia, Bitter Melon, kǔ guā
Ocimum sanctum, Sacred Basil, Tulsi
Platycodon grandiflorus, Balloon Flower, jié gěng
Prunella vulgaris, Heal All, xià kū cǎo
Rehmannia glutinosa, Chinese Foxglove, dì huáng
Rheum palmatum, Chinese Rhubarb, dà huáng
Salvia miltiorrhiza, *S. przewalskii*, *S. bowleyana*, Red Sage, dān shēn
Saposhnikovia divaricata, Siler, fáng fēng
Schizonepeta tenuifolia, Japanese Catnip, jīng jiè
Scrophularia buergeriana, Figwort, běi xuán shēn
Scutellaria baicalensis, Baikal Skullcap, huáng qín
Sophora flavescens, kǔ shēn
Trichosanthes kirilowii, Chinese Cucumber, guā lóu/tiān huā fěn
Withania somnifera, Ashwagandha
Ziziphus jujuba, Chinese Date, dà zǎo
Ziziphus jujuba var. *spinosa*, suān zǎo rén

Field Production

Plant out nursery stock that is at least one year old on ten-foot spacing in full sun to part shade. Soil should be well drained, but otherwise the plants tolerate clay and sand equally. Plants naturally form multi-trunked habits, which are easier to harvest than the single-trunk growth pattern that one sometimes sees. Fertilizer needs are low. Unless you harvest heavily, mulching with compost provides a sufficiently slow nutrient release. Provide irrigation in periods of drought.

Pests and Diseases

Deer browse on foliage.

Harvest and Yield

Plants need to grow for two to three seasons before they are old enough to harvest. Pick leaves with a few inches of woody stem before the flowers bloom in midsummer. Remember to wash leaves a few days prior to rinse off dust and impurities. Drying is easy, and there's no need to separate leaf from stem. "Good quality consists of green leaves with a fresh, aromatic fragrance and a bitter, astringent taste."[71] Yield varies greatly with the age of the plants. Ratio of fresh to dry is 3:1.

Codonopsis pilosula ([Franch.] Nannf.)
Common Name: Poor Man's Ginseng
Pinyin: Dǎng shēn
Family: Campanulaceae
Part Used: Root

Plant Description

An important and attractive herbaceous vining perennial, *Codonopsis pilosula* grows to seven feet tall. The roots have a fleshy whitish interior and are tan-skinned. If accidentally bruised, the foliage smells of burning tires and the stems exude white latex when broken. It is weak stemmed, and the one-inch ovate to cordate leaves are covered with downy fuzz. Many solitary pretty one-inch bell-shaped pale whitish and lavender flowers are borne in the leaf axils. *Codonopsis pilosula* grows well into Mongolia in the north and in southern China as well; it is cold hardy to approximately minus thirty degrees.[72] USDA hardiness zones 2–11.

Propagation

Start seeds indoors in fall or early spring and water gently—the seeds are very small. Emergence takes place in eight to fourteen days with bottom heat; expect good germination rates. Seeds also germinate well in cool soil, but germination times will be in the range of three to four weeks. Plants size up enough for field planting in three months. Do not allow them to become pot-bound because the roots will retain the form of the container even when planted out. Given enough root room, though, the plants tolerate containerization well. They are floriferous and produce a large quantity of very small seed.

Garden and Polyculture Planting

This primary Chinese medicinal herb is attractive and easy to grow, making it a must for the ornamental garden or border. Planted on one-foot spacing, poor man's ginseng should have a light trellis or other plants to clamber on in full sun (in hot climates, in a lightly shaded site). Not considered drought tolerant, poor man's ginseng requires soils that are at least fairly well drained and of average to moderate fertility. Poor man's ginseng prefers a cool location; avoid siting in a hot western or southern exposure. It has a rather delicate habit; place it away from paths or other locations where it may be damaged. Though the flowers are quite pretty, they don't last well as cut flowers.

Suitable Companions

Agastache rugosa, Korean Mint, tǔ huò xiāng
Allium macrostemon, xiè bái
Allium tuberosum, Garlic Chives, jiǔ cài zǐ
Angelica dahurica, baí zhǐ
Aster tataricus, Tartar Aster, zǐ wǎn
Belamcanda chinensis, Blackberry Lily, shè gān
Chrysanthemum morifolium, Mum, jú huā

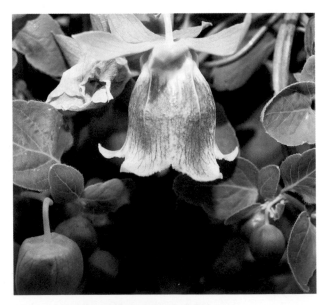

Codonopsis pilosula **has pretty bell flowers.**

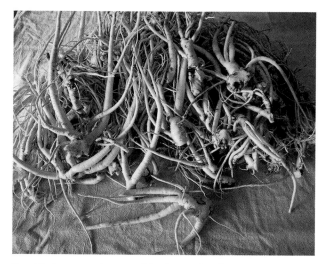

Freshly harvested roots of *Codonopsis pilosula*.

Cornus officinalis, Dogwood, shān zhū yú
Dianthus superbus, Fringed Pink, qú mài
Houttuynia cordata, yú xīng cǎo
Lilium lancifolium, *L. brownii*, Lily, bǎi hé
Ophiopogon japonicus, Lilyturf, mài mén dōng
Paeonia lactiflora, Chinese Peony, bái/chì sháo
Paeonia suffruticosa, Tree Peony, mǔ dān pí
Platycodon grandiflorus, Balloon Flower, jié gěng
Prunella vulgaris, Heal All, xià kū cǎo
Salvia miltiorrhiza, *S. przewalskii*, *S. bowleyana*,
  Red Sage, dān shēn
Saposhnikovia divaricata, Siler, fáng fēng
Scutellaria baicalensis, Baikal Skullcap, huáng qín
Scutellaria barbata, Barbat Skullcap, bàn zhī lián

Field Production

Poor man's ginseng enjoys a moist but well-drained, cool, sun-to-shady location in a soil that is deeply dug, somewhat sandy, and rich in organic matter. Transplant one foot on center, being careful not to break the fragile vine, into soil enriched with compost. Use a lightweight six-foot trellis; I have found bamboo poles simple as well as ideal for this twining grower. Weed to keep competition in check.

Pests and Diseases

If leaf stippling occurs, mites or thrips are most likely present. Do not use horticultural oils as they are phytotoxic to *Codonopsis pilosula*. Protect from slugs. Gophers are a major pest but deer seem repelled by the odoriferous nature of the foliage.

Medicinal Uses of Dǎng shēn

Dǎng shēn is the root of *Codonopsis pilosula*. Sweet and neutral, it tonifies the qi, strengthens the spleen and the lung, nourishes the blood, promotes the generation of fluids, and is sometimes used to restore the qi in the presence of pathogenic factors. It is gentle and effective, strengthening the qi without overstimulating the body. Because of this it is very commonly used to replace rén shēn or *Panax ginseng* in formulas. It is used to address issues such as fatigue, weakness, indigestion, diarrhea, coughing, wheezing, shortness of breath, weakness following illness, or chronic illness. It is now considered to have adaptogenic (helping the body to respond to stress) and immunostimulant functions and is used in Western herbal medicine as well as TCM. It is also edible and commonly used in dietary therapy.

Dǎng shēn is usually used in combination with other herbs. Common methods of administration include soups and other culinary dishes, decoctions, powders, concentrated granules, alcohol extracts, tablets, and pills. It is often used to replace ginseng in formulas such as Si Junzi Tang (Four Gentlemen Decoction), Ba Zhen Tang (Eight Treasures Decoction), Shen Ling Bai Zhu San (Ginseng, *Poria*, and *Atractylodes* Powder) and similar formulas.

Harvest and Yield

Dig roots in fall (when plants are dormant) after three years' growth. The pale yellow roots have no root bark, are flexible, and grow one foot deep, making for a relatively easy harvest by shovel or tractor-mounted potato digger. Washing is easy with a hose or power washer. If the herb is to be dried, cut the roots lengthwise to facilitate even drying. A traditional but labor intensive method (mentioned in *Herbal Emissaries*) that I have yet to try to dry the whole root involves putting a string through the crown and hanging until half dry. Then the roots are rubbed on a board (redistributing the moisture within), partially redried, and this is repeated three or four times before they are fully dry.[73] The best quality is said to be "thick, pliable roots with a thin outer bark, a 'chrysanthemum-heart' in cross section, and a sweet taste." The "chrysanthemum-heart" refers to a cross section of the root showing a radiating pattern.[74] Two-year-old root yields a half pound per plant fresh. Ratio of fresh to dry herb is 4:1.

Notes

Several other species of *Codonopsis* are serviceable as dǎng shēn.

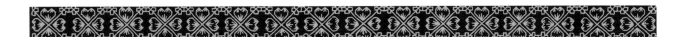

Coix lacryma-jobi (L.)
Common Name: Job's Tears
Pinyin: Yì yǐ rén
Family: Poaceae
Part Used: Seed

Plant Description

Coix lacryma-jobi is a water-loving temperate-region tender annual growing three to eight feet tall. The upright leaf blades are linear and green, as expected of a grass, and are two to four feet long by 1½ inches wide. Male or female flowering spikelets are separate but reside on the same plant. Females produce the quarter-inch green seed, which matures into a very hard fruit that ranges in color from lavender to pearl grey. Inside the hard testa is one flattened oval-shaped seed. Growing in streams and other wet areas throughout China (except the arid west) and many other Asian counties, it is cultivated in tropical and subtropical regions.[75] *Coix lacryma-jobi* self-seeds where it is sufficiently content and exhibits invasive qualities in warm areas. USDA hardiness zones 2–11.

Propagation

Sow seeds in spring, leaving the hard testa intact. In regions that have either short or cool summers, sow early with the aid of a heated greenhouse to make sure the crop has time to mature. Germination is two weeks, and it should be five weeks to sale date. Direct seeding in warm-summer or long-season climates is an easy option. Keep well watered; fertility needs are average.

Garden and Polyculture Planting

Grown for many years in this country as an ornamental, Job's tears is well suited to the shade garden and

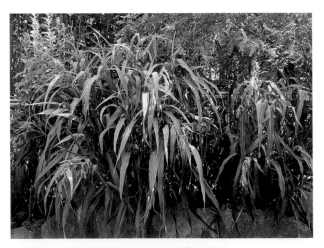

Coix lacryma-jobi in the ornamental garden.

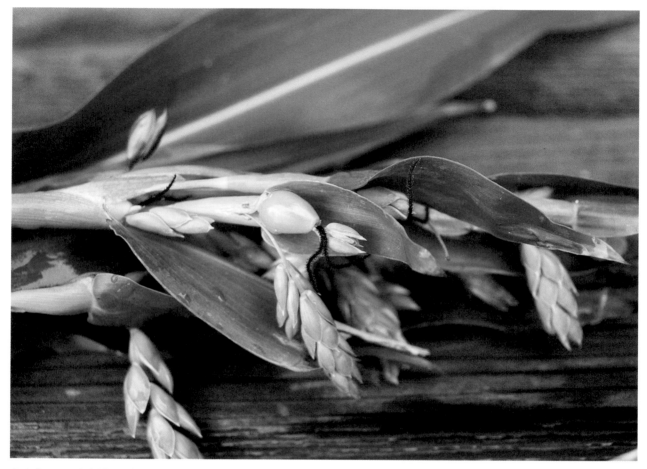

Coix lacryma-jobi **flowers.**

durable enough for a hedgerow. It can survive in a regularly watered garden, but it thrives in fertile, wet sites. Plant on one-foot spacing. When temperatures dip to twenty degrees the plant withers and dies.

Suitable Companions
Agastache rugosa, Korean Mint, tǔ huò xiāng
Alisma plantago-aquatica subsp. *orientale*, Water Plantain, zé xiè
Anemarrhena asphodeloides, zhī mǔ
Angelica dahurica, bái zhǐ
Bacopa monnieri, Brahmi
Cornus officinalis, Dogwood, shān zhū yú
Crataegus pinnatifida, Chinese Hawthorn, shān zhā
Eclipta prostrata, Eclipta, mò hàn lián
Eucommia ulmoides, Hardy Rubber Tree, dù zhòng
Ginkgo biloba, Ginkgo, bái guǒ

Gynostemma pentaphyllum, Sweet Tea Vine, jiǎo gǔ lán
Houttuynia cordata, yú xīng cǎo
Ligustrum lucidum, Chinese Privet, nǔ zhēn zǐ
Magnolia denudata, xīn yí huā
Mentha haplocalyx, Field Mint, bò hé
Ophiopogon japonicus, Lilyturf, mài mén dōng
Pinellia ternata, bàn xià
Plantago asiatica, Plantain, chē qián zǐ
Prunella vulgaris, Heal All, xià kū cǎo
Scrophularia buergeriana, Figwort, běi xuán shēn

Field Production
Transplant or direct seed Job's tears in part shade in a well-watered or wet location on one-foot spacing. Fertile soils result in better fruit production.

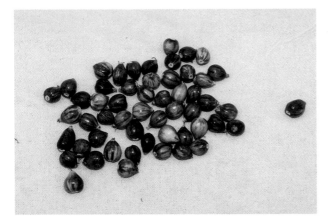

Dry seeds of *Coix lacryma-jobi*, **yì yǐ rén.**

Pests and Diseases

Gophers hollow out the root system, killing the plants—but eschew the grassy tops, leaving them toppled on the ground.

Harvest and Yield

I found harvesting by hand is too slow for any profitability; a better method needs to be explored for this to be a viable small-scale crop. Perhaps something like a blueberry or chamomile rake would make harvesting more time efficient. The seed coat needs to be pearled similar to rice processing, to yield the interior seed that the industry is accustomed to. The best quality is said to be a white, large, and plump seed.[76] The mature seed is about the same weight as dry; yield is 0.05–0.1 pounds per plant.

Notes

Coix lacryma-jobi var. *ma-yuen* is also used medicinally as yì yǐ rén. *Coix* seed is commonly made into beads used in jewelry.

Medicinal Uses of Yì yǐ rén

Yì yǐ rén is the seed of *Coix lacryma-jobi*. Sweet, bland, and cool, it strengthens the spleen, resolves dampness (particularly dampness due to spleen qi deficiency), addresses dampness in the muscles to relieve pain, clears heat, and dispels pus. Yì yǐ rén is relatively mild and is usually used in larger doses over time. It is edible and is commonly used in TCM dietary therapy. It is used to strengthen the digestion and address digestive disorders, loose stools, low appetite, water swelling, urinary difficulty, muscle and joint pain, spasms, muscle weakness, skin disorders such as acne, and for intestinal and lung abscesses.

Yì yǐ rén is used by itself and in combination with other herbs. Common methods of administration include powders, decoctions, concentrated granules, tablets, pills, and culinary dishes such as porridge and soup. It is in formulas such as Yi Yi Ren Tang (*Coix* Decoction) (of which there are several versions), Shen Ling Bai Zhu San (Ginseng, *Poria*, and *Atractylodes* Powder), Si Miao San (Four Marvels Powder), and Da Huang Mu Dan Tang (Rhubarb and *Moutan* Powder).

Cornus officinalis (Sieb. & Zucc.)
Common Name: Dogwood
Pinyin: Shān zhū yú
Family: Cornaceae
Part Used: Fruit

Plant Description

Attractive in all seasons, *Cornus officinalis* is a small deciduous tree growing up to twenty feet tall in a columnar to spreading manner. Smooth-margined, elliptically-shaped leaves are arranged opposite each other on the stems and grow to four inches long. Small, yellow-flowering umbels are surrounded by four prominent calyxes and bloom before leafing out in spring. Cherrylike clustered fruits are three-quarters of an inch long and half as wide, maturing in fall to a brilliant red. *Cornus officinalis* is native to Japan and Korea, where it can be found growing on hills and along wooded river areas; it is also cultivated in central to east central China.[77] USDA hardiness zones 4–9.

Propagation

Seeds or semihardwood cuttings taken in summer are the most common methods of propagation. The seed is a multicycle germinator; sow in the late summer to early fall for seed to receive three months or so of warm conditioning, then winter's chill of three months or more, finishing with germination the following spring. For best results, sow seeds in an eight-inch-deep flat with average media and vernalize the seed by exposing the flat to the winter. Where winters are very wet, protect the nascent seed from excessive moisture by moving the flat under cover.

Garden and Polyculture Planting

Dogwood is attractive as a specimen or in grouped plantings set on roughly ten-foot spacing. It has showy leaf color in fall, and the flower buds ornament the tree in winter. An orderly branching habit and handsome peeling bark make this tree welcome in sunny ornamental gardens and hedgerows.

Suitable Companions

Agastache rugosa, Korean Mint, tŭ huò xiāng
Albizia julibrissin, Mimosa, hé huān pí/huā
Allium macrostemon, xiè bái
Allium tuberosum, Garlic Chives, jiŭ cài zĭ
Anemarrhena asphodeloides, zhī mŭ

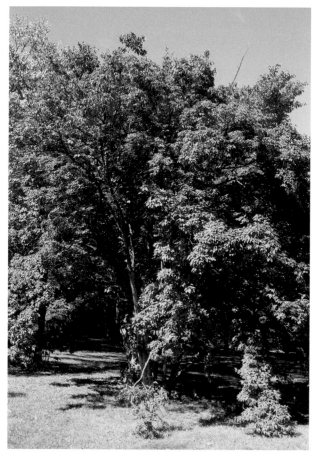

Several mature *Cornus officinalis* specimens full of fruit at the Arnold Arboretum of Harvard University, Massachusetts. Photo courtesy of Jean Giblette.

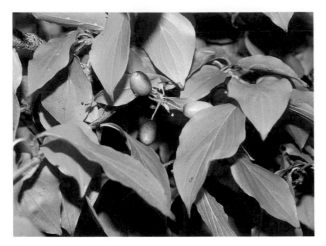

Cornus officinalis fruit.

Medicinal Uses of Shān zhū yú

Shān zhū yú is the fruit of *Cornus officinalis*. Sour and slightly warm, shān zhū yú tonifies the liver and the kidneys, retains the jing (essences), and stabilizes the body fluids. It is used to address issues such as weakness, dizziness, aching low back and knees, impotence, premature ejaculation, tinnitus (ringing in the ears), blurred vision, excessive sweating, excessive uterine bleeding, and urinary incontinence.

Shān zhū yú is usually used in combination with other herbs. Common methods of administration include decoctions, powders, concentrated granules, alcohol extracts, tablets, and pills. It appears in many important formulas, including Liu Wei Di Huang Wan (Six Flavor *Rehmannia* Pills) and its many derivatives, Zuo Gui Yin (Restore the Left Kidney Decoction), and You Gui Wan (Restore the Right Kidney Pills).

Angelica dahurica, bái zhǐ
Angelica pubescens, dú huó
Asparagus cochinchinensis, tiān mén dōng
Aster tataricus, Tartar Aster, zǐ wǎn
Atractylodes macrocephala, Chinese Thistle Daisy, bái zhú
Belamcanda chinensis, Blackberry Lily, shè gān
Bupleurum chinense, Hare's Ear, chái hú
Carthamus tinctorius, Safflower, hóng huā
Celosia argentea, qīng xiāng zǐ
Celosia cristata, Cockscomb, jī guān huā
Chrysanthemum morifolium, Mum, jú huā
Clerodendrum trichotomum, Glorybower, chòu wú tóng
Codonopsis pilosula, Poor Man's Ginseng, dǎng shēn
Crataegus pinnatifida, Chinese Hawthorn, shān zhā
Dianthus superbus, Fringed Pink, qú mài
Dioscorea opposita, Chinese Yam, shān yào
Dolichos lablab, Hyacinth Bean, bái biǎn dòu
Eriobotrya japonica, Loquat, pí pá yè
Eucommia ulmoides, Hardy Rubber Tree, dù zhòng
Forsythia suspensa, lián qiào
Ligusticum jeholense, Chinese Lovage, gǎo běn
Ligustrum lucidum, Chinese Privet, nǔ zhēn zǐ
Lilium lancifolium, *L. brownii*, Lily, bǎi hé
Lonicera japonica, Honeysuckle, jīn yín huā
Magnolia denudata, xīn yí huā
Ocimum sanctum, Sacred Basil, Tulsi
Platycodon grandiflorus, Balloon Flower, jié gěng

Prunella vulgaris, Heal All, xià kū cǎo
Rehmannia glutinosa, Chinese Foxglove, dì huáng
Rheum palmatum, Chinese Rhubarb, dà huáng
Salvia miltiorrhiza, *S. przewalskii*, *S. bowleyana*, Red Sage, dān shēn
Saposhnikovia divaricata, Siler, fáng fēng
Schizonepeta tenuifolia, Japanese Catnip, jīng jiè
Scrophularia buergeriana, Figwort, běi xuán shēn
Scutellaria baicalensis, Baikal Skullcap, huáng qín
Scutellaria barbata, Barbat Skullcap, bàn zhī lián
Sophora flavescens, kǔ shēn
Trichosanthes kirilowii, Chinese Cucumber, guā lóu/tiān huā fěn
Withania somnifera, Ashwagandha

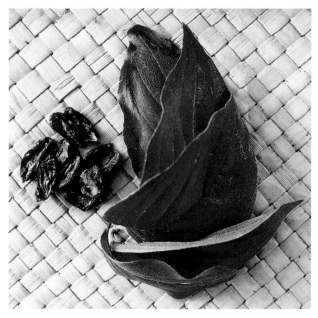

Freshly dried *Cornus officinalis* fruit (shān zhū yú) and fall leaves. Photo by Nina Zhito.

Field Production

For orchard production plant three-year-old nursery-grown stock on fifteen- to twenty-foot spacing. Dogwood prefers average to fertile well-draining soils and full sun. Expect flowers and fruit to set once trees are five to seven years old.

Pests and Diseases

I've never had problems with birds eating dogwood fruit, but keeping a vigilant eye on your trees in the fall would be prudent.

Harvest and Yield

Harvest the fruit when it is red and ripe in fall; if trees are tall use fruit or orchard ladders. Rinse and cut the fruit away from the seed and dry. Drying is easy and uneventful; the best quality is flexible and dark red. Yields vary by size and age of tree. Ratio of fresh to dry is unknown.

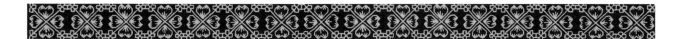

Crataegus pinnatifida (Bge.)
Common Name: Chinese Hawthorn
Pinyin: Shān zhā
Family: Rosaceae
Part Used: Fruit

Plant Description

Another edible medicinal, *Crataegus pinnatifida* (as well as various other *Crataegus* species) are used in Eastern as well as Western herbal traditions. *Crataegus pinnatifida* trees grow to twenty feet tall and spread ten to fifteen feet wide. Oftentimes multi-trunked, this species has fewer thorns than most hawthorns. The serrate-margined leathery leaves are dark green and rather irregular, but generally three- to seven-lobed and triangularly ovate to three to four inches long. White clustered flowers looking much like apple flowers bloom in spring after leaves make their return. Small, round, red, applelike fruits (did you know that *Crataegus pinnatifida* is an apple

relative?) around three-quarters of an inch in diameter follow in fall. Endemic to Asia, it is hardy in USDA hardiness zones 6–9.

Propagation

Propagate Chinese hawthorn by seed or rooted suckering stems. You'll need to remove the seeds from the fruit before sowing. If seed is fresh, germination should be quick; sow in a large, deep flat in fall. If seed is older it will have locked itself into a protective dormancy. The key to unlock this multicycle germinator is to sow it in a large deep flat and expose the flat to fall and winter weather. Only the amount of time will be different—fresh seed should germinate in spring and older seed might take up to two years. As an alternative, stratify the seed in the refrigerator. Many times the trees throw water-sprouts—fast growing upright branches—from the base of the tree. If these have roots they can be cut or pulled and replanted. Trees do well as potted plants for some years before needing to be planted out.

Garden and Polyculture Planting

A useful and charming tree that has beauty and function, Chinese hawthorn is ornamental in all phases: spring bloom, summer foliage (which often segues into orange fall coloration), fall's red fruit, and winter's attractive horizontal branching. It is also a desirable habitat plant, offering food to nectar-feeding and pollinating insects, while the fruits are attractive to songbirds and other wildlife. It is well suited to the hedgerow or back of the mixed ornamental border. Chinese hawthorn prefers full sun and well-draining soils and tolerates wind. Fertilizer needs are low; overfertilization encourages water-sprouts.

Suitable Companions

Acanthopanax gracilistylus, wǔ jiā pí
Achyranthes bidentata, Oxknee, huái niú xī
Agastache rugosa, Korean Mint, tǔ huò xiāng
Albizia julibrissin, Mimosa, hé huān pí/huā
Allium macrostemon, xiè bái
Allium tuberosum, Garlic Chives, jiǔ cài zǐ
Anemarrhena asphodeloides, zhī mǔ
Angelica dahurica, bái zhǐ
Angelica pubescens, dú huó
Aster tataricus, Tartar Aster, zǐ wǎn
Atractylodes macrocephala, Chinese Thistle Daisy, bái zhú
Belamcanda chinensis, Blackberry Lily, shè gān
Bupleurum chinense, Hare's Ear, chái hú
Carthamus tinctorius, Safflower, hóng huā
Celosia argentea, qīng xiāng zǐ
Celosia cristata, Cockscomb, jī guān huā
Chrysanthemum morifolium, Mum, jú huā
Clerodendrum trichotomum, Glorybower, chòu wú tóng
Cornus officinalis, Dogwood, shān zhū yú

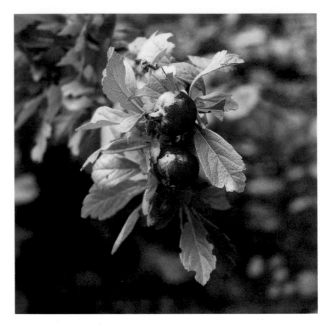

***Crataegus pinnatifida* fruit.**

Cyathula officinalis, Hookweed, chuān niú xī
Dianthus superbus, Fringed Pink, qú mài
Dolichos lablab, Hyacinth Bean, bái biǎn dòu
Eriobotrya japonica, Loquat, pí pá yè
Eucommia ulmoides, Hardy Rubber Tree, dù zhòng
Forsythia suspensa, lián qiào
Ligusticum jeholense, Chinese Lovage, gǎo běn
Ligustrum lucidum, Chinese Privet, nǚ zhēn zǐ
Lilium lancifolium, L. brownii, Lily, bǎi hé
Lonicera japonica, Honeysuckle, jīn yín huā
Lycium chinense, Chinese Wolfberry, gǒu qǐ zǐ/dì gǔ pí
Magnolia denudata, xīn yí huā
Mentha haplocalyx, Field Mint, bò hé
Momordica charantia, Bitter Melon, kǔ guā
Ocimum sanctum, Sacred Basil, Tulsi
Plantago asiatica, Plantain, chē qián zǐ
Platycodon grandiflorus, Balloon Flower, jié gěng
Prunella vulgaris, Heal All, xià kū cǎo
Rehmannia glutinosa, Chinese Foxglove, dì huáng
Rheum palmatum, Chinese Rhubarb, dà huáng
Salvia miltiorrhiza, S. przewalskii, S. bowleyana, Red Sage, dān shēn
Saposhnikovia divaricata, Siler, fáng fēng
Schizonepeta tenuifolia, Japanese Catnip, jīng jiè
Scrophularia buergeriana, Figwort, běi xuán shēn

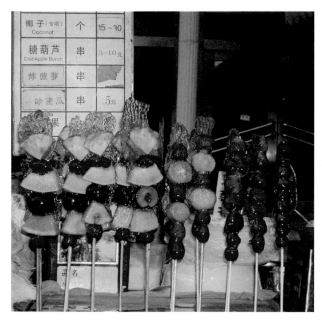

Beijing street vendor selling fresh candied fruit; the stick on the far right is 100 percent Chinese hawthorn.

Scutellaria baicalensis, Baikal Skullcap, huáng qín
Sophora flavescens, kǔ shēn
Trichosanthes kirilowii, Chinese Cucumber, guā lóu/tiān huā fěn
Withania somnifera, Ashwagandha

Field Production

Transplant Chinese hawthorn trees that are several years old into the medicinal orchard on fifteen-foot spacing. Prune out dead or infected wood in winter with clean pruning cutters, and sterilize them frequently as you work to lessen the potential spread of fireblight. Remove root suckers (water-sprouts) if desired. Water requirements are average.

Pests and Diseases

Like many members of the Rosaceae family, *Crataegus pinnatifida* is susceptible to the bacterial disease fireblight (it blackens and kills whole limbs). *Crataegus pinnatifida* is somewhat deer resistant.

Harvest and Yield

Trees need to be about five years old to fruit. Harvest fruits in fall when they are shiny, red, and ripe. Wash to remove dust or other impurities and use or sell

Medicinal Uses of Shān zhā

Shān zhā is the fruit of *Crataegus pinnatifida*. Sweet, sour, and slightly warm, shān zhā promotes digestion, disperses food stagnation, activates the blood, and disperses blood stagnation. It is used to support digestion and address issues such as abdominal fullness; pain and distention; diarrhea; difficulty digesting meat, fats, and oils; and general indigestion. In modern times its use has been expanded to encompass many cardiovascular disorders, and it is used to address high cholesterol, angina, high blood pressure, and coronary artery disorder.

Shān zhā is medicinally most commonly used in combination with other herbs. Common methods of administration include decoctions, powders, concentrated granules, alcohol extracts, tablets, and pills. It is in the well-known formulas Bao He Wan (Preserve Harmony Pills) and Jian Pi Wan (Strengthen the Spleen Pills) and many modern formulas that address high cholesterol and other cardiovascular issues.

fresh. For a dry product slice horizontally with the skin on, removing the seed, and dry at roughly one hundred degrees. The best quality is said to be "of large fruit (or slices) with a red or reddish brown surface and fleshy pulp."[78] Yield varies greatly with the age of the trees.

Notes

These small fruits have a dried, sour-apple flavor. Steep them in teas as you would rose hips, adding a bit of honey to sweeten the flavor. In China, they are preserved in sugar and served as a candied treat.

Cyathula officinalis (Kuan.)
Common Name: Hookweed
Pinyin: Chuān niú xī
Family: Amaranthaceae
Part Used: Root

Plant Description

Cyathula officinalis is an herbaceous perennial growing four to five feet tall and three feet wide. Light green leaves up to five inches long sit opposite on many branching green stems (also oppositely arranged). The elliptically shaped leaves are tomentose, or covered with a short thick wooly hair. The whole plant is a curious Dr. Seuss type, with its hooked seed all bunched in a ball on the stem terminals. Flowers are light green and rather inconspicuous. Seed dispersal is ingenious—they catch onto fabric, hair, dog fur, almost anything. Monitor for invasive qualities: we haven't noticed any at the Chinese Medicinal Herb Farm, but there are many other environments to consider for this little-known plant. *Cyathula officinalis* primarily grows in south central China in "waste places" above 5,000 feet.[79] USDA hardiness zones 7–10.

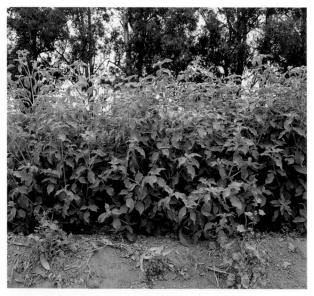

Field-cultivated *Cyathula officinalis*.

Propagation

Seed and crown divisions are the recommended methods of increasing stock. Sow seed shortly after harvesting for best results; otherwise germination is slow and sporadic. Hookweed most likely requires a chilling period for improved germination rates. Division, using even small pieces of root with some crown material, works well—especially on bottom heat in the greenhouse. Large sections of exposed cut roots, as long as there is some crown, also grow well. Grow seed-started or division stock for three months before transplanting to its final growing site. Hookweed is not a good permanent potted plant, and is not recommended for container sale.

Garden and Polyculture Planting

Easy to grow, hookweed prefers full sun in average well-draining soil. Place in the middle to back of the garden, border, or hedgerow—certainly away from pathways. In spring, after what is expected to be the last frost of the season (famous last words, eh?), cut back last year's brown shabby growth.

Suitable Companions

Acanthopanax gracilistylus, wǔ jiā pí
Achyranthes bidentata, Oxknee, huái niú xī
Agastache rugosa, Korean Mint, tǔ huò xiāng
Albizia julibrissin, Mimosa, hé huān pí/huā
Allium macrostemon, xiè bái
Allium tuberosum, Garlic Chives, jiǔ cài zǐ
Andrographis paniculata, Kalmegh, chuān xīn lián
Anemarrhena asphodeloides, zhī mǔ
Angelica dahurica, bái zhǐ
Angelica pubescens, dú huó
Aster tataricus, Tartar Aster, zǐ wǎn

Atractylodes macrocephala, Chinese Thistle Daisy, bái zhú

Belamcanda chinensis, Blackberry Lily, shè gān

Bupleurum chinense, Hare's Ear, chái hú

Carthamus tinctorius, Safflower, hóng huā

Celosia argentea, qīng xiāng zǐ

Celosia cristata, Cockscomb, jī guān huā

Chrysanthemum morifolium, Mum, jú huā

Clerodendrum trichotomum, Glorybower, chòu wú tóng

Cornus officinalis, Dogwood, shān zhū yú

Crataegus pinnatifida, Chinese Hawthorn, shān zhā

Dianthus superbus, Fringed Pink, qú mài

Dolichos lablab, Hyacinth Bean, bái biǎn dòu

Eriobotrya japonica, Loquat, pí pá yè

Eucommia ulmoides, Hardy Rubber Tree, dù zhòng

Forsythia suspensa, lián qiào

Ginkgo biloba, Ginkgo, bái guǒ

Houttuynia cordata, yú xīng cǎo

Ligusticum jeholense, Chinese Lovage, gǎo běn

Ligustrum lucidum, Chinese Privet, nǔ zhēn zǐ

Lilium lancifolium, *L. brownii*, Lily, bǎi hé

Lonicera japonica, Honeysuckle, jīn yín huā

Lycium chinense, Chinese Wolfberry, gǒu qǐ zǐ/dì gǔ pí

Magnolia denudata, xīn yí huā

Mentha haplocalyx, Field Mint, bò hé

Momordica charantia, Bitter Melon, kǔ guā

Ocimum sanctum, Sacred Basil, Tulsi

Platycodon grandiflorus, Balloon Flower, jié gěng

Prunella vulgaris, Heal All, xià kū cǎo

Rehmannia glutinosa, Chinese Foxglove, dì huáng

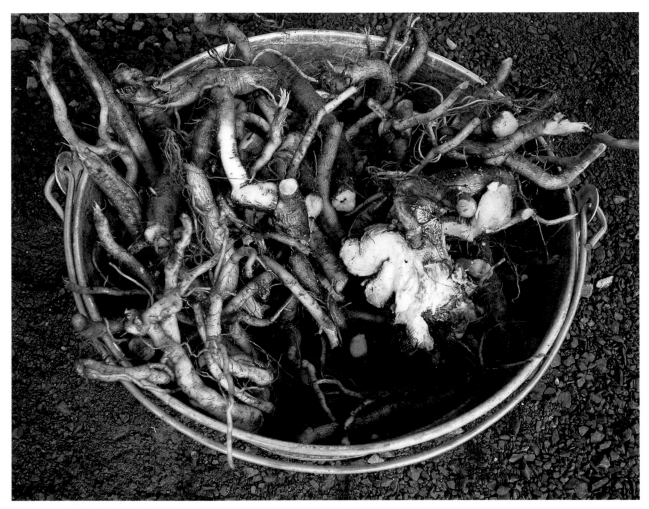

Freshly harvested *Cyathula officinalis*.

Rheum palmatum, Chinese Rhubarb, dà huáng

Salvia miltiorrhiza, *S. przewalskii*, *S. bowleyana*, Red Sage, dān shēn

Saposhnikovia divaricata, Siler, fáng fēng

Schizonepeta tenuifolia, Japanese Catnip, jīng jiè

Scutellaria baicalensis, Baikal Skullcap, huáng qín

Sophora flavescens, kǔ shēn

Trichosanthes kirilowii, Chinese Cucumber, guā lóu/tiān huā fěn

Withania somnifera, Ashwagandha

Ziziphus jujuba, Chinese Date, dà zǎo

Ziziphus jujuba var. *spinosa*, suān zǎo rén

Field Production

Transplant nursery-grown stock on two-foot spacing in full sun in soils with average fertility. Irrigate regularly and mulch to conserve water and suppress weeds.

Pests and Diseases

Gophers (happily, I assume) eat the roots.

Harvest and Yield

Grow hookweed for two to three years before harvesting roots in the fall or winter, when the plants are dormant. The large white roots have a thin brown skin, sometimes tinged with pink. Separate roots from crowns, and wash. A power washer is quick and easy—but do not remove the brown skin, just the dirt. You'll notice a thin layer of oil on the surface of the wash water, but this is normal. Cut roots lengthwise in quarter-inch slices and dry. The benchmark for quality of dry chuān niú xī is "thick, soft and oily, yellowish brown roots."[80] Yield for two-year-old roots is three pounds per plant fresh. Ratio of fresh to dry is 3:1.

Medicinal Uses of Chuān niú xī

Chuān niú xī is the root of *Cyathula officinalis*. Bitter, sour, and neutral it activates the blood, dispels blood stagnation, promotes urination, directs fire and blood downward, tonifies the kidney and liver, and strengthens the tendons and bones. It is used to address many gynecological issues, pain due to injury, painful urination, lower back and knee soreness, joint pain of the lower body, certain types of toothache and mouth ulcers, dizziness, and headache.

Chuān niú xī is usually used in combination with other herbs. Such formulas are administered by decoction, powder, concentrated granule, alcohol extract, tablets, and pills. It is in formulas such as Shen Tong Zhu Yu Tang (Eliminate Stasis from a Painful Body Decoction), Xue Fu Zhu Yu Tang (Eliminate Stasis from the Mansion of Blood Decoction), Tian Ma Gou Teng Yin (*Gastrodia* and *Uncaria* Decoction), and Zuo Gui Wan (Restore the Left Kidney Pills).

Chuān niú xī and huái niú xī (*Achyranthes bidentata*) have almost identical functions. Although there are some differences, in many older texts there is no distinction made between the two herbs.

Dianthus superbus (L.)
Common Name: Fringed Pink
Pinyin: Qú mài
Family: Caryophyllaceae
Part Used: Herb

Plant Description
Dianthus superbus, as well as the other three-hundred-plus species in this genus, are all commonly called "Pinks." This one is a short-lived herbaceous perennial growing three feet tall—or wide, as they have rather lax stems. Blue-green or glaucous linear-lanceolate leaves four inches long clasp the stem, forming sheaths that sit opposite each other on branching stems. The flowers of the five-petaled *Dianthus superbus* are surrounded by tubular calyxes, bloom in summer to autumn—and have either pink, white, or purple dissected one-inch flowers. These flowers are beautiful, but what is just as nice is their sweetly scented fragrance. *Dianthus superbus* can be found growing on mountain slopes, in woods, and in meadows near streams throughout China; *Dianthus superbus* is also extensively cultivated in China and world-wide.[81] Suitable for cultivating in USDA hardiness zones 3–9.

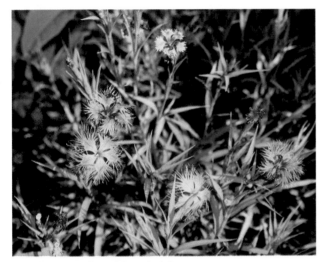

***Dianthus superbus*, Fringed Pink.**

Propagation
Seeds sown in early spring germinate readily in two to three weeks in warm soil in the nursery or indoors. Culture is easy; plants hold only somewhat well in nursery pots.

Garden and Polyculture Planting
Fringed pink generally grows best in cool, moist climates; avoid planting on a hot, exposed site. Sow seeds directly or set out transplants in spring or early summer. It prefers a light, sandy, well-drained fertile soil that is a little alkaline. Flower production is at its peak in the second season of growth.

Suitable Companions
Acanthopanax gracilistylus, wǔ jiā pí
Achyranthes bidentata, Oxknee, huái niú xī
Agastache rugosa, Korean Mint, tǔ huò xiāng
Albizia julibrissin, Mimosa, hé huān pí/huā
Allium macrostemon, xiè bái
Allium tuberosum, Garlic Chives, jiǔ cài zǐ
Anemarrhena asphodeloides, zhī mǔ
Angelica dahurica, bái zhǐ
Angelica pubescens, dú huó
Aster tataricus, Tartar Aster, zǐ wǎn
Belamcanda chinensis, Blackberry Lily, shè gān
Bupleurum chinense, Hare's Ear, chái hú
Celosia argentea, qīng xiāng zǐ
Celosia cristata, Cockscomb, jī guān huā
Chrysanthemum morifolium, Mum, jú huā
Clerodendrum trichotomum, Glorybower, chòu wú tóng
Cornus officinalis, Dogwood, shān zhū yú
Crataegus pinnatifida, Chinese Hawthorn, shān zhā

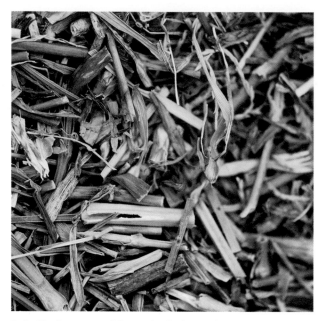

Dried leaf, stem, and flower bud of *Dianthus superbus*, qú mài. Photo by Jasmine Oberste.

Medicinal Uses of Qú mài

Qú mài is the herb or aerial portion of *Dianthus superbus*. Bitter and cold, it regulates the fluids, promotes urination, invigorates the blood, and regulates menstruation. It is an important herb for addressing many types of painful urination, including painful urination with burning, painful urination with blood in the urine, and painful urination due to stones. It is also used to address lack of menstruation (amenorrhea) and menstrual cramping with clots.

Qú mài is usually used in combination with other herbs. Common methods of administration include decoctions, powders, concentrated granules, alcohol extracts, herbal teas, tablets, and pills. It is a key ingredient in the important formula Ba Zheng San (Eight Rectifications Powder).

Cyathula officinalis, Hookweed, chuān niú xī
Dolichos lablab, Hyacinth Bean, bái biǎn dòu
Eriobotrya japonica, Loquat, pí pá yè
Eucommia ulmoides, Hardy Rubber Tree, dù zhòng
Forsythia suspensa, lián qiào
Ginkgo biloba, Ginkgo, bái guǒ
Houttuynia cordata, yú xīng cǎo
Ligusticum jeholense, Chinese Lovage, gǎo běn
Ligustrum lucidum, Chinese Privet, nǚ zhēn zǐ
Lilium lancifolium, L. brownii, Lily, bǎi hé
Lonicera japonica, Honeysuckle, jīn yín huā
Magnolia denudata, xīn yí huā
Mentha haplocalyx, Field Mint, bò hé
Momordica charantia, Bitter Melon, kǔ guā
Ocimum sanctum, Sacred Basil, Tulsi
Paeonia lactiflora, Chinese Peony, bái/chì sháo
Paeonia suffruticosa, Tree Peony, mǔ dān pí
Plantago asiatica, Plantain, chē qián zǐ
Platycodon grandiflorus, Balloon Flower, jié gěng
Prunella vulgaris, Heal All, xià kū cǎo
Rehmannia glutinosa, Chinese Foxglove, dì huáng
Rheum palmatum, Chinese Rhubarb, dà huáng
Salvia miltiorrhiza, S. przewalskii, S. bowleyana, Red Sage, dān shēn
Saposhnikovia divaricata, Siler, fáng fēng
Schizonepeta tenuifolia, Japanese Catnip, jīng jiè
Scrophularia buergeriana, Figwort, běi xuán shēn
Scutellaria barbata, Barbat Skullcap, bàn zhī lián
Sophora flavescens, kǔ shēn
Trichosanthes kirilowii, Chinese Cucumber, guā lóu/tiān huā fěn

Field Production

Transplant fringed pink into a full sun or part sun site in spring on eight-inch to one-foot spacing. Irrigate for best growth potential. Side dress with compost or fertilizer early in the second spring. Mulch or compost is beneficial to keep the soil and root zone cool, moist, and biologically healthy. After the second season the plants have run their course; retire them to the compost pile.

Pests and Diseases
None.

Harvest and Yield
Harvest will be small in the first season; you'll take the bulk of the crop in the second season. Harvest the aerial portions of the plant in summer and autumn when the flower bud is about to bloom; two or more harvests a year are possible.[82] The best quality is said to be "of tender yellowish green twigs and leaves, without rootlets or foreign matter. The flower buds should still be closed."[83] Yield is unknown but estimated to be in the range of a quarter-pound per plant per harvest fresh.

Dioscorea opposita (Thunb.)
Botanical Synonym: *D. polystachya* (Turcz.), *D. batatas* (Decne.) (latter name obsolete)
Common Name: Chinese Yam
Pinyin: Shān yào
Family: Dioscoreaceae
Part Used: Root

Plant Description
This perennial dioecious vine, climbing to fifteen feet, has fragrant cinnamon-scented insignificant flowers blooming in leaf axils from summer to fall. The dark green leaves are heart-shaped, opposite on the stem, and somewhat leathery. In warm climates, three-winged chambered brown seedpods form in the leaf axils (which also produce air bulbils, or air tubers). The cylindrical tan-skinned root grows up to three feet long and may have a one-foot-long underground stem before the true tuber begins. There is at least one other form than that of the cylindrical *Dioscorea opposita*, with a tuber that grows roughly in the shape of a hand. Herbaceous, durable, and persistent, *Dioscorea opposita* is cold tolerant to roughly minus ten degrees. In warm regions or areas with summer rainfall, air tuber production is prolific—making *Dioscorea opposita* invasive. In areas with cooler or shorter growing seasons neither air bulbils nor seeds are produced. With a wide potential geographic distribution, *Dioscorea opposita* is hardy in USDA hardiness zones 5–11.

Propagation
It's easier to propagate Chinese yam by bulbils (air tubers) or root pieces than by seed. Cut roots into segments with "eyes," similar to potatoes. To form a barrier against potential pathogens, I let the cut portions of root segments heal a day or two before planting. In the nursery keep the vines staked and

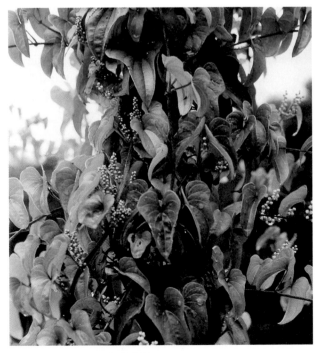

Dioscorea opposita in full bloom.

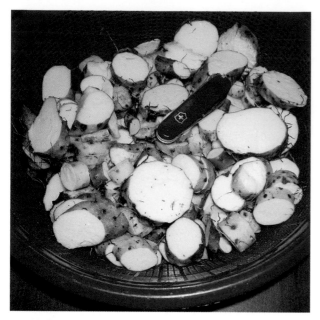

Freshly harvested and sliced root of *Dioscorea opposita* ready for drying.

separated—or they will become one huge tangled mass. Flat papery brown seeds (removed from their pods) sown in spring germinate in two to three weeks. They containerize well—and when they are more than ready to be repotted, the long root will eject the plant from its pot! Water sparingly while plants are winter dormant.

Garden and Polyculture Planting

Reliable and undemanding, Chinese yam is easy to cultivate and incorporate into the hedgerow, perennial vegetable garden, or ornamental border. Full sun, average fertility and drainage, and moderate watering are Chinese yam's minor cultural requirements. Plant on one-foot spacing and set up a trellis—or just allow the vines to clamber over and through trees and shrubs; they grow to fifteen feet in two seasons. When the weather is warm, the flowers produce a good semblance of a cinnamon scent.

Suitable Companions

Agastache rugosa, Korean Mint, tǔ huò xiāng
Angelica dahurica, baí zhǐ
Angelica pubescens, dú huó
Aster tataricus, Tartar Aster, zǐ wǎn

Belamcanda chinensis, Blackberry Lily, shè gān
Carthamus tinctorius, Safflower, hóng huā
Celosia argentea, qīng xiāng zǐ
Celosia cristata, Cockscomb, jī guān huā
Chrysanthemum morifolium, Mum, jú huā
Cyathula officinalis, Hookweed, chuān niú xī
Dianthus superbus, Fringed Pink, qú mài
Eucommia ulmoides, Hardy Rubber Tree, dù zhòng
Lilium lancifolium, *L. brownii*, Lily, bǎi hé
Lonicera japonica, Honeysuckle, jīn yín huā
Momordica charantia, Bitter Melon, kǔ guā
Ocimum sanctum, Sacred Basil, Tulsi
Prunella vulgaris, Heal All, xià kū cǎo
Rheum palmatum, Chinese Rhubarb, dà huáng
Salvia miltiorrhiza, *S. przewalskii*, *S. bowleyana*, Red Sage, dān shēn
Saposhnikovia divaricata, Siler, fáng fēng
Schizonepeta tenuifolia, Japanese Catnip, jīng jiè
Scutellaria baicalensis, Baikal Skullcap, huáng qín
Withania somnifera, Ashwagandha

Field Production

Plant out, after danger of frost has passed, on one-foot spacing. Provide full sun and soils that are friable, fertile, and well drained. On a farm scale, I recommend trellising to save space, for ease of soil cultivation, and ease of collection of bulbils or seed in the fall. Spring reemergence is very late.

Pests and Diseases

Waterlogged soils encourage root rot. Deer occasionally browse the leaves.

Harvest and Yield

The traditional time to harvest the root for medicine is after frost has encouraged dormancy; however, if Chinese yam is to be eaten as a food it can be harvested at other times. When fresh, the interior of the tan-skinned root is very white and mucilaginous, and handling it can cause temporary itching and in some people a rash. Harvest the first fall or leave in the ground for a future harvest. Most tubers grow straight down; keep in mind that they form as far as a foot below the soil surface and can be as long as three

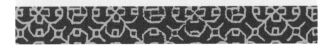

Chinese Yam Recipes

An excellent edible herb, Chinese yams have a color and texture more like the white Idaho potato than orange-fleshed yams. To serve them mashed, peel and cook them in water or vegetable stock until soft enough to mash. You may also bake them until soft, and serve them with a topping of chopped chives and olive oil. The raw tuber may feel slippery, but this texture disappears with cooking.

feet. The roots are brittle, too. The best way I have found to harvest them is to dig a large, deep hole at the head of a row, step in, and dig the roots laterally. If you don't initially find them, keep digging deeper! Washing is easy with a power washer. For dry herb, cut tubers into quarter-inch cross sections and dry in a single layer; when done they should be chalk-like and dense. Check your stored stock often, as they tend to mold if not thoroughly dried. The yield is variable ("mature tubers can weigh 8 to 10 pounds"[84]) but an average is ½–1½ pounds per fresh root in the first season, and 1–3 pounds per fresh root for tubers more than one season old. Ratio of fresh to dry is 4:1.

Notes

The names *Dioscorea opposita* (Thunberg) and *Dioscorea batatas* (Decne.) are nomenclaturally superfluous.[85] I use them here because they are most commonly known.

Medicinal Uses of Shān yào

Shān yào is the root of *Dioscorea opposita*. Sweet and neutral, shān yào tonifies the qi; nourishes the spleen; tonifies the stomach, lung, and kidney yin; and treats Xiao Ke (wasting and thirsting syndrome). Shān yào strengthens and restores the qi without being warming, overdrying, or overstimulating—making it suitable for a wide range of conditions. It is edible and is commonly used in dietary therapy. It is used to address a wide variety of problems, including lack of energy, weakness, poor appetite, low body weight, indigestion, loose stools, diarrhea, vaginal discharge, coughing, wheezing, soreness and weakness of the lower back and knees, frequent urination, premature ejaculation, and elevated blood glucose levels.

Shān yào is often used by itself as well as being used in many traditional and modern formulas. It is administered in congees (rice porridges), decoctions, powders, concentrated granules, alcohol extracts, tablets, and pills. It is in many important formulas including Shen Ling Bai Zhu San (Ginseng, *Poria*, and *Atractylodes* Powder), Jian Pi Wan (Strengthen the Stomach Pills), Liu Wei Di Huang Wan and all of its derivatives, You Gui Wan (Restore the Right Kidney Pills), Zuo Gui Yin (Restore the Left Kidney Decoction), Wan Dai Tang (End Discharge Decoction), and Jin Suo Gu Jing Wan (Gold Lock Pill to Stabilize the Essences).

Dolichos lablab (L.)

Common Name: Hyacinth Bean
Pinyin: Bái biǎn dòu
Family: Fabaceae
Part Used: Seed

Plant Description

Dolichos lablab is an attractive perennial vine often grown as an annual. In temperate regions this climbing twiner reaches ten to fifteen feet in a season; in the tropics it can reach more than twenty feet. Broadly ovate green trifoliate leaves have long petioles. There are many named cultivars, mostly found in the tropics; these cultivars are important food sources for people and livestock. In Chinese medicine the species, or unselected stock, is used—the primary one has white flowers and beans (bái biǎn dòu translates as "white flat bean"). Sometimes a variety with purple flowers, pods, and seed is used as well. Both bear loose five-inch panicles at vine terminals and leaf axils. Each panicle consists of about ten large pealike flowers that develop into smooth, five-inch-long seedpods. For summer cultivation as an annual in all zones; to winter over they tolerate a low of fifteen to twenty degrees. USDA hardiness zone 9.

Propagation

Direct sow from a half inch to one inch deep where plants are to grow, or transplant these fast-growing plants when young. Hot summer areas are ideal: in mild summer areas plant by June 1 to make sure there is enough time for beans to mature. Germination is quick and easy and takes place in a week. In the nursery it takes two to three weeks from spring sowing to four-inch transplant or containerized sale. Like all beans hyacinth bean is self-fertile; occasionally insects will cross-pollinate it with other bean varieties, but generally they come true to type.

Garden and Polyculture Planting

Hyacinth bean is as easy and undemanding to grow as a pole bean. It also works well as a very ornamental, fast, and functional summer screen; plant in warm soils and provide a trellis. Fertilize sparingly; like all legumes, hyacinth beans produce their own nitrogen. Plant at least a handful of beans for a good show in the garden. The pods, especially the beautiful purple variety, make excellent long-lasting cut "flowers."

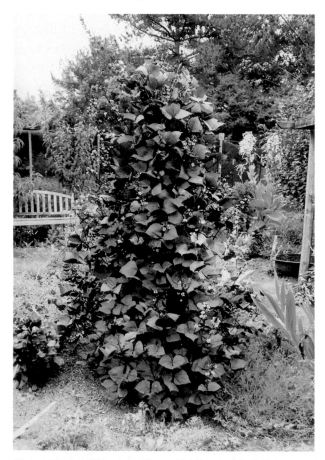

The gardenworthy purple-flowering form of *Dolichos lablab*, hyacinth bean.

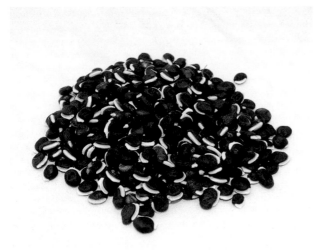

Dried seed of *Dolichos lablab*, biǎn dòu.

Suitable Companions

Agastache rugosa, Korean Mint, tǔ huò xiāng
Allium tuberosum, Garlic Chives, jiǔ cài zǐ
Angelica dahurica, baí zhǐ
Angelica pubescens, dú huó
Aster tataricus, Tartar Aster, zǐ wǎn
Astragalus membranaceus, Milk Vetch, huáng qí
Atractylodes macrocephala, Chinese Thistle Daisy, bái zhú
Belamcanda chinensis, Blackberry Lily, shè gān
Carthamus tinctorius, Safflower, hóng huā
Celosia argentea, qīng xiāng zǐ
Celosia cristata, Cockscomb, jī guān huā
Chrysanthemum morifolium, Mum, jú huā
Clerodendrum trichotomum, Glorybower, chòu wú tóng
Cornus officinalis, Dogwood, shān zhū yú
Crataegus pinnatifida, Chinese Hawthorn, shān zhā
Cyathula officinalis, Hookweed, chuān niú xī
Dioscorea opposita, Chinese Yam, shān yào
Eucommia ulmoides, Hardy Rubber Tree, dù zhòng
Forsythia suspensa, lián qiào
Lilium lancifolium, *L. brownii*, Lily, bǎi hé
Lycium chinense, Chinese Wolfberry, gǒu qǐ zǐ/dì gǔ pí
Magnolia denudata, xīn yí huā
Momordica charantia, Bitter Melon, kǔ guā
Ocimum sanctum, Sacred Basil, Tulsi
Platycodon grandiflorus, Balloon Flower, jié gěng

Medicinal Uses of Bái biǎn dòu

Bái biǎn dòu, also referred to as biǎn dòu, is the seed of *Dolichos lablab*. Sweet and slightly warm, it strengthens the spleen, dissolves dampness, clears summer heat, and eliminates toxins. It is used to address issues such as weakness, fatigue, decreased appetite, loose stools, diarrhea, vaginal discharge, and certain types of nausea and vomiting. It also has important applications in treating food poisoning and various toxins, such as pufferfish poisoning, poultry poisoning, and arsenic poisoning.

Bái biǎn dòu is used as a food by itself or medicinally in combination with other herbs. Common methods of administration include decoctions, powders, concentrated granules, tablets, and pills. It is in formulas such as Shen Ling Bai Zhu San (Ginseng, *Poria*, and *Atractylodes* Powder) and Xiang Ru Yin (*Elsholtzia* Decoction).

Dry-fried bái biǎn dòu is usually used to strengthen the spleen, and the unprocessed herb is used to eliminate toxins.

Other parts of *Dolichos lablab* are sometimes used medicinally as well, although less commonly. Biǎn dòu yi is the skin of the fruit, with similar but weaker functions than bái biǎn dòu. Bái biǎn huā is the flower and is primarily used to address fever, diarrhea or dysentery, and certain types of leukorrhea.

Rheum palmatum, Chinese Rhubarb, dà huáng
Salvia miltiorrhiza, S. przewalskii, S. bowleyana, Red Sage, dān shēn
Saposhnikovia divaricata, Siler, fáng fēng
Schizonepeta tenuifolia, Japanese Catnip, jīng jiè

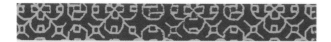

Hyacinth Bean Recipes

The immature pods of hyacinth beans may be steamed or stir-fried as you would green beans or edible pod peas. Widely consumed in the tropics, the mature beans may be taken out of their pods and dried, but they must be cooked for at least thirty minutes to destroy toxins that develop in mature beans.

Scutellaria baicalensis, Baikal Skullcap, huáng qín
Sophora flavescens, kǔ shēn
Trichosanthes kirilowii, Chinese Cucumber, guā lóu/tiān huā fěn
Withania somnifera, Ashwagandha

Ziziphus jujuba, Chinese Date, dà zǎo
Ziziphus jujuba var. *spinosa*, suān zǎo rén

Field Production

Plant one foot apart in row and provide a six-foot trellis. For best results provide soil that is well drained and is of average fertility; irrigate to maintain even moisture. Heat- and sun-loving, hyacinth bean is somewhat drought tolerant and if need be can manage in poor soils.

Pests and Diseases

In humid climates mildew can be a problem. Deer eat the foliage.

Harvest and Yield

Each floral panicle is a heavy producer and produces five to eight pods; each pod contains three to five beans. Collect when pods dry, shell the beans, and dry beans to roughly 10 percent moisture. Yield is 0.2 pounds per plant. Ratio of fresh to dry is 7:1.

Eclipta prostrata ([L.] L.)
Common Name: Eclipta
Pinyin: Mò hàn lián   Alternative Pinyin name: hàn lián cǎo
Family: Asteraceae
Part Used: Herb

Plant Description

This unassuming plant is used in Ayurvedic as well as Chinese herbal medicine. *Eclipta prostrata* is a many-branched annual growing two feet tall and just as wide. The simple leaves are lance-shaped with a wavy margin and are scratchy to the touch, owing to their many fine hairs. The green leaves sit opposite each other on pliant red stems that root where they come in contact with moist soil. Half-inch white flowers resemble daisies, with the center disk flowers maturing into grey faceted seed. Growing commonly in many parts of the world, this herb has naturalized in the eastern half of the United States, Texas, New Mexico, Arizona, and California—as well as India, China, South America, Australia, and so on.[86] In moist areas *Eclipta prostrata* has invasive qualities. All USDA hardiness zones.

Propagation

Seeds are easy to sow; plants are easy to grow. Spring germination is one to three weeks in the greenhouse. Keep well watered; average media is sufficient. Due

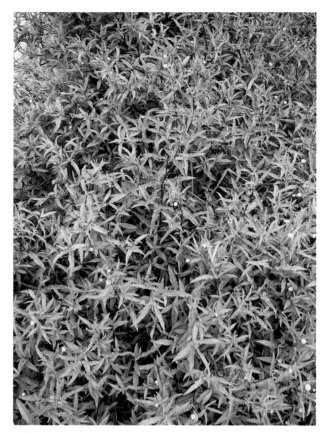

Eclipta prostrata.

Medicinal Uses of Mò hàn lián

Mò hàn lián is the herb or aerial portion of *Eclipta prostrata*. Sweet, sour, and cold, mò hàn lián nourishes the yin, tonifies the kidneys, cools the blood, and stops bleeding. It is used to address issues such as weakness, dizziness, blurred vision, prematurely grey hair, soreness of the back and knees, and menopausal symptoms. It is also used to address bleeding issues such as excessive menstrual bleeding, blood in the urine, and external bleeding due to injury.

Mò hàn lián is used as a single herb and in combination with other herbs. It is administered in decoctions, powders, concentrated granules, as a juice, and in tablet and pill form. Mò hàn lián makes up half of the formula Er Zhi Wan (Two Solstices Pills).

Fresh mò hàn lián is generally used to stop bleeding while the dry herb is used for more nourishing functions.

to its self-sowing properties it is best not to offer this herb for sale as transplants. Eclipta does not hold well in pots.

Garden and Polyculture Planting

Eclipta prefers a moist, humid site in part shade. Place near the front of the border or under a tree. It has a mounding habit, blooms in summer through fall, and is very frost tender.

Suitable Companions

Andrographis paniculata, Kalmegh, chuān xīn lián
Anemarrhena asphodeloides, zhī mǔ
Angelica dahurica, bái zhǐ
Angelica pubescens, dú huó
Asparagus cochinchinensis, tiān mén dōng
Bacopa monnieri, Brahmi
Centella asiatica, Gotu Kola, jī xuě cǎo
Codonopsis pilosula, Poor Man's Ginseng, dǎng shēn

Coix lacryma-jobi, Job's Tears, yì yǐ rén
Gentiana scabra, lóng dǎn cǎo
Gentiana straminea, qín jiāo
Gynostemma pentaphyllum, Sweet Tea Vine, jiǎo gǔ lán
Houttuynia cordata, yú xīng cǎo
Pinellia ternata, bàn xià
Plantago asiatica, Plantain, chē qián zǐ
Schisandra chinensis, Five Flavored Fruit, wǔ wèi zǐ
Scrophularia buergeriana, Figwort, běi xuán shēn
Scutellaria barbata, Barbat Skullcap, bàn zhī lián

Field Production

At the Chinese Medicinal Herb Farm we transplant ten-week-old seedlings to one-foot spacing in a shady, well-irrigated site. A row crop cover

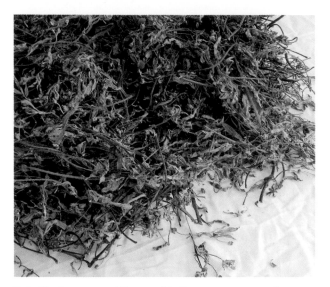

Dried leaf, stem, and flower of *Eclipta prostrata*, mò hàn lián.

can suffice for shade in a field situation and boost humidity as well. Weed to facilitate clean, quick harvests. Apply mulch to suppress weeds and keep soil moist.

Pests and Diseases
None.

Harvest and Yield
Depending on the length of the warm season, at least one and sometimes two harvests are possible. Plants are ready when they are in flower. Use gas-powered hedge shears to cut above the network of stems, many of which lie prostrate on the ground. Cut the top foot of material, leaving the network of stems to regrow for another harvest come fall. Wash and cut to manageable lengths of four to six inches and dry. Drying is quick and easy; the dried product should be green. Yield is a quarter-pound per fresh plant with potentially two harvests in a season. Ratio of fresh to dry is high for this water-loving herb, 7:1.

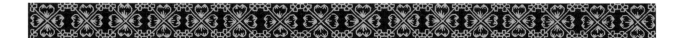

Ephedra sinica (Stapf.)
Common Name: Ephedra
Pinyin: Má huáng/Má huáng gēn
Family: Ephedraceae
Part Used: Herb, root

Plant Description
This unusual-looking but important perennial herb is a slow-growing shrub up to fifteen inches high. The bright green modified leaves are small and pointed to lessen water loss, giving the plant a look of being mostly prostrately arranged branch material. Floral cones that emerge at leaf axils or branch terminals mature in late summer into red fruits that yield two seeds each. Rare in cultivation, *Ephedra sinica* is found growing in full sun in arid regions in sandy, very well-drained soils. Endemic to northern China and Russia, *Ephedra sinica* grows in "waste and sandy places, plains, mountain slopes; 700–1600 m. Gansu, Hebei, Heilongjiang, Jilin, Liaoning, Nei Mongol, Ningxia, Shaanxi, Shanxi [Mongolia]."[87] Obviously this herb is very drought and cold tolerant. USDA hardiness zones 3–9.

Propagation
I have had my best germination results by lightly covering the seed with sand and keeping it in a heated greenhouse. Add sand to both the germination and potting mix to provide excellent drainage. If seed is of good quality, high germination rates can be expected in one week. Average water is fine while plants are young: water less frequently as the plants mature. You can also propagate ephedra by division or layering of its adventitious stems.

Garden and Polyculture Planting

If massed or allowed to expand, ephedra forms a ground cover. Surprisingly enough, it is companionable with many other plants, and with some habitat modification, it will grow well even in areas with an annual rainfall of forty inches or so. Sandy and well-drained soils are important; raised growing areas can facilitate water movement away from plants. Ephedra tolerates overhead watering as long as drainage conditions are met. Rock gardens are ideal planting areas. Plant one foot apart in moderately nutrient-deficient soil.

Suitable Companions

Astragalus membranaceus, Milk Vetch, huáng qí
Belamcanda chinensis, Blackberry Lily, shè gān
Eucommia ulmoides, Hardy Rubber Tree, dù zhòng
Lilium lancifolium, L. brownii, Lily, bǎi hé
Salvia miltiorrhiza, S. przewalskii, S. bowleyana, Red Sage, dān shēn
Saposhnikovia divaricata, Siler, fáng fēng
Scutellaria baicalensis, Baikal Skullcap, huáng qín
Withania somnifera, Ashwagandha

Ziziphus jujuba, Chinese Date, dà zǎo
Ziziphus jujuba var. *spinosa*, suān zǎo rén

Field Production

Drainage is of the utmost importance. If you can provide excellent drainage, you may be able to succeed with this herb even if your climate is not arid. Set out transplants in full sun one to two feet apart. Unamended soil should be sandy and very well drained. Ephedra is drought tolerant; do not overwater.

Pests and Diseases

None.

Harvest and Yield

Pick the foliage/stem material from August through October and remove the nodes.[88] The quality criteria for stem portions are "light green or yellowish green stems with a reddish brown center. The stems cannot be pulled apart."[89] Cut branch material into manageable lengths for drying. The root is also used; traditionally harvest time is fall or winter.[90] Roots

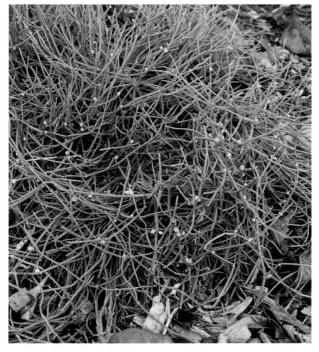

Ephedra sinica growing at the University of California Berkeley Botanical Garden.

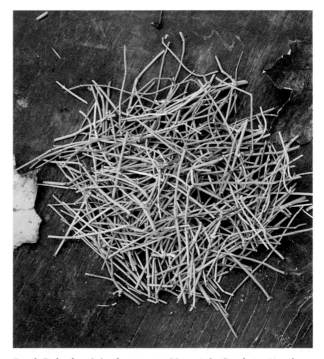

Fresh *Ephedra sinica* harvest at Mountain Gardens, North Carolina. Photo courtesy of Jean Giblette.

Medicinal Uses of Má huáng/Má huáng gēn

Má huáng is the herb or aerial portion of *Ephedra sinica*. Acrid, bitter, and warm, it releases the surface (through diaphoresis), relieves wheezing, stops cough, and regulates water circulation. It is used to address issues such as upper respiratory tract infection with chills, fever, absence of sweating, headache, body ache, and nasal congestion. It is also used to address acute wheezing due to colds with cough or other exterior causes, edema, and muscle aches and pain made worse by exposure to cold, wind, and damp.

Má huáng is usually combined with other herbs. It is usually administered by decoction; traditionally, it is decocted before other herbs and the foam that rises is removed. It is also administered by concentrated granules, tablets, and pills. Má huáng is in many well-known formulas, including Ma Huang Tang (*Ephedra* Decoction) and all of its derivative formulas, Ma Xing Gan Shi Tang (*Ephedra*, Apricot Kernel, Licorice, and Gypsum Decoction), Xiao Qing Long Tang (Minor Bluegreen Dragon Decoction), and Yue Bi Tang (Maidservant from Yue Decoction).

Traditionally má huáng is for short term use, is not used for chronic wheezing, and is never taken over long periods of time. Modern research has shown it to have a stimulating effect on the sympathetic nervous system, which may lead to adverse reactions, particularly when used inappropriately.

The root of *Ephedra sinica*, má huáng gēn, is used in TCM to stop sweating. It is interesting to note that within the same plant the root has an opposite function as the aerial portion (má huáng).

that are ruddy brown with a yellow to white interior are considered to be of good quality.[91] Plants that are three seasons old are harvestable. A grower in northern New Mexico relates a yield of three pounds fresh from a ten-by-four-foot bed, and that the crop spreads readily.

Notes

Legal restrictions apply to this herb, specifying that it can only be sold to licensed acupuncturists. *Ephedra intermedia*, *E. monosperma*, and *E. equisetina*, as well as a few other species, are also used as má huáng/má huáng gēn.

Eriobotrya japonica ([Thunb.] Lindl.)
Common Name: Loquat
Pinyin: Pí pá yè
Family: Rosaceae
Part Used: Leaf

Plant Description

Eriobotrya japonica is one of the few evergreen plants in the Chinese materia medica. A small tree growing up to twenty-five feet tall with a dense rounded crown, which also spreads up to twenty-five feet across, it has dark-green, bold, leathery leaves with prominent venation. Leaves grow ten inches long and three inches wide. The undersides of the leaves are covered with brown fuzz; topside they are smooth and shiny. Fall flowers are borne from fuzzy brown clusters and are small, white, and fragrant. The yellow to peachy-orange two-inch fruit matures in early spring. Although it's the leaves that are primarily used in Chinese medicine, the ovate fruit is edible fresh—and pieworthy to boot. This plant is native to south central China and is cultivated throughout the south of China and in southeast Asia.[92] USDA hardiness zones 7 or 8–11.

Propagation

Seeds or cuttings work well to increase stock. Fresh seed germinates readily, while seed that is older requires one to four months to sprout. Keep on the dry side; media should drain well. Cuttings are generally taken in summer; since the leaves are large, remove part of each leaf to keep the plants from transpiring to death. To do this simply cut off the top half or third of the leaf portion sticking out of the cutting flat. Loquat is a good container plant. Fertilize frequently with a diluted solution of fertilizer.

Garden and Polyculture Planting

Since loquat is very ornamental and suitable as a specimen, there are many cultivars in the nursery trade, mostly bred for fruit production. Planting in the back of the border or as a hedgerow is ideal.

Eriobotrya japonica tree with **Crataegus pinnatifida** in the foreground at the University of California Berkeley Botanical Garden.

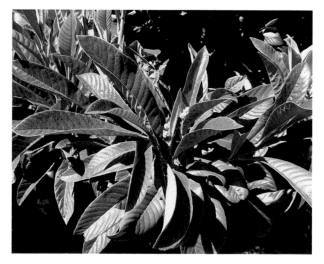

Eriobotrya japonica leaf.

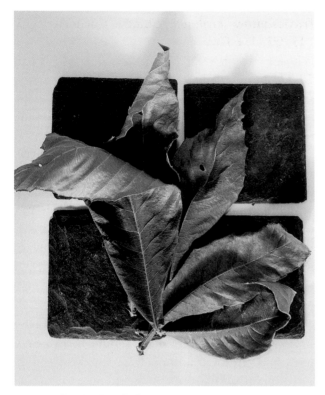

Pí pá yè, the dried leaf of *Eriobotrya japonica*. Photo by Nina Zhito.

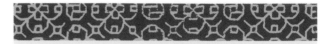

Loquat Recipes

Loquats are yellow, small, refreshing fruits with large seeds. Because they bruise easily, they are not widely available in stores, although they may be found in Asian markets. To pit, cut them in half, and the seed will easily slip out. Try them preserved or as a snack eaten fresh, add them to smoothies with bananas and orange juice, or stew them briefly in a simple sugar or honey syrup.

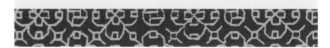

Suitable Companions

Acanthopanax gracilistylus, wǔ jiā pí
Achyranthes bidentata, Oxknee, huái niú xī
Agastache rugosa, Korean Mint, tǔ huò xiāng
Albizia julibrissin, Mimosa, hé huān pí/huā
Allium macrostemon, xiè bái
Allium tuberosum, Garlic Chives, jiǔ cài zǐ
Anemarrhena asphodeloides, zhī mǔ
Angelica dahurica, bái zhǐ
Angelica pubescens, dú huó
Aster tataricus, Tartar Aster, zǐ wǎn
Atractylodes macrocephala, Chinese Thistle Daisy, bái zhú
Belamcanda chinensis, Blackberry Lily, shè gān
Bupleurum chinense, Hare's Ear, chái hú
Carthamus tinctorius, Safflower, hóng huā
Celosia argentea, qīng xiāng zǐ
Celosia cristata, Cockscomb, jī guān huā
Chrysanthemum morifolium, Mum, jú huā
Clerodendrum trichotomum, Glorybower, chòu wú tóng

Coix lacryma-jobi, Job's Tears, yì yǐ rén
Cornus officinalis, Dogwood, shān zhū yú
Crataegus pinnatifida, Chinese Hawthorn, shān zhā
Cyathula officinalis, Hookweed, chuān niú xī
Dianthus superbus, Fringed Pink, qú mài
Dolichos lablab, Hyacinth Bean, bái biǎn dòu
Eucommia ulmoides, Hardy Rubber Tree, dù zhòng
Forsythia suspensa, lián qiào
Houttuynia cordata, yú xīng cǎo
Ligusticum jeholense, Chinese Lovage, gǎo běn
Ligustrum lucidum, Chinese Privet, nǔ zhēn zǐ
Lilium lancifolium, *L. brownii*, Lily, bǎi hé
Lonicera japonica, Honeysuckle, jīn yín huā
Lycium chinense, Chinese Wolfberry, gǒu qǐ zǐ/dì gǔ pí
Magnolia denudata, xīn yí huā
Mentha haplocalyx, Field Mint, bò hé
Momordica charantia, Bitter Melon, kǔ guā
Ocimum sanctum, Sacred Basil, Tulsi
Platycodon grandiflorus, Balloon Flower, jié gěng
Prunella vulgaris, Heal All, xià kū cǎo
Rehmannia glutinosa, Chinese Foxglove, dì huáng
Rheum palmatum, Chinese Rhubarb, dà huáng
Salvia miltiorrhiza, *S. przewalskii*, *S. bowleyana*, Red Sage, dān shēn

Medicinal Uses of Pí pá yè

Pí pá yè is the leaf of *Eriobotrya japonica*. Bitter and cool, pí pá yè dissolves phlegm, stops cough, harmonizes the stomach, and directs qi downward. It is primarily used to address coughs. Depending on what it is combined with, it may be used to address a cough with thick yellow mucus or a cough with dry sticky phlegm that is difficult to expectorate. It is sometimes also used to address nausea, vomiting, and acid regurgitation.

Pí pá yè is usually used in combination with other herbs. Common methods of administration include decoctions (with the herb usually wrapped in cheesecloth to minimize irritation from hairlike particles), syrups, concentrated granules, and pills. It is one of the primary ingredients in the widely available over-the-counter Honey Loquat Cough Syrup (Chuan Bei Pi Pa Lu).

To address coughs pí pá yè is usually prepared with honey, and to treat nausea and vomiting it is unprocessed.

Saposhnikovia divaricata, Siler, fáng fēng
Schizonepeta tenuifolia, Japanese Catnip, jīng jiè
Scutellaria baicalensis, Baikal Skullcap, huáng qín
Sophora flavescens, kǔ shēn

Trichosanthes kirilowii, Chinese Cucumber, guā lóu/tiān huā fěn
Withania somnifera, Ashwagandha
Ziziphus jujuba, Chinese Date, dà zǎo
Ziziphus jujuba var. *spinosa*, suān zǎo rén

Field Production

This is a plant for a full sun location; place in the orchard on twenty-foot spacing. Loquat is a nectar source for bees. Water at regular intervals, especially when young, and make sure soil is moderately fertile and well drained. The fruit produces well under warm conditions, and the trees are somewhat fast growing.

Pests and Diseases

Loquat is susceptible to the bacterial disease fireblight (it blackens and kills whole limbs). There are no known preventive measures.

Harvest and Yield

This is one of the few herbs that is traditionally harvested any time of the year. The best quality leaves are bright green and unbroken; sustainable leaf collection is 10–20 percent during any single year. Yields for leaf and fruit vary according to the age of the trees. Ratio of fresh to dry is 2½:1.

Notes

• This small tree is not only attractive due to its good looks, but having a dual crop adds to the interest potential.

Eucommia ulmoides (Oliv.)
Common Name: Hardy Rubber Tree
Pinyin: Dù zhòng
Family: Eucommiaceae
Part Used: Bark

Plant Description
Important to Chinese herbal medicine, this large tree stands up to sixty feet tall with an equally wide spread. Handsome grey-furrowed bark is the medicine: dù zhòng. Leaves are elliptic with serrate margins and three to four inches long; they resemble elm leaves. They have the curious distinction of producing rubbery latex threads that hold the leaves together when the leaves are slowly torn. This latex is also present in the bark. The spring flowers are insignificant but form one-inch-long samaras, winged

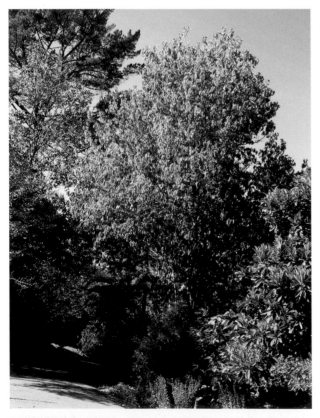

Eucommia ulmoides **growing at the University of California Berkeley Botanical Garden.**

seed-dispersing agents of the winds, not unlike those of maple trees. Endemic in lower-elevation mountains and widely cultivated in central China.[93] USDA hardiness zones 5–10.

Propagation
Hardy rubber tree is a multicycle germinator; sow seed in large flats and leave outside to stratify, or place in moist (not wet) sand and refrigerate to stratify for roughly three months. Check regularly, starting at two months, for germinating seeds; when found, plant in the nursery. Taking hardwood cuttings and replanting of root suckers initiated by root disturbance are other methods of increasing stock.[94] When growing nursery stock prune off side branches to encourage straight stems free of lower branching.

Garden and Polyculture Planting
An attractive large-scale shade tree with a rounded habit, hardy rubber tree unfortunately lacks fall color. It behaves well near sidewalks and patios; the roots do not disturb concrete. It's also a suitable street tree that tolerates air pollution and periods of drought. Plant in full sun in well-drained, fertile soil.

Suitable Companions
Codonopsis pilosula, Poor Man's Ginseng, dǎng shen
Eclipta prostrata, Eclipta, mò hàn lián
Gentiana scabra, lóng dǎn cǎo
Gentiana straminea, qín jiāo
Houttuynia cordata, yú xīng cǎo
Ligustrum lucidum, Chinese Privet, nǚ zhēn zǐ
Ophiopogon japonicus, Lilyturf, mài mén dōng

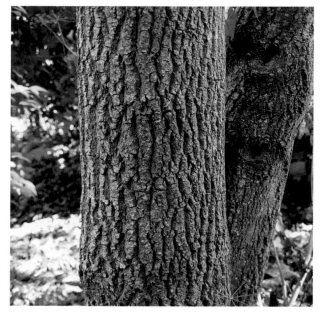

Tree bark of *Eucommia ulmoides* at the University of California Berkeley Botanical Garden.

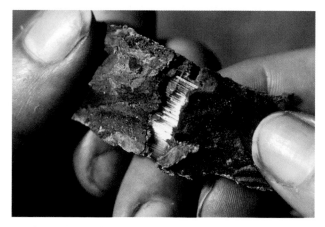

Dù zhòng, bark of the *Eucommia ulmoides* tree. Photo by Steven Foster ©2011.

Plantago asiatica, Plantain, chē qián zǐ
Schisandra chinensis, Five Flavored Fruit, wǔ wèi zǐ
Scrophularia buergeriana, Figwort, běi xuán shēn

Field Production

Good drainage is essential, but hardy rubber tree tolerates a wide spectrum of soil types. It prefers full sun and irrigation for vigorous growth in summer. Transplant three-year-old (or older) trees twenty-five feet or more apart. In preparation for harvests, continue pruning to keep the central trunk branch free.

Medicinal Uses of Dù zhòng

Dù zhòng is the bark of *Eucommia ulmoides*. Sweet and warm, dù zhòng tonifies the liver and kidney, strengthens the bones and sinews, tonifies kidney yang, and calms the fetus. It is used to address issues such as low back pain, dizziness, weakness, impotence, urinary incontinence, threatened miscarriage (when due to liver and kidney deficiency), and broken bones. In modern times its use has been expanded to include treating high blood pressure.

Dù zhòng is usually used in combination with other herbs. Common methods of administration include decoctions, concentrated granules, tablets, and pills. It is in formulas such as Du Huo Ji Sheng Tang (*Angelica pubescens* and *Loranthus* Decoction), You Gui Wan (Restore the Right Kidney Pills), San Bi Tang (Three Painful Obstructions Decoction), and Zan Yu Dan (Special Pill to Aid Fertility).

Dù zhòng is usually salt-fried to treat low back pain, impotence, and threatened miscarriage and dry-fried to treat hypertension.

Modern research has shown that the leaves of *Eucommia ulmoides*, dù zhòng yè, have the same constituents as the bark, and dù zhòng yè is beginning to be accepted as a substitute for dù zhòng.

Pests and Diseases
None.

Harvest and Yield

According to Steven Foster the bark is harvested in April or May from trees that are at least fifteen years old. In order not to girdle—and thus kill—the tree, cut strips of bark from only one side of the tree. If you let the tree heal before harvesting strips from other sections of the tree, you can rest assured that you are harvesting sustainably. After harvesting the bark, remove the outer, rough bark and dry.[95] Commercially the inner bark is scored and can be rolled or can lie in flat sheets. An indicator of good quality is a thick bark with an inner surface that is purplish-brown and, upon breaking, pieces with elastic threads connecting them together.[96]

Notes

Eucommia ulmoides is an important Chinese herb and considered a high value crop. Uncommonly it may be sold by specialty tree nurseries.

Fallopia multiflora ([Thunb.] Heraldson)
Botanical Synonym: *Polygonum multiflorum* (Thunb.)
Common name: Fo Ti
Pinyin: Shǒu wū/Yè jīao téng
Family: Polygonaceae
Part Used: Root, stem

Plant Description

Fallopia multiflora is a fast-growing and long-lived perennial; it is a hardy twining climber, vigorously growing up to thirty feet a year. The vine sports four-inch-long, light green cordate leaves and, rarely, small white or light pink flowers in panicles in the autumn. This important botanical has been widely cultivated in China and more recently in the United States. The many branching stems root wherever they touch ground: no doubt about it—this plant is invasive. When temperatures drop to about twenty degrees, the vine loses its leaves and enters dormancy. It grows throughout China except in the arid west.[97] USDA hardiness zones 5–10.

Propagation

The easiest method to increase stock is to take semi-hardwood stem cuttings in the late spring. Place them in water and they take root in about three weeks—or you can stick the cuttings in a rooting medium, such as a peat and perlite mixture, and place them on a propagation heat mat. When roots form, transplant to containers and grow out for several months until they are ready to transplant. Use bamboo stakes in pots to keep the vines separated. Because it is such a vigorous grower, fo ti frequently needs to be potted up to the next size. Spring-sown seed germinates in two weeks with the aid of a warm greenhouse or heat mat.

Garden and Polyculture Planting

Fo ti is not a community-minded plant; it tends to smother everything in its path. I only mention it as it is commonly available—and it is an important medicinal herb. Its long stems run and climb;

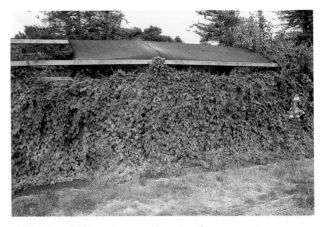
Fallopia multiflora **vine growing on a fence.**

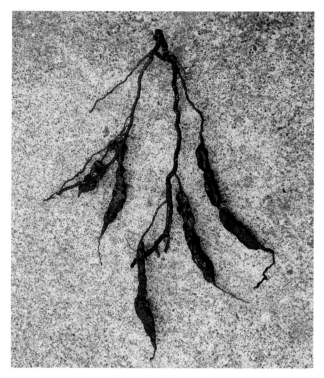

Three-foot-long roots grow straight down and are representational of this species' root growth pattern.

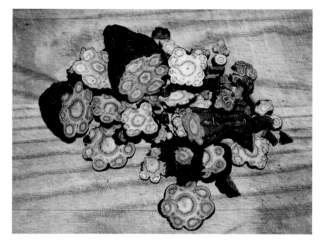

Fallopia multiflora **roots have a beautiful flowerlike pattern when sliced.**

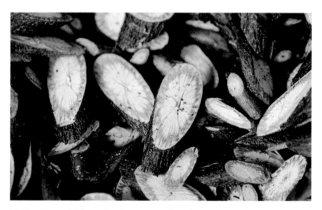

Fallopia multiflora **fresh stems sliced on an angle and ready to dry.**

any stems on the ground will take root, creating a massive vine patch. To control this plant, trellis it and cut back running stems. If grown against a building it will grow underneath it and out the other side, travelling long distances; it will also grow through buildings and into roof shingles. Fo ti is hard to eradicate once established.

Suitable Companions

None.

Field Production

Fo ti enjoys a full sun situation, but in hot climates part shade is recommended. It is tolerant of diverse soil types, even fairly wet winter clay, but prefers a moist fertile soil amended with organic matter. Sandy soil makes for easier root harvesting. Transplant onto two- or three-foot centers; trellis for support and to keep the runners off the ground. Placing landscape fabric around the row facilitates stem control. Fo ti can produce roots from the leaf axils far from the mother plant, so keep an eye out. If the stems root

they draw energy away from the main tuber and make for a poorer quality herb.

Pests and Diseases

Fo ti growing in containers experiences the occasional attack of spring aphids.

Harvest and Yield

Harvest the roots in the autumn after three or more years of growth. Larger roots are valued more than smaller. The stems are usually harvested in the winter or fall after a few years' growth, when they have a woody bark and are at least the thickness of a pencil. Stems tend to fall to the ground and root; these are not shǒu wū tubers. The true tubers are swollen and yamlike and can be found as deep as three feet

Medicinal Uses of Shǒu wū/Yè jīao téng

Shǒu wū is the root of *Fallopia multiflora*. Sweet, bitter, astringent, and slightly warm, it replenishes the jing (essences), nourishes the blood, tonifies the liver and kidney, moistens the intestines, unblocks the bowels, eliminates toxins, and addresses malarial disorders. Shǒu wū is one of the most commonly used tonics and is especially well known for treating signs of early aging such as prematurely grey hair, blurred vision, ringing in the ears, fatigue, infertility, dizziness, and weakness of the lower back and knees. It is also used to address anemia, abnormal uterine bleeding, irregular menstruation, dry stools, and constipation. In its unprocessed form it is used to address abscesses, goiter, swellings and nodules, and malarial disorders. Its use has recently been expanded to address cardiovascular disorders such as high cholesterol, angina, and high blood pressure.

Shǒu wū is used as an individual herb and in combination with other herbs. Common methods of administration include decoctions, alcohol extracts, syrups, powders, concentrated granules, tablets, and pills. It is in the formula Qi Bao Mei Ran Dan (Seven Treasures Special Pill for Beautiful Whiskers).

When used for its nourishing functions, the raw root is usually processed by steaming with black bean juice. When unprocessed it is primarily used for eliminating toxins, treating malarial disorders, and promoting bowel movement. The recent cardiovascular applications typically mix both processed and unprocessed shǒu wū.

The vine of *Fallopia multiflora*, yè jīao téng, is also used in TCM. Sweet, slightly bitter, and neutral it nourishes the heart, calms the shen, opens the channels, and dispels wind. It is a gentle herb that is primarily used for blood deficiency causing insomnia, soreness, and numbness and tingling in the extremities.

---

down. The aboveground stem grows down to root to tuber to a tendril of a root, then to tuber again—kind of like swimming pool rope and float lane dividers. Having said that, I also must say that I've heard reports of—and alas have also experienced the frustration of—finding no tubers, even after many years' growth and much excavation.

Both roots and stems are sliced crosswise and dried. Pruning saws are handy for this task. Both root and stem display a radiating pattern from the center outward. Desirable roots are large, dense, and reddish-brown, but not fibrous or pithy. Good quality stem material should have brown crackled bark and be thick and uniform.[98] The yield for three-year roots is two to five pounds per plant fresh; for stem it is four to six pounds per plant fresh. Root weight ratio of fresh to dry is 3:1; stem ratio of fresh to dry is 4:1.

Notes
- It is economically handy to have one plant that produces two herbs. Even though shǒu wū is the more important Chinese botanical, there is a market for yè jīao téng as well.
- Roots are not often used raw and should be further processed.

Forsythia suspensa ([Thunb.] Vahl)
Common Name: None
Pinyin: Lián qiào
Family: Oleaceae
Part Used: Fruit

Plant Description

Forsythia suspensa is an important herb in the Chinese materia medica, and is a close relative of a common hedge plant in the eastern United States, *Forsythia × intermedia* (border forsythia). *Forsythia suspensa* is a densely branching deciduous shrub growing eight to ten feet tall with arching branches that root where they touch ground. Stem and seed capsules are stippled with lenticels (openings for gas exchange). This shrub can be invasive, creating dense expanding thickets. Simple ellipticovate medium-green leaves that are three inches long sit opposite each other on the stem. Flowers are borne in the leaf axils before foliage leafs out in early spring. Showy golden yellow bells are three-quarters of an inch long, eventually becoming green pointed seed capsules one inch long that mature to brown by early fall. In China *Forsythia suspensa* grows from central to eastern China in moist grassy areas from 1,000–7,000 feet in elevation.[99] USDA hardiness zones 5–9.

Propagation

Seeds, cuttings, and layering are good methods of increasing stock. Seed, of course, yields the most genetic diversity and thus is the most desirable method. Sow seed in the fall in a deep flat and let winter stratify it for germination in the spring. Alternately cold stratify in the refrigerator for one month and sow in deep flats; this way germination occurs in two to three weeks. Warm soils are not necessary for germination to take place. Stem cuttings taken from May through September generally have a high rate of success. Layering just happens—especially if you don't want it to! When branches touch the soil, roots form, and voila!—a new plant is born . . . and real estate is lost. *Forsythia suspensa* holds relatively well as container stock.

Garden and Polyculture Planting

If you need an attractive large-scale groundcover or hillside erosion-control, this is your ticket, as long as it has defensible boundaries. You can also espalier this *Forsythia* against a fence or wall. Plant in full sun in the hedgerow as it may be too ungainly for the garden. Use control techniques as described in the Field Production section. There are many suitable companions for *Forsythia suspensa*, assuming it is managed to prevent its thicket-forming qualities; otherwise it is too aggressive except with trees. Flowering branches make good floral material.

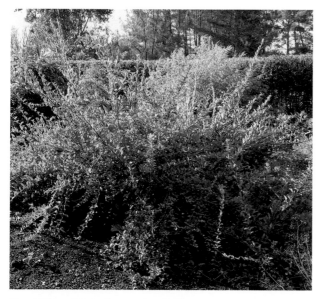

***Forsythia suspensa* in summer leaf.**

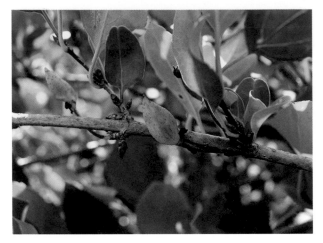

Young fruit of *Forsythia suspensa* on stem.

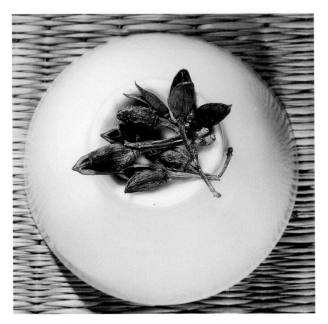

**Mature fruit of Forsythia suspensa, lián qiào.
Photo by Nina Zhito.**

Suitable Companions

Acanthopanax gracilistylus, wŭ jiā pí
Achyranthes bidentata, Oxknee, huái niú xī
Agastache rugosa, Korean Mint, tŭ huò xiāng
Albizia julibrissin, Mimosa, hé huān pí/huā
Angelica dahurica, bái zhĭ
Angelica pubescens, dú huó
Aster tataricus, Tartar Aster, zĭ wăn
Belamcanda chinensis, Blackberry Lily, shè gān
Celosia argentea, qīng xiāng zĭ
Celosia cristata, Cockscomb, jī guān huā
Chrysanthemum morifolium, Mum, jú huā
Clerodendrum trichotomum, Glorybower, chòu wú tóng
Cornus officinalis, Dogwood, shān zhū yú
Crataegus pinnatifida, Chinese Hawthorn, shān zhā
Cyathula officinalis, Hookweed, chuān niú xī
Dianthus superbus, Fringed Pink, qú mài
Dolichos lablab, Hyacinth Bean, bái biăn dòu
Eriobotrya japonica, Loquat, pí pá yè
Eucommia ulmoides, Hardy Rubber Tree, dù zhòng
Ginkgo biloba, Ginkgo, bái guŏ
Houttuynia cordata, yú xīng căo
Ligusticum jeholense, Chinese Lovage, găo běn
Ligustrum lucidum, Chinese Privet, nŭ zhēn zĭ
Lilium lancifolium, *L. brownii*, Lily, băi hé
Lonicera japonica, Honeysuckle, jīn yín huā
Lycium chinense, Chinese Wolfberry, gŏu qĭ zĭ, dì gŭ pí
Magnolia denudata, xīn yí huā
Mentha haplocalyx, Field Mint, bò hé
Momordica charantia, Bitter Melon, kŭ guā
Ocimum sanctum, Sacred Basil, Tulsi
Platycodon grandiflorus, Balloon Flower, jié gěng
Prunella vulgaris, Heal All, xià kū căo
Rehmannia glutinosa, Chinese Foxglove, dì huáng
Rheum palmatum, Chinese Rhubarb, dà huáng
Salvia miltiorrhiza, *S. przewalskii*, *S. bowleyana*, Red Sage, dān shēn
Saposhnikovia divaricata, Siler, fáng fēng
Schizonepeta tenuifolia, Japanese Catnip, jīng jiè
Scrophularia buergeriana, Figwort, běi xuán shēn
Scutellaria baicalensis, Baikal Skullcap, huáng qín
Sophora flavescens, kŭ shēn
Trichosanthes kirilowii, Chinese Cucumber, guā lóu/tiān huā fěn

Field Production

Transplant *Forsythia suspensa* in full sun, on six-to eight-foot spacing, in well-drained moist soils, and provide drip irrigation (overhead irrigation or summer rainfall provides optimal rooting opportunities for branches). Prune lower limbs while dormant to keep branches up off the soil; this will keep them from expanding their territory. Another method to keep plants in bounds is to surround them with landscape fabric and deny them soil access. *Forsythia suspensa* tolerates a wide range of soil types. For fruit production (the goal being the seed capsule) it may be necessary to plant several different plants, not clones with the same genetics.

Pests and Diseases

Deer resistant.

Harvest and Yield

Fruit production occurs in plants that are roughly five years old. Green as well as brown (mature) fruiting capsules are utilized as lián qiào, with the brown capsule considered superior. Check on the crop in late August and pick ripe fruits by hand. Further dry them; the ideal moisture content is 10 percent. The best quality lián qiào is considered to be "thick, clean fruit without seeds."[100] After the shrubs reach fruiting age, the amount of available herb probably will not be the limiting factor. That distinction will go to the time it takes to harvest any amount of crop, as they are hand-picked one or two at a time—that is slow going, and they are lightweight. Consideration of the importance of the crop will come into play with this essential herb. Yield varies greatly with the age of the stock.

Notes

There are several named cultivars of *Forsythia suspensa* that are in the nursery trade; for medicinal purposes choose the original unnamed species.

Medicinal Uses of Lián qiào

Lián qiào is the fruit of *Forsythia suspensa*. Bitter and cool, it clears heat and eliminates toxins. In addition, it is used to address a variety of heat disorders, including external wind heat, interior heat affecting the heart, heat at the ying level, and hot type lin (painful urination syndrome). It is one of the most commonly used herbs for addressing upper respiratory tract infections with sore throat, cough, and fever, as well as being used for issues such as skin sores, lesions, abscesses, nodules, and painful urination with burning.

Lián qiào is usually used in combination with other herbs. Common methods of administration include decoctions, powders, concentrated granules, alcohol extracts, tablets, and pills. It is a key ingredient in the widely used formula Yin Qiao San (*Lonicera* and *Forsythia* Powder) as well as formulas such as Sang Ju Yin (Mulberry Leaf and Chrysanthemum Decoction), Bao He Wan (Restore Harmony Pills), Gan Lu Xiao Du Dan (Sweet Dew Special Pill to Eliminate Toxins), and Pu Ji Xiao Du Yin (Universal Benefit Decoction to Eliminate Toxin).

Gentiana scabra (Bge.)

Medicinal Synonym: *Gentiana manshurica* (Kitag.)
Common Name: None
Pinyin: Lóng dǎn cǎo
Family: Gentianaceae
Part Used: Root

Plant Description

This is one of the more robust Gentians, exhibiting the classic outrageous blue flowers, and is a must-have for northern growers and others in locations without summer heat. *Gentiana scabra* is herbaceous and perennial to one foot tall. Leathery six-inch-long lanceolate foliage is shiny and dark green on top and pale green and dull below; leaves attach directly to erect stems without a petiole or leaf stalk. Campanulalike flowers are usually dark blue and frequently spotted (but sometimes not, as in the striking blue specimen shown in the photograph below). Corollas are 1½ inches long by ¾ inch across each, clustered terminally or off leaf axils lower on the stalk. Bloom and seed formation occur summer through fall, with seed maturing in late fall. It grows endemically in northern and eastern China as well as Japan, Korea, and eastern Russia.[101] USDA hardiness zones 5–9.

Gentiana scabra; **one of the most bitter of roots has one of the sweetest flowers.**

Propagation

Not surprisingly, *Gentiana scabra* is a cool-soil germinator. Rust-colored seeds are very tiny; sow them with just a thin cover of media in fall to early spring in deep flats. Place fall-sown flats outside for winter weather to naturally stratify the seed, and expect germination in the spring. If the seed is not fresh, be sure to stratify it; seed viability may not be long. Use very well-draining media but do not allow the soil to dry out. Transplant very carefully, and avoid handling or disturbing the new roots. *Gentiana scabra* holds very well in pots. Give minimal water while winter dormant.

Garden and Polyculture Planting

Gentiana scabra has an amazing flower so saturated with blue that it doesn't seem real. The plant prefers cool sites in cool climes and does not tolerate heat well; avoid placing in hot exposures. Plant one foot apart (carefully, as the roots resent disturbance) in sun to part shade and water regularly during the summer. Place toward the front of the border; it is a good plant for rock gardens.

Suitable Companions

Acanthopanax gracilistylus, wǔ jiā pí
Anemarrhena asphodeloides, zhī mǔ
Angelica dahurica, bái zhǐ
Angelica pubescens, dú huó
Asparagus cochinchinensis, tiān mén dōng
Bupleurum chinense, Hare's Ear, chái hú
Codonopsis pilosula, Poor Man's Ginseng, dǎng shēn

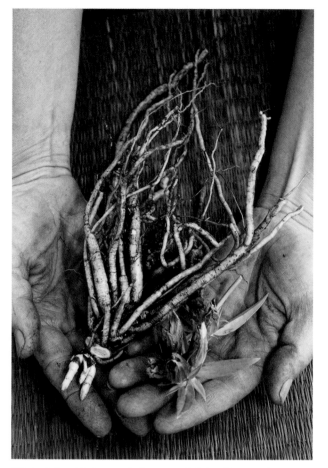

Winter's freshly harvested root and dying flower of *Gentiana scabra*. Photo by Nina Zhito.

Medicinal Uses of Lóng dǎn cǎo

Lóng dǎn cǎo is the root of *Gentiana scabra*. Bitter and cold, it clears heat, dries dampness, and sedates liver fire. It is one of the most important herbs for treating damp heat in the liver and gallbladder and their associated channels and for clearing liver fire. It is used to address issues such as redness and irritation of the eyes, tinnitus, headaches, constipation, jaundice, eczema, skin rashes, sores around the genitals, pain under the ribs, infectious hepatitis, and sexually transmitted diseases.

Lóng dǎn cǎo is usually used in combination with other herbs. It is used both internally and externally. Externally it is generally applied as a powder or paste in the treatment of skin conditions. Common methods of administration include decoctions, powders, concentrated granules, tablets, and pills. It is the chief herb in the formula Long Dan Xie Gan Tang (*Gentiana*, Drain the Liver Decoction).

Cornus officinalis, Dogwood, shān zhū yú
Crataegus pinnatifida, Chinese Hawthorn, shān zhā
Eucommia ulmoides, Hardy Rubber Tree, dù zhòng
Gentiana straminea, qín jiāo
Ginkgo biloba, Ginkgo, bái guǒ
Gynostemma pentaphyllum, Sweet Tea Vine, jiǎo gǔ lán
Lilium lancifolium, *L. brownii*, Lily, bǎi hé
Magnolia denudata, xīn yí huā
Paeonia lactiflora, Chinese Peony, bái/chì sháo
Paeonia suffruticosa, Tree Peony, mǔ dān pí
Pinellia ternata, bàn xià
Rheum palmatum, Chinese Rhubarb, dà huáng
Saposhnikovia divaricata, Siler, fáng fēng
Schisandra chinensis, Five Flavored Fruit, wǔ wèi zǐ
Scrophularia buergeriana, Figwort, běi xuán shēn

Field Production

Transplant one-season-old *Gentiana scabra* in part shade or full sun on one-foot spacing in moist but freely draining soil. Take care while planting, because of the roots' sensitivity. Deeply irrigate in summer at even time intervals; these plants are not considered drought tolerant. However, they are durable once established.

Pests and Diseases

None.

Harvest and Yield

Harvest light yellow roots that are at least four years old; they should be one foot or more long. The traditional time to lift the roots is when the plants are dormant in fall or early spring. The flavor is an intensely clear bitter taste. Wash and dry them whole; they will dry to a darker yellow. The best quality of lóng dǎn cǎo is said to be "thick, full, long, straight roots. The texture should be soft, the color yellow, and the taste extremely bitter."[102] Yield for fresh four-year-old root is a quarter-pound per plant. Ratio of fresh to dry is 2:1.

Notes

Gentiana crassa subsp. *rigescens* is another standard herb used as lóng dǎn cǎo. Its origins are in southern China, and it may be more heat tolerant in warmer climates; however, the seed does not currently appear to be on the market.

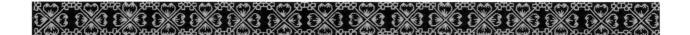

Gentiana straminea (Maxim.)
Common Name: None
Pinyin: Qín jiāo
Family: Gentianaceae
Part Used: Root

Plant Description

It seems that everyone has something to say about gentians; it just happens that they're all something different. "Needing perfect drainage"[103] says one source; another, "readers may be surprised to learn that . . . Gentians occupy distinctly marshy conditions in nature."[104] But their beauty alone should inspire cultivators to do their bidding. Growing from 1–1½ feet tall, foliage being the first foot and flowers the rest, the basal leaves of this herbaceous perennial are lanceolate and parallel veined. Rigid flower stalks are branched and terminate in clusters of white flowers that are finely spotted with green inside the flaring corolla. Bloom time is late summer, and light brown seed is set in late autumn. *Gentiana straminea* is native along rocky stream banks, in alpine meadows, and in forest areas in the western high altitude mountains of China and Nepal from 6,000–14,000 feet in elevation.[105] Very hardy; USDA hardiness zones 3–9.

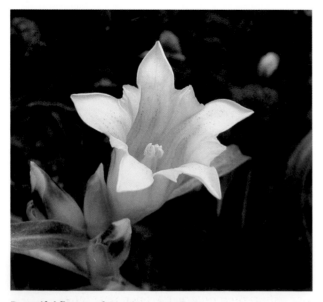

Beautiful flower of *Gentiana straminea*.

Propagation

I sow the small seeds in deep flats in fall and leave them to winter's devices to naturally stratify. Alternately you can place the seed in the refrigerator for one to two months to stratify and then sow it in the nursery in deep flats. Use very well-draining media but do not allow the soil to dry out, and expect germination in spring. Transplant very carefully, and avoid handling or disturbing the new roots. *Gentiana straminea*

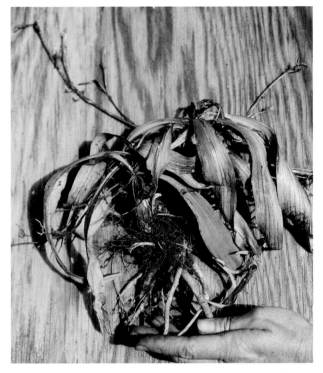

Late fall whole plant sample of *Gentiana straminea*. Photo by Nina Zhito.

holds very well in pots. Give it minimal water while winter dormant.

Garden and Polyculture Planting

All gentians prefer cool climates and a slightly acidic soil that drains well. Plant these beauties eight inches apart (carefully, as the roots resent disturbance) in part shade, and supply irrigation. Placement in the front of the border or under tree cover works well; it is a good plant for rock gardens. *Gentiana straminea* is a slow grower and will not thrive where summers are hot.

Suitable Companions

Acanthopanax gracilistylus, wǔ jiā pí
Anemarrhena asphodeloides, zhī mǔ
Angelica dahurica, bái zhǐ
Angelica pubescens, dú huó
Asparagus cochinchinensis, tiān mén dōng
Bupleurum chinense, Hare's Ear, chái hú
Codonopsis pilosula, Poor Man's Ginseng, dǎng shēn
Cornus officinalis, Dogwood, shān zhū yú

Medicinal Uses of Qín jiāo

Qín jiāo is the root of *Gentiana straminea*. Bitter, acrid, and cool, qín jiāo dispels wind damp, opens the channels, relaxes the sinews, clears deficiency heat, and has secondary functions of clearing damp heat jaundice. It is an important herb for treating bi (painful obstruction) syndrome. It is used to address issues such as chronic and acute joint and musculoskeletal pain, stiffness and tightness of the joints, paralysis, poststroke complications, night sweats, afternoon fever, steaming bone sensations, and jaundice.

Qín jiāo is usually used in combination with other herbs. Common methods of administration include decoctions, powders, concentrated granules, tablets, and pills. It is in formulas such as Da Qin Jiao Tang (Major *Gentiana* Decoction), Du Huo Ji Sheng Tang (*Angelica pubescens* and *Loranthus* Decoction), Juan Bi Tang (Remove Painful Obstruction Decoction), and Shen Tong Zhu Yu Tang (Eliminate Stasis from a Painful Body Decoction).

Crataegus pinnatifida, Chinese Hawthorn, shān zhā
Eucommia ulmoides, Hardy Rubber Tree, dù zhòng
Gentiana scabra, lóng dǎn cǎo
Ginkgo biloba, Ginkgo, bái guǒ
Gynostemma pentaphyllum, Sweet Tea Vine, jiāo gǔ lán
Lilium lancifolium, *L. brownii*, Lily, bǎi hé
Magnolia denudata, xīn yí huā
Paeonia lactiflora, Chinese Peony, bái/chì sháo
Paeonia suffruticosa, Tree Peony, mǔ dān pí
Pinellia ternata, bàn xià
Rheum palmatum, Chinese Rhubarb, dà huáng
Saposhnikovia divaricata, Siler, fáng fēng

Schisandra chinensis, Five Flavored Fruit, wǔ wèi zǐ
Scrophularia buergeriana, Figwort, běi xuán shēn

Field Production

Grow *Gentiana straminea* in part shade or full sun on eight-inch spacing in freely draining soil. Deeply irrigate at even time intervals; they are not considered drought tolerant. However, they are tough and durable once established.

Pests and Diseases

None.

Harvest and Yield

Harvest the barkless white roots in fall or early spring. Good quality is said to be "of large, solid, and heavy roots that are aromatic."[106] Large is a relative term here: roots from China or the United States are hard to see as "large." Indeed, they are quite aromatic, and bitter as the day is long, too (which is good, as that is part of their function). Roots grow slowly—all I can say is that it is years to harvest. In my experience, the root weight for a five-year-old plant is a mere quarter-pound fresh weight.

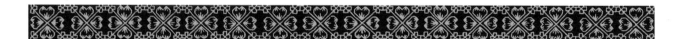

Ginkgo biloba (L.)
Common Name: Ginkgo
Pinyin: Bái guǒ
Family: Ginkgoaceae
Part Used: Seed, Leaf

Plant Description

A prehistoric relic tree of legend and lore, *Ginkgo biloba* once grew the world around, then was found only in China, and now it grows the world around—again! Deciduous fan-shaped leaves, oftentimes partially split on the outside margin, adorn columnar to spreading trees growing slowly to more or less sixty feet tall. Trees are dioecious; females produce a malodorous fruit and males provide DNA and leaves. Bark is a greyish brown, exhibiting bark fissures along the length of the trunk. These slow growing trees are very rare in the wild but are widely cultivated. USDA hardiness zones 3–10.

Propagation

Seed must be fresh; remove any flesh that may still be clinging onto the seed. Stratify by sowing one inch deep in deep nursery flats in fall and leave the flats exposed to the winter elements. It is also easy to stratify the seed in the refrigerator for one to two months and plant in the early spring. Germination occurs in one to two months. Semihardwood cuttings taken in summer are another method of propagation. There are many named cultivars offered as planting stock in the nursery trade; avoid them as they are all males and will not produce any fruit.

Garden and Polyculture Planting

Graceful while winter dormant or in leaf, Ginkgo is especially nice in fall when the green leaves turn to gold, making it eminently ornamental. Ginkgo is adaptable to many soil types and growing conditions, but provide water especially when the trees are young. Flowers are unisexual; for fruit production both sexes must be present. Companionable in the garden, landscape, and hedgerow, and a popular street tree, Ginkgo tolerates air pollution.

Suitable Companions

Agastache rugosa, Korean Mint, tǔ huò xiāng
Albizia julibrissin, Mimosa, hé huān pí/huā
Allium macrostemon, xiè bái

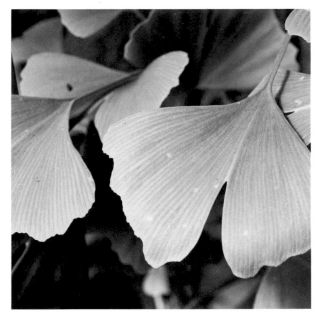

***Ginkgo biloba* leaf.**

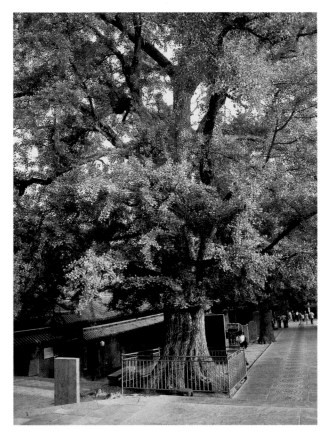

Ancient *Ginkgo biloba* tree at the Shaolin Temple at Song Shan, China.

Allium tuberosum, Garlic Chives, jiǔ cài zǐ

Anemarrhena asphodeloides, zhī mǔ

Angelica dahurica, bái zhǐ

Angelica pubescens, dú huó

Asparagus cochinchinensis, tiān mén dōng

Aster tataricus, Tartar Aster, zǐ wǎn

Atractylodes macrocephala, Chinese Thistle Daisy, bái zhú

Bacopa monnieri, Brahmi

Belamcanda chinensis, Blackberry Lily, shè gān

Bupleurum chinense, Hare's Ear, chái hú

Carthamus tinctorius, Safflower, hóng huā

Celosia argentea, qīng xiāng zǐ

Celosia cristata, Cockscomb, jī guān huā

Chrysanthemum morifolium, Mum, jú huā

Clerodendrum trichotomum, Glorybower, chòu wú tóng

Codonopsis pilosula, Poor Man's Ginseng, dǎng shēn

Cornus officinalis, Dogwood, shān zhū yú

Crataegus pinnatifida, Chinese Hawthorn, shān zhā

Dianthus superbus, Fringed Pink, qú mài

Eclipta prostrata, Eclipta, mò hàn lián

Eriobotrya japonica, Loquat, pí pá yè

Eucommia ulmoides, Hardy Rubber Tree, dù zhòng

Forsythia suspensa, lián qiào

Gentiana scabra, lóng dǎn cǎo

Gentiana straminea, qín jiāo

Gynostemma pentaphyllum, Sweet Tea Vine, jiǎo gǔ lán

Houttuynia cordata, yú xīng cǎo

Ligusticum jeholense, Chinese Lovage, gǎo běn

Ligustrum lucidum, Chinese Privet, nǚ zhēn zǐ

Lilium lancifolium, *L. brownii*, Lily, bǎi hé

Lonicera japonica, Honeysuckle, jīn yín huā

Lycium chinense, Chinese Wolfberry, gǒu qǐ zǐ/dì gǔ pí

Magnolia denudata, xīn yí huā

Mentha haplocalyx, Field Mint, bò hé

Ocimum sanctum, Sacred Basil, Tulsi

Ophiopogon japonicus, Lilyturf, mài mén dōng

Paeonia lactiflora, Chinese Peony, bái/chì sháo

Paeonia suffruticosa, Tree Peony, mǔ dān pí

Pinellia ternata, bàn xià

Plantago asiatica, Plantain, chē qián zǐ

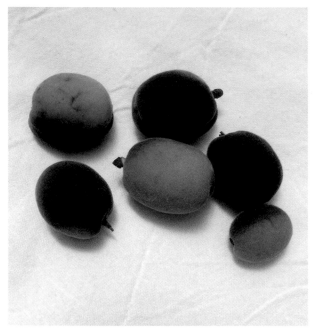

Fresh *Ginkgo biloba* fruit.

Platycodon grandiflorus, Balloon Flower, jié gěng
Prunella vulgaris, Heal All, xià kū cǎo
Rehmannia glutinosa, Chinese Foxglove, dì huáng
Rheum palmatum, Chinese Rhubarb, dà huáng
Salvia miltiorrhiza, *S. przewalskii*, *S. bowleyana*,
  Red Sage, dān shēn
Saposhnikovia divaricata, Siler, fáng fēng
Schisandra chinensis, Five Flavored Fruit, wǔ wèi zǐ
Schizonepeta tenuifolia, Japanese Catnip, jīng jiè
Scrophularia buergeriana, Figwort, běi xuán shēn
Scutellaria baicalensis, Baikal Skullcap, huáng qín
Scutellaria barbata, Barbat Skullcap, bàn zhī lián
Sophora flavescens, kǔ shēn
Withania somnifera, Ashwagandha

Field Production
Ginkgo is generally a carefree grower, managing well in acid and alkaline soils. It is drought-tolerant once established. Well-drained soil of average fertility is best. Spacing is variable depending on harvesting methodology and the resulting pruning techniques used.

Pests and Diseases
Gophers will eat the roots.

Medicinal Uses of Bái guǒ

Bái guǒ is the seed of *Ginkgo biloba*. Sweet, bitter, astringent, and neutral, it stops wheezing, dispels phlegm, and restrains leakage of fluids from the lower body. It is an important herb for treating asthma due to lung qi deficiency, phlegm, or heat and addresses issues such as wheezing, shortness of breath, cough, rapid breathing with phlegm, loss of voice, vaginal discharge, and cloudy urine.

Bái guǒ is usually used in combination with other herbs. Common methods of administration include decoctions, powders, concentrated granules, tablets, and pills. It is in formulas such as Ding Chuan Tang (Arrest Wheezing Decoction) and Yi Huang Tang (Change Yellow Decoction).

In order to reduce its mild toxicity, bái guǒ is usually processed by dry-frying before use.

The leaf of *Ginkgo biloba* (bái guǒ yè) is sometimes used in Chinese herbal medicine to relieve wheezing and shortness of breath and to improve the circulation. Some modern applications of yin gou ye include angina, high blood pressure, and high cholesterol. Although ginkgo leaf is quite popular as an over-the-counter dietary supplement for memory enhancement, it is not generally used for that purpose in TCM.

Harvest and Yield
Collect ripe fruits in fall from the tree (or collect the recently fallen fruit). "The best time to harvest *Ginkgo* seeds is around Thanksgiving. At this time the weather has softened the fleshy outer seed coat to such a degree that a slight pressure applied to the seed would separate the juicy smelly portion from the inner white hard cover. This fleshy portion . . . may

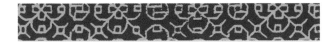

Ginkgo Recipes

The nuts from this tree are harvested in the fall. After removing the pulpy odiferous fruit (using gloves), gently crack the outer shell of the fresh nuts to uncover the kernel inside. Like almonds, the brown skin of the nut can be peeled off after a brief blanching in boiling water. Try toasting the nuts briefly in oil flavored with curry powder as a snack or toast them, chop them, and sprinkle a small portion on top of a noodle dish as you would peanuts. Be aware they have a slight bitter flavor, and some people are sensitive to them. Eat only small portions at any one time.

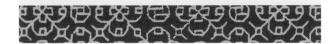

cause contact dermatitis in some people."[107] Wear gloves when harvesting and handling Ginkgo fruit. The best quality is said to be comparatively large, white, heavy nuts.[108] The shell is removed before use; however, some processing takes place at the pharmacy, and the nuts with white shells are delivered intact.[109] For the Western herb trade, the leaves are the marketable crop; collect leaves in fall when they are turning from green to gold. Drying is easy and should be uneventful.

Notes

- The Western herb trade in leaf and Chinese trade in nuts offer dual market opportunities.
- Some people may experience toxic side effects if too many Ginkgo nuts are consumed.
- Due to fruit odor, think twice before planting near a neighbor's fence line.

Glycyrrhiza uralensis (Fisch.)
Common Name: Chinese Licorice
Pinyin: Gān cǎo
Family: Fabaceae
Part Used: Root

Plant Description

This important Chinese medicinal blooms in summer, producing light purplish pealike flowers in spikes up to three feet tall. *Glycyrrhiza uralensis* is a deciduous perennial with pinnate leaves up to eight inches long. The ropy, three-foot-long rhizomes are many-branched and persistent; in some areas it is considered invasive. The very sweet tasting roots are grown for four years before harvesting. In the second or subsequent years they can send up shoots from distal points. Consider this a cold hardy perennial,

as it grows as far north as Mongolia. USDA hardiness zones 3–10.

Propagation

Sow seed in spring, or divide rhizomes in spring or fall. If using seed, direct sow or assist germination by scarifying the hard seed coat with sandpaper or soaking overnight in water. As it is calcium-loving, add calcium to the germination mix. Seeds have ongoing germination, ranging from five days to four or more weeks. For the rhizome cuttings cut so that there are

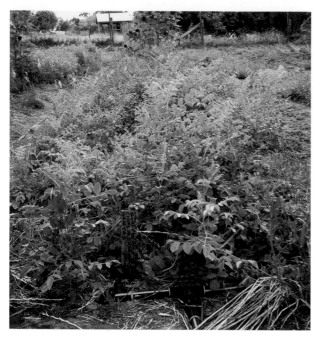

Two-year-old *Glycyrrhiza uralensis*.

two buds, or eyes, on each piece of root, and replant them. Take care not to overwater potted stock.

Garden and Polyculture Planting

Chinese licorice has stolons that run around the garden intermingling with other plants; this makes harvest difficult. You might have to dig up other plants to obtain the roots. You can try to control it with some degree of effectiveness by taking a shovel to sprouting runners, but these are not old enough to be suitable as medicine (although they do have food applications). This is one herb best grown by itself in a block area.

Suitable Companions

None.

Field Production

Chinese licorice is a four-year crop most easily grown by transplanting in the spring in full sun on one- to two-foot spacing into blocks rather than rows. Provide supplemental irrigation if needed; plants are somewhat drought tolerant. This genus has a reputation for liking alkaline soil, but it also grows successfully—and makes good medicine—in slightly acid

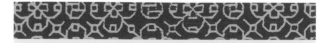

Chinese Licorice Recipes

Chinese licorice belongs to the Fabaceae or legume family, which is the family of plants that supplies all the naturally derived licorice used in candies and confections. Naturally sweet, the dried slices of Chinese licorice roots are often brewed with ginseng to make a healing tea. Although delicious it is for occasional use only; Chinese licorice should not be consumed on a continual basis.

Licorice Root and Ginseng Tea

   1 cup ginseng roots
   ½ cup dried Chinese licorice roots

Place the roots in a teapot, and fill with boiling water. Let steep for eight to ten minutes. Continue to refresh the pot with boiling water until the tea seems too weak.

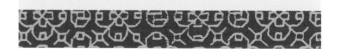

soil. Whatever the type of soil, it should be at least somewhat well drained; fertilizer requirements are low. Slow to break dormancy in the spring, Chinese licorice emerges around April in northern California. The runners sometimes pop up twelve feet from the crown, making rows superfluous. Since this important medicinal can be invasive, plant the blocks in areas that are surrounded by an open margin of at least twenty feet. This will enable a tractor-mounted chisel to cut deep enough to control the runners. You can also try rototilling stolons that are making a run for it. The main taproots grow up to three feet deep but the runners tend to be shallower. It is a persistent plant and may win the test of wills, so an initial block setup planting and strong boundary control may be the key to managing this crop.

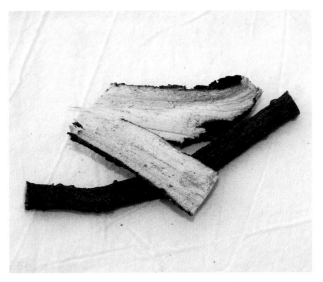

Gān cǎo, the dry roots of _Glycyrrhiza uralensis._

Pests and Diseases
None.

Harvest and Yield
Dig roots in the spring or fall of their third or fourth year while they are dormant. Just outside the harvest area dig a three-cubic-foot hole, get in, and dig laterally to unearth all the roots—or dig between the rows in the block and leave the crowns of the original plants if the bed is to remain in production. Rest assured that the side roots will regrow. A power washer is an effective tool for cleaning the roots. Cut roots of a quarter-inch or less on a diagonal to dry. Good quality roots should be heavy and light yellow inside with a thin reddish brown bark and a sweet taste. Dark brown to black root bark with a dark interior and bitter taste is not suitable as gān cǎo.[110] Since the peeled roots are considered to be of superior quality, the use of a power washer will facilitate this. Four-year roots yield 0.8 pounds per plant fresh. Fresh to dry ratio is 2:1.

Notes
Even though Chinese licorice is known to be invasive in many regions, efforts should be made to responsibly cultivate it, where appropriate, because gān cǎo is such an important herb to Chinese traditional medicine.

Medicinal Uses of Gān cǎo

Gān cǎo is the root of _Glycyrrhiza uralensis._ It is one of the most widely used herbs in TCM. Sweet (gān cǎo literally means "Sweet Herb") and neutral, it tonifies the spleen, benefits the qi, moistens the lung, stops cough, relieves spasm and pain, treats poisoning, clears heat toxins, and harmonizes other herbs in a formula. It has a wide range of applications and is used to address issues such as fatigue, loose stools, decreased appetite, palpitations, cough, wheezing, sore throat, muscle spasms, sores, burns, and poisoning (including food, pesticide, lead, and arsenic poisoning) and to harmonize the effects of multiple herbs in herbal formulas.

Gān cǎo is used in combination with other herbs and by itself. Common methods of administration include decoctions, powders, concentrated granules, alcohol extracts, syrups, tablets, and pills. It is in over 150 of the primary commonly used formulas in TCM. There is a saying in Chinese about someone who is not glamorous but acts in such a way that everything gets accomplished: "They are the gān cǎo in the formula."

Unprocessed gān cǎo is used primarily for clearing heat toxins, treating poisoning, and stopping cough. Processing gān cǎo with honey (zhi gān cǎo) enhances the tonifying functions of the herb.

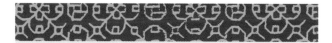

Gynostemma pentaphyllum ([Thunb.] Makino)
Common Name: Sweet Tea Vine
Pinyin: Jiǎo gǔ lán
Family: Cucurbitaceae
Part Used: Herb

Plant Description

Gynostemma pentaphyllum is an understory riparian plant growing as a mounding and climbing vine to twelve feet or more. The supple stems have grasping forked tendrils and palmately compound, lightly haired bright green leaves. Small and delicate white flowers bloom in summer all along the stems—followed by round, equally bright green seedpods almost half an inch in diameter. Indigenous to the humid mountainous areas of China, Japan, and Vietnam,[111] this semiherbaceous perennial is cold hardy to an estimated ten degrees. It grows at 300–3,200 meters in elevation.[112] USDA hardiness zones 7–9 or 10.

Propagation

The plants produce tiny, whitish-green, unisexual flowers; if seed is desired a male and female must be present. Seed sown in spring with heated soil germinates in two to five weeks. Alternately, it's easy to propagate by division in spring, or fall if grown in the cool greenhouse. Stock multiplies rapidly and requires frequent transplanting to the next size container. Plants hold their health and vigor fairly well in containers.

Garden and Polyculture Planting

For a mounding plant that will grow several feet tall, prune to keep the vigorous running stems in check. Plant the vine beside a light trellis and it will populate that. Grow with other shade and water-loving plants. If growing several or as a groundcover, plant them 1–1½ feet apart; if set out in spring they will fill in any gaps in six weeks or so, depending on the size of the transplants. They are not so vigorous as to smother other plants, but do give them a few feet of room to grow.

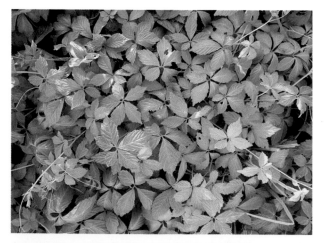
Gynostemma pentaphyllum **growing in the field.**

Sweet Tea Vine Recipes

The common name, sweet tea vine, gives voice to its primary use. The leaves are often combined with black teas.

Pour boiling water over the fresh or dried leaves and steep for two to three minutes. Use a larger quantity of fresh leaves to dried; adjust the amounts to your taste. If desired, stir in a teaspoon of honey per cup. Chilled, the tea makes a refreshing hot weather drink.

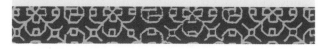

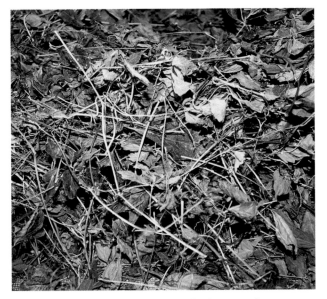

Dry jiǎo gǔ lán–the leaves, stems, and flowers of
Gynostemma pentaphyllum.

Suitable Companions

Albizia julibrissin, Mimosa, hé huān pí/huā
Andrographis paniculata, Kalmegh, chuān xīn lián
Asparagus cochinchinensis, tiān mén dōng
Bacopa monnieri, Brahmi
Centella asiatica, Gotu Kola, jī xuě cǎo
Codonopsis pilosula, Poor Man's Ginseng,
  dǎng shēn
Coix lacryma-jobi, Job's Tears, yì yǐ rén
Eclipta prostrata, Eclipta, mò hàn lián
Gentiana scabra, lóng dǎn cǎo
Gentiana straminea, qín jiāo
Houttuynia cordata, yú xīng cǎo
Ophiopogon japonicus, Lilyturf, mài mén dōng
Pinellia ternata, bàn xià
Plantago asiatica, Plantain, chē qián zǐ
Prunella vulgaris, Heal All, xià kū cǎo
Scutellaria barbata, Barbat Skullcap, bàn zhī lián

Field Production

Sweet tea vine is shade-loving and requires a fair
amount of water and at least somewhat well-draining,
average fertility soil. It will tolerate both clay and
sandy soil. Plug greenhouse transplants out on one-
foot spacing. It is important to keep the vines weeded,
as the tendrils will grab and hold weeds or debris

Medicinal Uses of Jiǎo gǔ lán

Jiǎo gǔ lán is the aerial portion of
Gynostemma pentaphyllum. Cool, slightly
bitter, and sweet, it tonifies the qi, generates fluids, clears heat, dispels phlegm, and
addresses heat toxins. Originally from the
south of China, it is sometimes known as
"southern ginseng" for its strong function of
supplementing the qi. It is used to strengthen
the body and to address asthma, migraines,
chronic headaches, chronic bronchitis, gastric ulcers, compromised immune function,
herpes zoster, hypertension, high cholesterol,
and as a part of therapy for many types of
cancer.

It is commonly used by itself and in
combination with other herbs. Common
methods of administration include as a
beverage, in decoctions, powders, alcohol
extracts, infusions, concentrated granules,
and pills.

Until relatively recently jiǎo gǔ lán was
famous in its local region but not well known
in the rest of China. It has now been included
in the Chinese materia medica and, due to its
effectiveness, has become widely used around
the world.

that can contaminate the harvest. Another option is
to plant through holes cut or burned through landscape fabric. Set up a drip line on the planting area
before laying the fabric. Trellising is not required.
If managed as a multiyear or permanent planting,
it will require fertilizer inputs, or production will
dramatically decrease.

Pests and Diseases

None.

Harvest and Yield

It is possible to get two to three harvests in the first season with spring transplanting. Monitor the crop and take the first harvest in midsummer when the mounded foliage is 1½ feet tall, before the lower material exhibits etiolation and loses leaves due to light exclusion. For successive harvests and the best quality herb, cut the crop just above the previous harvest cuts. Drying requires the long stems to be cut into three- to five-inch segments before drying;

otherwise, if you expose the leaves to drying conditions while attempting to dry the stem material, the leaves will be overdried while the stems will remain not quite dry. Jiǎo gǔ lán generates internal heat upon cutting, so do not allow the harvest to sit; chill or put to dry without delay. The best quality is still green when dry and has no extraneous material. Note that herb weight ratio from fresh to dry is very high. The yield is a half pound per plant fresh per season. Ratio of fresh to dry is 10:1.

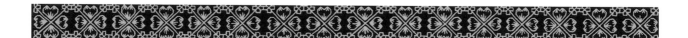

Houttuynia cordata (Thunb.)

Common Name: None
Pinyin: Yú xīng cǎo
Family: Saururaceae
Part Used: Herb

Plant Description

Yú xīng cǎo means "fish-smelling herb"; crushing a fresh leaf brings on a cannot-deny olfactory illustration. This herbaceous perennial groundcover grows one foot tall, has red stems, and spreads. *Houttuynia cordata* has dark green, heart-shaped leaves up to three inches long below insignificant flowers with two-inch-wide ornamental rounded white bracts. It is invasive in wet soils. The endemic geographic distribution is central to southern China as well as Bhutan, India, Indonesia, Japan, Korea, Myanmar, Nepal, and Thailand.[113] USDA hardiness zones 5–9.

Propagation

Propagate *Houttuynia cordata* by seed or division. Sow the seed in spring, expect germination in two to three months, overwinter, and transplant the following spring. Those adventitious rhizomes and stems that root? They can be simply dug up and replanted or potted to increase stock. *Houttuynia cordata* makes an excellent potted plant. Keep it well watered.

Garden and Polyculture Planting

Very attractive as a groundcover, *Houttuynia cordata* has made its way into the horticultural trade in both the green species form used in Chinese

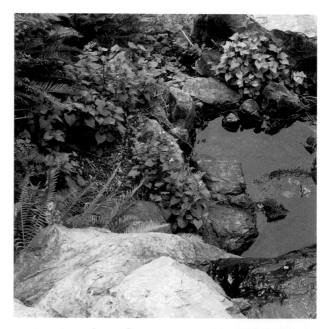

Houttuynia cordata in flower enjoys a moist shady location at Quarryhill Botanical Garden.

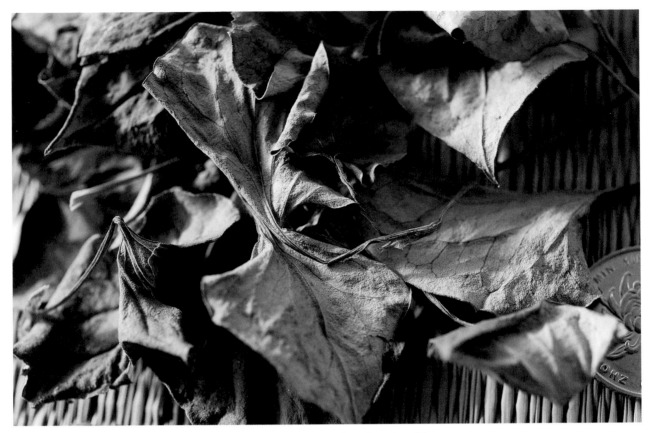

Yú xīng cǎo is the dried leaves and stems of *Houttuynia cordata*. Photo by Nina Zhito.

medicine and as ornamental cultivars. Place it at the front of the border; it is quick to establish growth and can be rampant in moist soils (which need to be somewhat well drained). *Houttuynia cordata* is not a bad candidate to grow in shade. Curb its growth by withholding water in summer or by solid bed edging such as bender board, rock, or other barriers—or employ a raised bed.

Suitable Companions
Agastache rugosa, Korean Mint, tǔ huò xiāng
Alisma plantago-aquatica subsp. *orientale*, Water Plantain, zé xiè
Anemarrhena asphodeloides, zhī mǔ
Angelica dahurica, bái zhǐ
Angelica pubescens, dú huó
Asparagus cochinchinensis, tiān mén dōng
Aster tataricus, Tartar Aster, zǐ wǎn
Bacopa monnieri, Brahmi
Centella asiatica, Gotu Kola, jī xuě cǎo

Codonopsis pilosula, Poor Man's Ginseng, dǎng shēn
Coix lacryma-jobi, Job's Tears, yì yǐ rén
Eclipta prostrata, Eclipta, mò hàn lián
Gynostemma pentaphyllum, Sweet Tea Vine, jiǎo gǔ lán
Mentha haplocalyx, Field Mint, bò hé
Ocimum sanctum, Sacred Basil, Tulsi
Ophiopogon japonicus, Lilyturf, mài mén dōng
Pinellia ternata, bàn xià
Plantago asiatica, Plantain, chē qián zǐ
Prunella vulgaris, Heal All, xià kū cǎo
Schisandra chinensis, Five Flavored Fruit, wǔ wèi zǐ
Schizonepeta tenuifolia, Japanese Catnip, jīng jiè
Scrophularia buergeriana, Figwort, běi xuán shēn
Scutellaria barbata, Barbat Skullcap, bàn zhī lián

Field Production
Transplant one-season-old established container plants on one-foot spacing. Grow in full sun to part

shade; regular irrigation is required, as is a freely draining moist soil of average fertility. Plants will fill in and at least one harvest is feasible in the first season.

Pests and Diseases
None.

Harvest and Yield
Two harvests a season are possible—the first in the early summer and the second in early fall. Harvesting is easy: the leaves and stems are soft and fleshy. I've used electric hedge pruners or whole-bed lettuce hand harvesters (they look like a saw with a bag) to harvest this crop. Wash after harvest to remove any impurities; drying is quick and easy. The best quality yú xīng cǎo has a bright green leaf and red stem without roots. Whole leaves are more appropriate than broken as the cell walls are still intact and the product has not degraded via the damaged areas (or in practitioner-speak, the vital qi has not leaked away). Yield estimate for fresh leaf and stem is one pound per square foot per season. Ratio of fresh to dry is 7:1.

Notes
- *Houttuynia cordata* may be more valuable to the ornamental Chinese herb garden than as a medicinal crop, as it is not frequently requested.
- The popular, pretty, tricolored nursery-trade cultivar 'Chameleon' is considered less medicinally appropriate than the species form.

Medicinal Uses of Yú xīng cǎo

Yú xīng cǎo is the herb or aerial portion of *Houttuynia cordata*. Acrid and cool, it clears heat, eliminates toxins, drains pus, and normalizes urination. It is used to address issues such as lung infections, lung abscesses, cough, pneumonia, acute and chronic bronchitis, urinary tract infection, and sores and skin lesions.

Yú xīng cǎo is used as a single herb and in combination with other herbs. It is used topically (or topically and internally) for skin conditions and internally otherwise. For topical use it is administered as a paste made from the crushed fresh herb, or infused and used as a rinse. Internally, yú xīng cǎo is most typically administered in decoctions (fresh or dried, it should only be decocted for a short time), concentrated powders, tablets, and pills.

Yú xīng cǎo can be used as a fresh or dried herb. If fresh, the dosage is usually doubled.

The name yú xīng cǎo literally means "fish-smelling herb" due to the smell when it is harvested. It typically does not have a particularly unpleasant odor or taste once it is decocted or otherwise prepared.

Ligusticum jeholense (Nakai & Kitag.)

Common Name: Chinese Lovage
Pinyin: Găo běn
Family: Apiaceae
Part Used: Root

Plant Description

There is much confusion and not much consensus when it comes to deciphering the taxonomy of *Ligusticum jeholense* and its closely related, genetically complex botanical allies. There may be a change in nomenclature when it gets a good scientific review—but don't hold your breath.[114] This is not to say that there is confusion on the current market; the name may simply change as many others have recently. Botany as a science is evolving faster than the plants. But speaking of plants, *Ligusticum jeholense* is an herbaceous perennial up to 2½ feet tall with branching stems up to 1½ feet wide. Leaves are four to six inches long, including the petiole, and are comprised of three parts; each part is divided again and has lobed margins. Summer-blooming, white-flowered umbels are four inches in diameter and yield many tan to brown flattish seeds in fall. Roots have a brown exterior and a white interior. *Ligusticum jeholense* grows in the central region of eastern China from 3,000–8,000 feet in elevation, in moist sites along streams, in meadows, and in forested areas.[115] USDA hardiness zones 4–9.

Propagation

Seeds or plant division are the preferred techniques for increasing stock. Seeds sown in early fall will yield plants ready to set out in the spring; germination is in two to three weeks. For division, separate in the fall and replant. Chinese lovage holds well in pots. Fertilizer requirements are low.

Garden and Polyculture Planting

For those of you who have grown only western lovage, you'll find that Chinese lovage is much more diminutive and not nearly as vigorous. It is, however, somewhat durable. Plant in the middle to front of the border in masses on one- to two-foot spacing. Chinese lovage is a good source of food for nectar feeders of all kinds.

Suitable Companions

Acanthopanax gracilistylus, wŭ jiā pí
Achyranthes bidentata, Oxknee, huái niú xī
Agastache rugosa, Korean Mint, tŭ huò xiāng
Allium macrostemon, xiè bái
Allium tuberosum, Garlic Chives, jiŭ cài zĭ
Anemarrhena asphodeloides, zhī mŭ

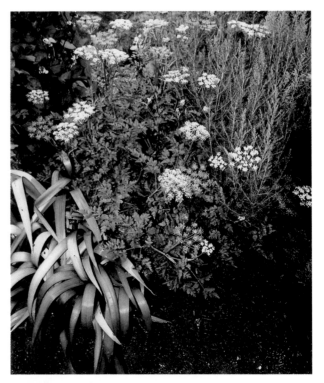

White flowers of *Ligusticum jeholense* are attractive to pollinators.

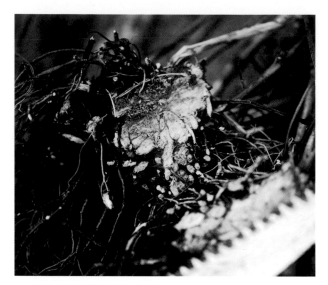

Cross-section of a fresh *Ligusticum jeholense* root in the harvesting process. Photo by Nina Zhito.

Angelica dahurica, bái zhǐ
Angelica pubescens, dú huó
Aster tataricus, Tartar Aster, zǐ wǎn
Belamcanda chinensis, Blackberry Lily, shè gān
Celosia argentea, qīng xiāng zǐ
Celosia cristata, Cockscomb, jī guān huā
Chrysanthemum morifolium, Mum, jú huā
Coix lacryma-jobi, Job's Tears, yì yǐ rén
Cornus officinalis, Dogwood, shān zhū yú
Crataegus pinnatifida, Chinese Hawthorn, shān zhā
Cyathula officinalis, Hookweed, chuān niú xī
Dianthus superbus, Fringed Pink, qú mài
Dolichos lablab, Hyacinth Bean, bái biǎn dòu
Eriobotrya japonica, Loquat, pí pá yè
Eucommia ulmoides, Hardy Rubber Tree, dù zhòng
Forsythia suspensa, lián qiào
Houttuynia cordata, yú xīng cǎo
Ligustrum lucidum, Chinese Privet, nǔ zhēn zǐ
Lilium lancifolium, *L. brownii*, Lily, bǎi hé
Lonicera japonica, Honeysuckle, jīn yín huā
Magnolia denudata, xīn yí huā
Mentha haplocalyx, Field Mint, bò hé
Momordica charantia, Bitter Melon, kǔ guā
Ocimum sanctum, Sacred Basil, Tulsi
Plantago asiatica, Plantain, chē qián zǐ
Platycodon grandiflorus, Balloon Flower, jié gěng
Prunella vulgaris, Heal All, xià kū cǎo

Medicinal Uses of Gǎo běn

Gǎo běn is the root of *Ligusticum jeholense*. Acrid and warm, it releases the exterior, dispels cold, dispels wind-damp-cold, and relieves pain. It is often included in formulas as an envoy, to guide the functions upward to the head. It is used to address issues such as vertex (top of the head) headaches, migraines, colds, fever, muscle aches, lower back pain, and pain in the muscles and joints that is made worse by exposure to damp and cold.

Gǎo běn is usually used in combination with other herbs. Common methods of administration include decoctions, powders, concentrated granules, alcohol extracts, tablets, and pills. It is in formulas such as Qiang Huo Sheng Shi Tang (*Notopterygium* Decoction to Overcome Dampness) and Xin Yi San (Magnolia Flower Powder).

Rheum palmatum, Chinese Rhubarb, dà huáng
Salvia miltiorrhiza, *S. przewalskii*, *S. bowleyana*, Red Sage, dān shēn
Saposhnikovia divaricata, Siler, fáng fēng
Schizonepeta tenuifolia, Japanese Catnip, jīng jiè
Scrophularia buergeriana, Figwort, běi xuán shēn
Scutellaria baicalensis, Baikal Skullcap, huáng qín
Sophora flavescens, kǔ shēn
Trichosanthes kirilowii, Chinese Cucumber, guā lóu/tiān huā fěn

Field Production

Plant on one-foot spacing in full sun in soils that are of average fertility and at least somewhat well draining. Irrigate regularly in the growing season. Too much water in heavy soils can promote root decay. In sandy soils provide mulch—and in all soils, a yearly topdressing of compost.

Pests and Diseases

Gophers will eat the roots.

Harvest and Yield

Wait to harvest until plants are at least three years old. The best time is in the autumn after plants express dormancy, and the second best time is in the spring when the plants are breaking dormancy and foliage is emerging.[116] Digging the roots is relatively simple; they are not very large nor very deep.

They have a strong celery smell, as you might expect from their family affiliation: "Good quality consists of big rhizomes with only a few hairy roots, and is intensely aromatic."[117] Wash to remove the majority of the clinging soil and, utilizing a saw, cut from the crown down in quarter-inch-thick slabs. Wash to remove any remaining soil and dry. Yield is a half pound per plant fresh at three years old. Ratio of fresh to dry is 3:1.

Ligustrum lucidum (Ait.)

Common Name: Chinese Privet
Pinyin: Nǔ zhēn zǐ
Family: Oleaceae
Part Used: Fruit

Plant Description

Ligustrum lucidum is a widespread and popular hedging plant. Left as an unpruned tree it can grow thirty to forty feet tall and has a spreading crown. The evergreen, simple, five-inch-long, dark-green leaves are leathery and elliptically shaped. Ten-inch terminal panicles of small, white, scented flowers bloom in late spring or early summer and mature in summer or fall into masses of half-inch-long, teardrop-shaped, black fruit. Invasive by way of seed drop or bird dispersal, it is widely distributed from central to eastern China and throughout all of southern China.[118] USDA hardiness zones 7–11.

Propagation

Both seeds and cuttings are easy; expect high rates of success with either method. Seed sown in spring germinates in as little as eight days. Take stem cuttings anytime from June through March.[119] Start the year before any expected transplant or sale. Plants hold well in containers and will bear fruit and make good permanent potted specimens or porch plants.

Garden and Polyculture Planting

Use for screening or as a windbreak in the garden—or find Chinese privet ideally suited to the hedgerow or medicinal orchard. Plant it away from paths and other areas where its messy dropped fruit would be unwelcome. Chinese privet is durable and very adaptable to different soils, thriving in sun or shade. Average well-draining soils are recommended.

Suitable Companions

Acanthopanax gracilistylus, wǔ jiā pí
Achyranthes bidentata, Oxknee, huái niú xī
Agastache rugosa, Korean Mint, tǔ huò xiāng
Albizia julibrissin, Mimosa, hé huān pí/huā
Allium macrostemon, xiè bái
Allium tuberosum, Garlic Chives, jiǔ cài zǐ
Andrographis paniculata, Kalmegh, chuān xīn lián
Anemarrhena asphodeloides, zhī mǔ
Angelica dahurica, bái zhǐ
Angelica pubescens, dú huó
Aster tataricus, Tartar Aster, zǐ wǎn
Astragalus membranaceus, Milk Vetch, huáng qí

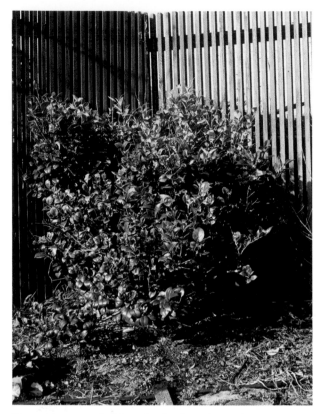

Young *Ligustrum lucidum* shrub. Photo by Andrew Jacobson.

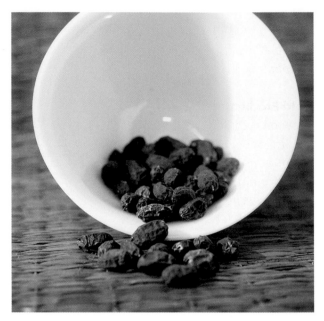

Nǔ zhēn zǐ, the dried fruit of *Ligustrum lucidum*. Photo by Nina Zhito.

Atractylodes macrocephala, Chinese Thistle Daisy, bái zhú

Belamcanda chinensis, Blackberry Lily, shè gān

Bupleurum chinense, Hare's Ear, chái hú

Carthamus tinctorius, Safflower, hóng huā

Celosia argentea, qīng xiāng zǐ

Celosia cristata, Cockscomb, jī guān huā

Chrysanthemum morifolium, Mum, jú huā

Clerodendrum trichotomum, Glorybower, chòu wú tóng

Cornus officinalis, Dogwood, shān zhū yú

Crataegus pinnatifida, Chinese Hawthorn, shān zhā

Cyathula officinalis, Hookweed, chuān niú xī

Dianthus superbus, Fringed Pink, qú mài

Eclipta prostrata, Eclipta, mò hàn lián

Eriobotrya japonica, Loquat, pí pá yè

Eucommia ulmoides, Hardy Rubber Tree, dù zhòng

Forsythia suspensa, lián qiào

Ginkgo biloba, Ginkgo, bái guǒ

Ligusticum jeholense, Chinese Lovage, gǎo běn

Lilium lancifolium, *L. brownii*, Lily, bǎi hé

Lonicera japonica, Honeysuckle, jīn yín huā

Lycium chinense, Chinese Wolfberry, gǒu qǐ zǐ/dì gǔ pí

Magnolia denudata, xīn yí huā

Mentha haplocalyx, Field Mint, bò hé

Momordica charantia, Bitter Melon, kǔ guā

Ocimum sanctum, Sacred Basil, Tulsi

Ophiopogon japonicus, Lilyturf, mài mén dōng

Plantago asiatica, Plantain, chē qián zǐ

Platycodon grandiflorus, Balloon Flower, jié gěng

Prunella vulgaris, Heal All, xià kū cǎo

Rehmannia glutinosa, Chinese Foxglove, dì huáng

Rheum palmatum, Chinese Rhubarb, dà huáng

Salvia miltiorrhiza, *S. przewalskii*, *S. bowleyana*, Red Sage, dān shēn

Saposhnikovia divaricata, Siler, fáng fēng

Schisandra chinensis, Five Flavored Fruit, wǔ wèi zǐ

Schizonepeta tenuifolia, Japanese Catnip, jīng jiè

Scrophularia buergeriana, Figwort, běi xuán shēn

Scutellaria baicalensis, Baikal Skullcap, huáng qín

Scutellaria barbata, Barbat Skullcap, bàn zhī lián

Sophora flavescens, kǔ shēn

Trichosanthes kirilowii, Chinese Cucumber, guā lóu/tiān huā fěn

Withania somnifera, Ashwagandha
Ziziphus jujuba, Chinese Date, dà zǎo
Ziziphus jujuba var. *spinosa*, suān zǎo rén

Field Production
Grow on eight-foot spacing in full sun to part shade, and irrigate during periods of drought or where summer rainfall is scarce. Chinese privet can take hard pruning, which should be employed to keep plants low enough to maintain harvesting heights within OSHA (i.e., safe) standards.

Pests and Diseases
None.

Harvest and Yield
Plants produce fruit about five years after sowing. In fall when the fruit matures, harvest by stripping the clusters into a collecting vessel. Little stem pieces from the fruit are vexingly hard to separate from the crop. Fruit set is the highest in warm and humid regions, and "good quality consists of large, full, solid, greyish black fruit."[120] Yield will vary depending on the size of the plant. Ratio of fresh to dry fruit is 2:1.

Notes
- There are many cultivars in the nursery trade; choose one that has not been selected for its ornamental quality.
- In the nursery industry *Ligustrum lucidum* is often offered as *Ligustrum japonicum*, which is not considered medicinal but can be identified by both a smaller flowering panicle up to six inches long and by being more densely floral.

Medicinal Uses of Nǚ zhēn zǐ

Nǚ zhēn zǐ is the fruit of *Ligustrum lucidum*. Sweet, bitter, and cool, it tonifies the liver and kidney yin and essences, clears empty heat, and brightens the eyes. It is a mild tonic herb suitable for use over an extended period of time. It is used to address issues such as hot flashes, night sweats, high thirst, mood swings, irritability, dizziness, ringing in the ears, low back weakness and soreness, prematurely grey hair, constipation, blurred vision, and red and painful eyes. In modern China it is also used to treat patients with tuberculosis that present with similar symptoms.

Nǚ zhēn zǐ is most commonly used in combination with other herbs. Common methods of administration include decoctions, powders, concentrated granules, tablets, and pills. It is one-half of the well-known formula Er Zhi Wan (Two Solstices Pill).

Nǚ zhēn zǐ is often processed by steaming it with grain-based alcohol in order to enhance its tonic effects on the liver and the kidney. Unprocessed nǚ zhēn zǐ has a stronger overall moistening effect and is used for addressing constipation and other dryness issues.

Lilium lancifolium (Thunb.)
Medicinal Synonym: *L. brownii* (F.E.Br. ex Miellez)
Common Name: Lily
Pinyin: Bǎi hé
Family: Liliaceae
Part Used: Bulb

Plant Description

Revered for their beauty, these two Asian species are exceptionally gorgeous. Herbaceous leaves of both species are narrowly lanceolate with parallel veining. *Lilium lancifolium* is a real looker with numerous reflexed bold orange, maroon-speckled flowers blooming in nodding racemes atop six-foot stems. This type of tiger lily blooms from midsummer to late summer. Categorized in the Asian group of lilies,

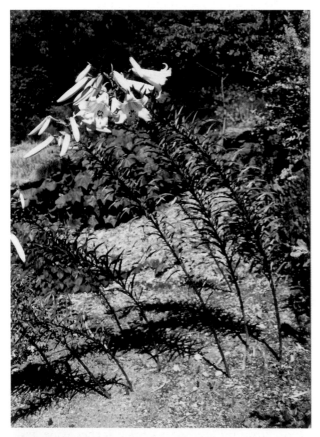

Lilium brownii **growing five feet tall at the University of California Berkeley Botanical Garden.**

Lilium lancifolium is one of the species that form air bulbils in the leaf axils. *Lilium brownii*, of the Oriental Lily category, is truly lovely, with its single, terminal, purple-blushed buds opening into large, white, trumpet-shaped flowers. These late summer floral performers dance on five-foot-tall upright stems. *Lilium brownii* is often cultivated in China for food and medicine; it grows in the central region and up and down the eastern seaboard.[121] USDA hardiness zones 6–10.

Originally from China, *Lilium lancifolium* is one of the hardiest of lilies and was introduced—and occasionally has escaped—domestic cultivation, becoming invasive in eastern North America in the Canadian provinces of New Brunswick, Nova Scotia, Ontario, and Quebec. In the United States it is feral in most of the states east of the Mississippi River as well as Iowa, Missouri, Nebraska, and the Dakotas.[122] USDA hardiness zones 4-9.

Propagation

Lilies can be produced by seed, bulb scales, bulb offsets, or air bulbils. Both species named above produce hundreds of light tan seed per plant. The seeds look like sacks of sliced bread, in their three-chambered pods. Easy to grow; if seed is fresh, there is no delay in germination—it takes place in only a week or two. In the case of *Lilium brownii*, if the seed is older, germination can take up to three months. These seed-sown lilies take three years of growth to flower. The other methods are asexual (vegetative) and thus clonal; the genetics will be the same, and if disease is present in the parent it will be present in the offspring. However, these methods increase stock more rapidly than seed culture. The fleshy bulb scales can be separated from the mother bulb, rooted as single leaflike scales in perlite (or another suitable media), kept moist and warm, and will grow roots in a few weeks and can be potted. Bulbs may produce offsets near the mother bulb, which can be separated and replanted to increase stock; there is no need to wait for roots to develop. In the case of *Lilium lancifolium* the use of air bulbils is the easiest method of propagation. In mid to late summer simply remove the small dark purple bulbs that have formed in the leaf axils and plant them. Lilies hold well in pots and make excellent permanently containerized specimens. Let containers dry out between waterings.

Garden and Polyculture Planting

The lily is one of the quintessential garden flowers. How lucky we are that it is not only easy to grow but has a long-lasting floral show and is edible as well! Eat your medicine! In the midborder these flowers bring grace and beauty and work well with many other plants. For dramatic displays plant them massed on one-foot spacing. *Lilium lancifolium* naturalizes almost too easily (by air bulbils) in the garden and may be difficult to eradicate. These are full sun to part shade plants, but be mindful not to plant in hot exposures in hot summers. Both species have strong erect stems and do not need staking.

Suitable Companions

Acanthopanax gracilistylus, wǔ jiā shēn/pí
Achyranthes bidentata, Oxknee, huái niú xī
Agastache rugosa, Korean Mint, tǔ huò xiang
Allium tuberosum, Garlic Chives, jiǔ cài zǐ
Anemarrhena asphodeloides, zhī mǔ
Angelica dahurica, baí zhǐ
Angelica pubescens, dú huó
Aster tataricus, Tartar Aster, zǐ wǎn
Atractylodes macrocephala, Chinese Thistle Daisy, bái zhú
Belamcanda chinensis, Blackberry Lily, shè gān
Carthamus tinctorius, Safflower, hóng huā
Celosia argentea, qīng xiāng zǐ
Celosia cristata, Cockscomb, jī guān huā

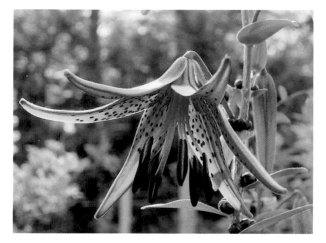

Flowers and air bulbils of *Lilium lancifolium*.

Chrysanthemum morifolium, Mum, jú huā
Cornus officinalis, Dogwood, shān zhū yú
Crataegus pinnatifida, Chinese Hawthorn, shān zhā
Cyathula officinalis, Hookweed, chuān niú xī
Dianthus superbus, Fringed Pink, qú mài
Eriobotrya japonica, Loquat, pí pá yè
Eucommia ulmoides, Hardy Rubber Tree, dù zhòng
Ginkgo biloba, Ginkgo, bái guǒ
Paeonia lactiflora, Chinese Peony, bái/chì sháo
Paeonia suffruticosa, Tree Peony, mǔ dān pí
Platycodon grandiflorus, Balloon Flower, jié gěng
Prunella vulgaris, Heal All, xià kū cǎo
Rehmannia glutinosa, Chinese Foxglove, dì huáng
Rheum palmatum, Chinese Rhubarb, dà huáng
Salvia miltiorrhiza, *S. przewalskii*, *S. bowleyana*, Red Sage, dān shēn
Saposhnikovia divaricata, Siler, fáng fēng
Schizonepeta tenuifolia, Japanese Catnip, jīng jiè
Scrophularia buergeriana, Figwort, běi xuán shēn
Scutellaria baicalensis, Baikal Skullcap, huáng qín
Sophora flavescens, kǔ shēn
Withania somnifera, Ashwagandha

Field Production

Here at the Chinese Medicinal Herb Farm we plant these lilies in and between rows on one-foot spacing in full sun to light shade. The soil should be well drained and fairly fertile. At maturity the bulbs of *Lilium brownii* are one to three inches wide and *Lilium lancifolium* two to five inches wide; both

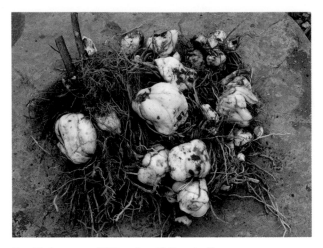

Freshly harvested *Lilium lancifolium* bulb.

prefer acid soils (*Lilium lancifolium* dislikes lime).[123] Plants can handle short durations of drought; mulching will ameliorate the condition.

Pests and Diseases

Lilies have a reputation for susceptibility to viruses, but I haven't seen any symptoms on the plants in my gardens. Gophers eat lily bulbs, and rabbits eat everything.

Harvest and Yield

Harvest bulbs aged two years or more in the late fall or winter. Washing is easy as soil doesn't adhere to the smooth scales, although some scales will need to be separated to remove clinging soil. For even drying separate the rest of the scales. More trials and investigation need to be done on how to keep scales from turning brown—without the use of sulfur: "Good quality consists of fleshy, hard, white scales, uniform in size, with leaf veins."[124] For *Lilium lancifolium* average harvest for two-year bulbs grown from bulbils are 0.6 pounds per plant fresh. Ratio of fresh to dry is 3:1.

Medicinal Uses of Bǎi hé

Bǎi hé is the bulb of *Lilium brownii* or *Lilium lancifolium*. Sweet and cool, it moistens the lung, stops cough, calms the heart and shen, and nourishes the stomach yin. It is often used in dietary therapy as a nourishing food in soups, congees (porridges), and other dishes. It is a gentle tonic herb suitable for use over an extended period of time. Bǎi hé is used to strengthen and nourish the lungs and stomach and address issues such as chronic dry cough, night sweats, asthma, tuberculosis, lung abscess, insomnia, palpitations, inability to concentrate, stomach ulcers, and gastritis. It is also used topically for sores.

Bǎi hé is commonly used by itself as well as in combination with other herbs. Common methods of administration include decoctions, powders, concentrated granules, pills, pastes (topically), and as a therapeutic food. It is in the formula Bai He Gu Jin Tang (Lily Bulb Decoction to Preserve Metal).

Typically, the fresh herb is crushed to make a paste or the dry herb is powdered for topical applications. The dried, unprocessed herb is used for all other applications.

Notes

There are many other lilies, all of them *Lilium* species, that are well accepted as bǎi hé. *Lilium pumilum* is a standard species used as well; however, its bulbs are much smaller, about 50 percent by weight for the same age as some of the others, especially *Lilium lancifolium*.

Lonicera japonica (Thunb.)
Medicinal Synonym: *Lonicera hypoglauca* (Miq.)
Common Name: Honeysuckle
Pinyin: Jīn yín huā
Family: Caprifoliaceae
Part Used: Flower

Plant Description

An increasingly important and valuable herb in the Chinese materia medica, *Lonicera japonica* is a vigorous, perennial, woody vine reaching thirty feet in length. This rampant grower can be invasive and weedy in the eastern and southern areas of the United States as well as Hawaii. Invasive by rooting stem material as well as propagation by seed-eating birds, *Lonicera japonica* appears on various northeastern US state or county noxious weed lists but shows few aggressive properties in the northwest or northern prairie states. Interestingly enough, this species of honeysuckle is commonly sold by US nurseries. It is evergreen in mild winter regions, and semideciduous to deciduous in four-season climates. Dark green three-inch leaves are oval and, like the flowers, appear in pairs on the stem. White two-lipped flowers open to 1½ inches long, are tinged with purple turning to gold, and are wonderfully fragrant. The native extent of this species of honeysuckle is throughout much of eastern Asia. USDA hardiness zones 5–11.

Propagation

Seeds, vegetative cuttings, and layering all work well to propagate this easy-to-grow vine. Seeds need two to three months of cold treatment; sow in deep flats and expose to the winter elements, or stratify in the refrigerator for the same length of time. Hardwood stem cuttings taken in spring root readily. The layering technique is the easiest yet—in the garden, roots will form wherever the vines are buried in moist soil. If propagated by vegetative means, plant starts can be either transplanted or sold in the first season. Long-term containerized stock will require occasional fertilization.

Garden and Polyculture Planting

This species of honeysuckle is a common garden vine offering attractive screening, scented flowers, and nectar for hummingbirds. Take care not to plant where it may escape cultivation and become weedy. Transplant on a fence or sturdy, large-scale trellis on three- to four-foot spacing. Train stems up and off the soil. Prune in early spring to keep plants within bounds and to keep buildup of stem material to a minimum. If the vigorous nature of honeysuckle growth can be managed, the following are compatible.

Suitable Companions

Acanthopanax gracilistylus, wŭ jiā pí
Achyranthes bidentata, Oxknee, huái niú xī
Agastache rugosa, Korean Mint, tŭ huò xiāng
Albizia julibrissin, Mimosa, hé huān pí/huā

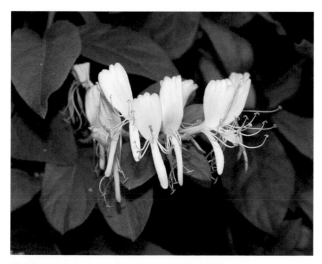

The flowering vine of *Lonicera hypoglauca*.

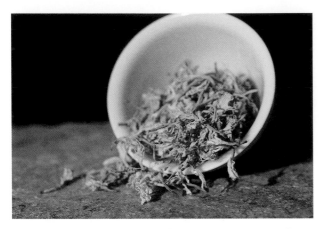

Jīn yín huā, the dried flowers of *Lonicera hypoglauca*. Photo by Nina Zhito.

Honeysuckle Recipes

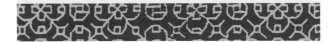

Fresh or dried honeysuckle flowers and flower buds are often used as a tea. You can add them to your favorite green tea mix for a pleasant change in flavor. Try a tea made with honeysuckle as well as the flowers of *Chrysanthemum morifolium* (Mum, jú huā).

Pour boiling water over the dried or fresh flowers and steep for two to three minutes. Use a larger quantity of fresh flowers or buds to dried; adjust the amount to your taste.

Allium tuberosum, Garlic Chives, jiǔ cài zǐ

Andrographis paniculata, Kalmegh, chuān xīn lián

Anemarrhena asphodeloides, zhī mǔ

Angelica dahurica, bái zhǐ

Angelica pubescens, dú huó

Aster tataricus, Tartar Aster, zǐ wǎn

Astragalus membranaceus, Milk Vetch, huáng qí

Atractylodes macrocephala, Chinese Thistle Daisy, bái zhú

Belamcanda chinensis, Blackberry Lily, shè gān

Bupleurum chinense, Hare's Ear, chái hú

Carthamus tinctorius, Safflower, hóng huā

Celosia argentea, qīng xiāng zǐ

Celosia cristata, Cockscomb, jī guān huā

Chrysanthemum morifolium, Mum, jú huā

Clerodendrum trichotomum, Glorybower, chòu wú tóng

Cornus officinalis, Dogwood, shān zhū yú

Crataegus pinnatifida, Chinese Hawthorn, shān zhā

Cyathula officinalis, Hookweed, chuān niú xī

Dianthus superbus, Fringed Pink, qú mài

Dolichos lablab, Hyacinth Bean, bái biǎn dòu

Eriobotrya japonica, Loquat, pí pá yè

Eucommia ulmoides, Hardy Rubber Tree, dù zhòng

Forsythia suspensa, lián qiào

Ginkgo biloba, Ginkgo, bái guǒ

Houttuynia cordata, yú xīng cǎo

Ligusticum jeholense, Chinese Lovage, gǎo běn

Ligustrum lucidum, Chinese Privet, nǔ zhēn zǐ

Lilium lancifolium, *L. brownii*, Lily, bǎi hé

Lycium chinense, Chinese Wolfberry, gǒu qǐ zǐ/dì gǔ pí

Magnolia denudata, xīn yí huā

Mentha haplocalyx, Field Mint, bò hé

Momordica charantia, Bitter Melon, kǔ guā

Ocimum sanctum, Sacred Basil, Tulsi

Paeonia lactiflora, Chinese Peony, bái/chì sháo

Paeonia suffruticosa, Tree Peony, mǔ dān pí

Platycodon grandiflorus, Balloon Flower, jié gěng

Prunella vulgaris, Heal All, xià kū cǎo

Rehmannia glutinosa, Chinese Foxglove, dì huáng

Rheum palmatum, Chinese Rhubarb, dà huáng

Salvia miltiorrhiza, *S. przewalskii*, *S. bowleyana*, Red Sage, dān shēn

Saposhnikovia divaricata, Siler, fáng fēng

Schizonepeta tenuifolia, Japanese Catnip, jīng jiè

Scrophularia buergeriana, Figwort, běi xuán shēn

Scutellaria baicalensis, Baikal Skullcap, huáng qín

Sophora flavescens, kǔ shēn

Trichosanthes kirilowii, Chinese Cucumber, guā lóu/tiān huā fěn

Withania somnifera, Ashwagandha

Ziziphus jujuba, Chinese Date, dà zǎo

Ziziphus jujuba var. *spinosa*, suān zǎo rén

Field Production

Plant nursery-grown material in full sun with three-to five-foot spacing along a fence or trellis. Prune yearly and train vines onto the support structure. Regular irrigation is preferred but they will tolerate some short-term drought. Honeysuckle likes clay soils that are at least moderately draining. Fertilization is not necessary.

Pests and Diseases

Deer occasionally browse this plant.

Harvest and Yield

Vines will bloom in their second year during the spring or summer. Pick flowers that are just starting to open when they are still white. Do not pick the more mature orange ones, as they dry to an undesirable brown. To maximize the yield, pick flowers every other day; the average harvest season lasts for a month to six weeks. The flowers are fragile and discolor easily; pick them in the morning before they warm up. Immediately put to dry on a low to medium heat (not exceeding one hundred degrees). The best quality is described as "unfragmented, yellow flower buds that are just opening."[125] The flowers are lightweight, and it may be difficult to find a buyer willing to pay for domestic labor costs. It is, however, an important herb; just how important will determine if the crop is grown and harvested or wild-crafted. Yields will vary with the age of the plant; two-year-old plants gave 0.05 pounds per plant each day fresh. Ratio of fresh to dry is 5:1.

Notes

- Where this species of honeysuckle is invasive, collect from existing stands.
- There are many named cultivars in the nursery trade; choose a species that is unselected (has not been selected for an ornamental property).
- The stem, rěn dōng téng, is also a Chinese herb, but I've never had a buyer request it.

Medicinal Uses of Jīn yín huā

Jīn yín huā is the flower of *Lonicera japonica*. Sweet and cold, it clears heat, including wind heat, early stage febrile disorders, heat at any of the four levels (wei, qi, ying, and xue), summer heat, and heat toxins. It is used to address a relatively wide range of issues including upper respiratory tract infections, bronchitis, pneumonia, fever, sore throat, heat stroke, skin sores and lesions, intestinal abscess, diarrhea with mucus or blood, and dysentery.

Jīn yín huā is usually used in combination with other herbs. Common methods of administration include decoctions, powders, concentrated granules, alcohol extracts, infusions, tablets, and pills. It is one of the key ingredients in the very widely used formula Yin Qiao San (*Lonicera* and *Forsythia* Powder) as well as formulas such as Wu Wei Xiao Du Yin (Five Ingredient Decoction to Eliminate Toxins) and Qing Ying Tang (Clear the Nutritive Level Decoction).

Some modern research indicates that fresh flowers have a stronger effect than dried and that the leaves may have stronger properties than the flowers for certain functions.

Lycium chinense (Mill.)
Alternate Species: *L. barbarum* (L.)
Common Name: Chinese Wolfberry
Pinyin: gǒu qǐ zǐ/dì gǔ pí
Family: Solanaceae
Part Used: Fruit, root bark

Plant Description
Lycium chinense is a deciduous shrub up to five feet tall. The arching branches are multiple stemmed; the two-inch bright green leaves are simple, and ovate to linear-lanceolate. Some plants sport thorns. Pretty bee- and wasp-pollinated purple star-shaped flowers bloom in summer and fade to tan before falling off, yielding a half- to one-inch red fruit that is variable from plant to plant in its size and sweetness. *Lycium chinense* has a very wide geographic distribution in China and is vigorous and grows well from -10 to 110 degrees. USDA hardiness zones 3–10 or 11.

Propagation
Propagate Chinese wolfberry by seeds, cuttings, and layering. For sowing, remove the seed from the fruit

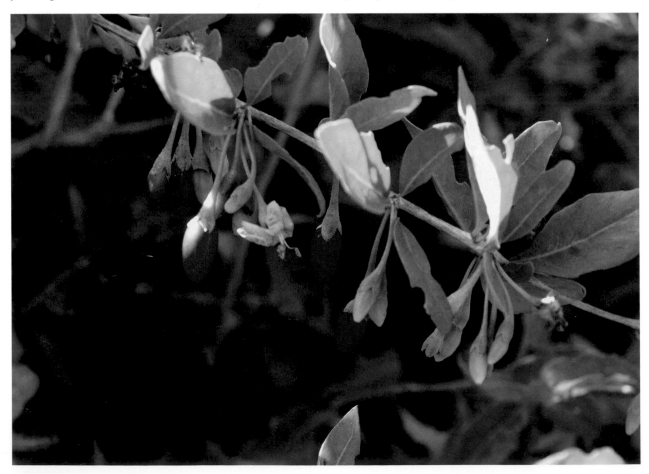

Lycium chinense **fruit in the garden.**

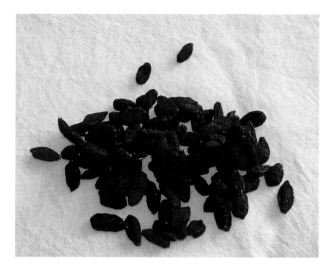

Freshly dried gǒu qǐ zǐ fruit.

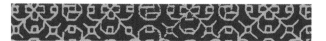

Chinese Wolfberry Recipes

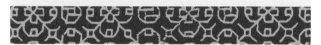

The reddish-orange berries, dried, may be used like raisins—served over cereal or added to congee. Fresh fruit can be juiced and is traditionally added to Chinese pork and chicken dishes. The leaves are also used as a classic herbal tea.

(if not previously cleaned) and sow seed in spring or fall in a heated greenhouse; germination takes place in about two weeks. Plant out, or sell, the following season. Fruiting occurs when plants are two to three years old. Cuttings yield fruit more quickly. If you need clonal material in order to eliminate genetic variables, then take hardwood cuttings in the fall. The stems are adventitious, and layering in the garden happens wherever the branches touch the soil. They hold well as a container plant.

Garden and Polyculture Planting

Chinese wolfberry shows heat and drought tolerance and does well in alkaline as well as slightly acid soils; plant stock in full sun in well-drained soil. Plant spacing is three to five feet; Chinese wolfberry is an excellent hedgerow shrub. Frequent removal of naturally layered stems is necessary to keep plants from expanding; unchecked, this expansion results in an impenetrable thicket. To encourage fruiting, prune back the plants while winter dormant. Besides pruning terminal branches, prune low branches hard (bringing growth higher, which facilitates fruit harvest and lessens stem layering).

Suitable Companions

Aster tataricus, Tartar Aster, zǐ wǎn
Astragalus membranaceus, Milk Vetch, huáng qí

Belamcanda chinensis, Blackberry Lily, shè gān
Carthamus tinctorius, Safflower, hóng huā
Chrysanthemum morifolium, Mum, jú huā
Dolichos lablab, Hyacinth Bean, bái biǎn dòu
Ephedra sinica, Ephedra, má huáng/má huáng gēn
Ligustrum lucidum, Chinese Privet, nǚ zhēn zǐ
Momordica charantia, Bitter Melon, kǔ guā
Salvia miltiorrhiza, S. przewalskii, S. bowleyana,
  Red Sage, dān shēn
Scutellaria baicalensis, Baikal Skullcap, huáng qín
Sophora flavescens, kǔ shēn
Trichosanthes kirilowii, Chinese Cucumber, guā
  lóu/tiān huā fěn
Withania somnifera, Ashwagandha
Ziziphus jujuba, Chinese Date, dà zǎo
Ziziphus jujuba var. *spinosa*, suān zǎo rén

Field Production

Chinese wolfberry enjoys a sunny and summer-hot location, and a good winter chill. Row crop spacing is three feet in row. Pruning back to one to two feet tall when dormant not only encourages fruiting but makes the plants more manageable. You can install a trellis to hold sprawling plants upright to facilitate harvesting of fruit, and to keep plants from layering and expanding out of control. Fertilizer is not necessary for fruit or root production.

Medicinal Uses of Gŏu qĭ zĭ/Dì gŭ pí

Gŏu qĭ zĭ is the fruit of *Lycium chinense*. Sweet and neutral, it tonifies the liver and kidney yin, brightens the eyes, and moistens the lung yin. It is often used in dietary therapy as a nourishing food in soups, congees (porridges), and other dishes. It is a gentle tonic herb suitable for use over an extended period of time. It is used to address issues such as fatigue, dizziness, blurry vision and other visual disturbances, weakness of the back and knees, infertility, night sweats, steaming bones sensation, prematurely grey hair, and dry cough.

Gŏu qĭ zĭ is commonly used by itself as well as in combination with other herbs. Methods of administration include decoctions, powders, alcohol extracts, concentrated powders, tablets, and pills—and as a food in soups, congee, and other rice dishes. It is sometimes mixed with oil and used topically to treat burns. It is in formulas such as Qi Ju Di Huang Wan (*Lycium*, Chrysanthemum, and *Rehmannia*), Yi Guan Jian (Linking Decoction), Zuo Gui Wan (Restore the Left Kidney Pill), and You Gui Wan (Restore the Right Kidney Pill). Recently, gŏu qĭ zĭ, sold as "goji berries," has become popular as a "super-food" in health-food stores.

Gŏu qĭ yè, the leaf of *Lycium chinense*, is sometimes used as a substitute for the fruit.

Dì gŭ pí is the bark of *Lycium chinense*. Sweet, bland, and cold, it cools the blood, clears lung heat, and stops bleeding. It is used to address steaming bones sensation, night sweats, high thirst, frequent urination, toothache, cough, wheezing, constipation, and many bleeding disorders.

Gŏu qĭ gēn is the root of *Lycium chinense*. Sweet and cold, it clears liver fire and is used to address eye disorders, hepatitis, and tendonitis in combination with other herbs. It is a less commonly used herb.

Pest and Diseases
Birds eat the fruit, so covering plants with netting may be helpful.

Harvest and Yield
Harvest bright red fruit when fully ripe in fall. Chinese wolfberry has ongoing ripening. To maximize yield, plan on weekly harvests for a month or so in the fall. Fruit is in full production by the third or fourth year. Drying fruit in a dehydrator works better than a passive drying system, since it dries faster and leaves less opportunity for the fruit to oxidize. The best quality is a large, fleshy, red fruit that is sweet and has few seeds.[126] Roots are dug from the third year on, from winter dormant plants. Wash, peel to remove the bark, cut into sections, and dry. The best quality root bark is large and thick, without any heartwood.[127] Fruit yield is one to two pounds per fresh plant with four harvests per fall possible. Ratio of fresh to dry fruit is 3:1.

Notes
- Both *Lycium* species exhibit invasive qualities and have escaped cultivation in the eastern U.S. and England.
- Some *Lycium* cultivars were developed for leaf rather than fruit production.

Magnolia denudata (Desr.)

Medicinal Synonym: *Magnolia sprengeri* (Pamp.)*, Magnolia biondii* (Pamp.)
Common Name: None
Pinyin: Xīn yí huā
Family: Magnoliaceae
Part Used: Flower bud

Plant Description

Magnolia denudata has simply some of the most stunning flowers ever to ornament a tree. It is a deciduous tree up to forty feet tall by thirty feet wide; the bark is grey and the six-inch tulip-shaped flowers are elegant, white- to cream-colored, and with a blush of purple at the base of each petal. They are very fragrant and emerge from the fuzzy desirable buds before the spring leaf-out. The green leathery leaves are five to seven inches long with simple smooth margins. Seeds are produced in the typical fashion for this genus—five-inch-long brown fruits containing numerous seeds. *Magnolia denudata* is not suitable in hot dry regions but otherwise has a wide geographic distribution. This native of China, almost extinct in the wild, is currently cultivated worldwide. USDA hardiness zones 6–11.

Propagation

Seeds of *Magnolia denudata* need stratification to break dormancy and germinate. The secret code to unlock this beauty is three months of cold. Either sow in deep flats and leave for winter to chill naturally or take matters into your own . . . refrigerator, packed in moist sand. Germination occurs in the first spring after a fall sowing. Semihardwood cuttings are also an option to increase stock; the best time is late spring or early summer.

Garden and Polyculture Planting

Functional beauty at its finest! This tree is unrivaled as an informal specimen. Plant singly in the garden or hedgerow—mass plantings do not show the beautiful flowers to their best advantage. Plant in the full sun in slightly acidic to neutral soils that are well drained and of average fertility. Prune in spring to manage form. Late spring frosts may damage flowers. It is best to leave an area around the root zone free from competing plants. Place any companion plantings near the drip line, or near where the branching ends.

Suitable Companions

Acanthopanax gracilistylus, wǔ jiā pí
Achyranthes bidentata, Oxknee, huái niú xī
Agastache rugosa, Korean Mint, tǔ huò xiāng
Allium macrostemon, xiè bái
Allium tuberosum, Garlic Chives, jiǔ cài zǐ
Andrographis paniculata, Kalmegh, chuān xīn lián
Anemarrhena asphodeloides, zhī mǔ
Angelica dahurica, bái zhǐ
Angelica pubescens, dú huó
Asparagus cochinchinensis, tiān mén dōng
Aster tataricus, Tartar Aster, zǐ wǎn

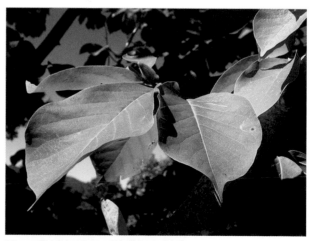

Magnolia denudata **with flower bud.**

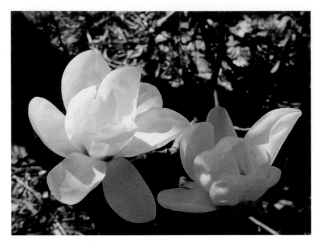

Beautiful flowers of *Magnolia denudata* at Quarryhill Botanical Garden. Photo courtesy of Jesika Jennings.

Medicinal Uses of Xīn yí huā

Xīn yí huā is the flower bud of *Magnolia denudata* (and several other magnolia species). Acrid and warm, it dispels wind cold and opens the nasal orifices. It is one of the most frequently used herbs for addressing nasal obstruction and is used to address sinusitis, allergic and nonallergic rhinitis, and the common cold.

Xīn yí huā is usually used in combination with other herbs, although it is sometimes used by itself as an essential oil or powder for topical application. Common methods of administration include decoctions, powders, concentrated granules, oils, alcohol extracts, tablets, and pills. It is a key ingredient in formulas such as Xin Yi San (Magnolia Flower Powder), Cang Er Zi San (*Xanthium* Seed Powder), Qing Bi Tang (Clear the Nose Decoction), and Xin Yi Qing Fei Tang (Magnolia Flower to Clear the Lung Decoction).

Atractylodes macrocephala, Chinese Thistle Daisy, bái zhú

Bacopa monnieri, Brahmi

Belamcanda chinensis, Blackberry Lily, shè gān

Bupleurum chinense, Hare's Ear, chái hú

Carthamus tinctorius, Safflower, hóng huā

Celosia argentea, qīng xiāng zǐ

Celosia cristata, Cockscomb, jī guān huā

Centella asiatica, Gotu Kola, jī xuě cǎo

Chrysanthemum morifolium, Mum, jú huā

Clerodendrum trichotomum, Glorybower, chòu wú tóng

Codonopsis pilosula, Poor Man's Ginseng, dǎng shēn

Cornus officinalis, Dogwood, shān zhū yú

Crataegus pinnatifida, Chinese Hawthorn, shān zhā

Cyathula officinalis, Hookweed, chuān niú xī

Dianthus superbus, Fringed Pink, qú mài

Dioscorea opposita, Chinese Yam, shān yào

Dolichos lablab, Hyacinth Bean, bái biǎn dòu

Eclipta prostrata, Eclipta, mò hàn lián

Eriobotrya japonica, Loquat, pí pá yè

Eucommia ulmoides, Hardy Rubber Tree, dù zhòng

Forsythia suspensa, lián qiào

Gentiana scabra, lóng dǎn cǎo

Gentiana straminea, qín jiāo

Ginkgo biloba, Ginkgo, bái guǒ

Ligusticum jeholense, Chinese Lovage, gǎo běn

Ligustrum lucidum, Chinese Privet, nǚ zhēn zǐ

Lilium lancifolium, *L. brownii*, Lily, bǎi hé

Lonicera japonica, Honeysuckle, jīn yín huā

Lycium chinense, Chinese Wolfberry, gǒu qǐ zǐ/dì gǔ pí

Mentha haplocalyx, Field Mint, bò hé

Momordica charantia, Bitter Melon, kǔ guā

Ocimum sanctum, Sacred Basil, Tulsi

Ophiopogon japonicus, Lilyturf, mài mén dōng

Paeonia lactiflora, Chinese Peony, bái/chì sháo

Paeonia suffruticosa, Tree Peony, mǔ dān pí

Pinellia ternata, bàn xià

Plantago asiatica, Plantain, chē qián zǐ

Platycodon grandiflorus, Balloon Flower, jié gěng

Prunella vulgaris, Heal All, xià kū cǎo

Rehmannia glutinosa, Chinese Foxglove, dì huáng

Rheum palmatum, Chinese Rhubarb, dà huáng

Salvia miltiorrhiza, S. przewalskii, S. bowleyana, Red Sage, dān shēn

Saposhnikovia divaricata, Siler, fáng fēng

Schisandra chinensis, Five Flavored Fruit, wǔ wèi zǐ

Schizonepeta tenuifolia, Japanese Catnip, jīng jiè

Scrophularia buergeriana, Figwort, bĕi xuán shēn

Scutellaria baicalensis, Baikal Skullcap, huáng qín

Scutellaria barbata, Barbat Skullcap, bàn zhī lián

Sophora flavescens, kǔ shēn

Trichosanthes kirilowii, Chinese Cucumber, guā lóu/tiān huā fĕn

Withania somnifera, Ashwagandha

Field Production

Plant out three- to four-year-old saplings into a medicinal orchard or hedgerow on thirty-foot spacing in full sun in moderately fertile, well-draining soil. Provide irrigation, and mulch to keep weed competition low and conserve and moderate water availability. Do not overfertilize or leaf burning may ensue. Provide even water.

Pests and Diseases

None.

Harvest and Yield

Harvest young buds in spring before any floral petals are present. Floral buds may form on trees as young as seven years but may not bloom until trees reach eleven years of age. Dry and cut some open to check for doneness. The best quality is said to be "of unfragmented, compact flower buds with dense perianth [floral parts] segments, short stalks, soft, glossy hair, and an aromatic fragrance."[128] The *Magnolia denudata* trees at the Chinese Medicinal Herb Farm are still too young for analysis of yield, and I did not find yield data from any other source.

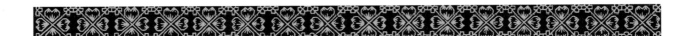

Mentha haplocalyx, (Briq.)
Common Name: Field Mint
Pinyin: Bò hé
Family: Lamiaceae
Part Used: Herb

Plant Description

Mentha haplocalyx is a rhizomatous and creeping herbaceous perennial. It is similar in growth habit to other mints, such as peppermint and spearmint, but distinctly different in fragrance; it smells less like food and more like medicine. Plants are many-branched and up to two feet tall and spreading. Coarsely toothed, hairy, ovate, medium-green leaves are arranged in spikes that have many small, light, purple flowers in whorled clusters in the leaf axils. This species exhibits invasive properties similar to several other similar species native to the United States. It is commonly cultivated and naturalized across China, and many other Eastern regions, from sea level to almost 10,000 feet.[129] USDA hardiness zones 5–9.

Propagation

You can increase your stock of this easy-to-grow plant by seed or division. The plants readily cross-pollinate, so take care if collecting seed for replanting. Sow seed in spring on the medium surface (it is a light-dependent germinator); with heat, emergence takes place in two weeks. Division is quick and trouble-free; simply dig or cut sections of plants that have roots and replant or repot. Water well and provide average soil fertility. Because of its fast growth it does not hold well in pots. Renew often and supplement with fertilizer.

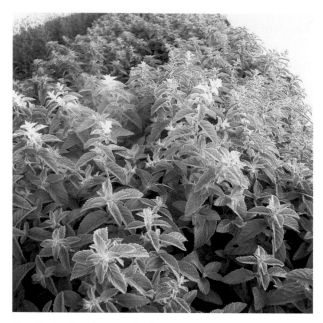

Mentha haplocalyx as a field crop.

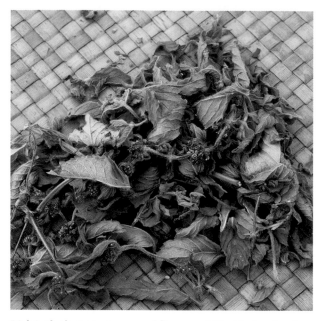

Bò hé—the leaves, stems, and flowers of *Mentha haplocalyx*.

Garden and Polyculture Planting

Field mint can be an invasive groundcover via runners or stolons. To incorporate in a garden without risking a minty invasion, confine to control. Plant in a fifteen-gallon pot and sink it most of the way into the soil, or plant in a large pot and use as an accent or dooryard pot. Mints like a full sun to part shade exposure in moist fertile soils. Because they are a bit aggressive, mints do not have many plant friends. They do not outcompete trees, though.

Suitable Companions

Clerodendrum trichotomum, Glorybower, chòu wú tóng
Cornus officinalis, Dogwood, shān zhū yú
Crataegus pinnatifida, Chinese Hawthorn, shān zhā
Eucommia ulmoides, Hardy Rubber Tree, dù zhòng
Forsythia suspensa, lián qiào
Ginkgo biloba, Ginkgo, bái guǒ

Field Production

Transplant field mint on one-foot spacing in and between rows. Plants will tolerate some drought, but they prefer a moist fertile environment. In spring, after the first season, cut down any winter or errant stems to prepare for a clean harvest; a tractor-mounted mower, gas string trimmer, or gas hedge shears work well. Top-dress permanent plantings in early spring with compost. To control the invasive tendencies I plant where a rototiller can keep runners in check. In arid areas it will not grow beyond the irrigated zone.

Pests and Diseases

Occasionally spring aphids or fall spider mites occur on nursery stock. On a small scale an insecticidal soap should knock back these pests to manageable populations.

Harvest and Yield

You may be able to harvest field mint in the first season if you plant it early enough in the spring. Harvest leaf and stem the first of two times per season in the heat of summer when flowers are coming into full bloom, and the second time in the early fall. Prewash the crop a day or two before harvest to remove any dust or any other unwanted elements such as old yellowing leaves. Gas hedge shears make quick work of the woody stems. Reap the crop early in the day to minimize interaction with bees. The herb should be deeply aromatic. Be sure to include the stems, as they are used in Chinese medicine. After cutting the crop at more or less one foot, either place on drying

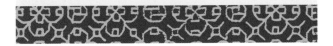

Field Mint Recipes

Use the leaves of this mint in tea. The flowers are edible and can be scattered over salads and on top of soups as a garnish.

Pour boiling water over the dried or fresh leaves and steep for two to three minutes. Use a larger quantity of fresh leaves to dried, adjust the amounts to your taste if desired, and stir a teaspoon of honey into each individual cup. Chilled, the tea makes a refreshing hot-weather drink.

screens or bundle and hang. Field mint generates internal heat upon cutting—do not allow harvest to sit; chill or put to dry without delay. When dry, riddle on a screen by holding the bundle perpendicular to one-inch hardware cloth and rake back and forth to break up the herb. Yield is 0.35 pounds per square foot fresh. Ratio of fresh to dry is 5:1.

Notes

- Harvest timing for field mint is best in the summer when the weather is hot, which yields a crop high in desirable essential oils. Harvest in the cool of the morning to avoid heat stressing the crop—and the harvesters, too!
- Do not plant field mint in riparian or wetland areas where there is any connection to natural bodies of water.

Medicinal Uses of Bò hé

Bò hé is the herb or aerial portion of *Mentha haplocalyx*. Acrid and cool, it releases the exterior, dispels wind heat, clears the head, brightens the eyes, benefits the throat, vents rashes, relieves liver stagnation, and disperses turbid qi from the abdomen. It is used to address a variety of issues including upper respiratory tract infection with sore throat and fever, headache, red eyes, rash, eczema, measles, irritability, and discomfort and fullness in the chest and abdomen—and certain types of abdominal pain, vomiting, and diarrhea.

It is usually used in combination with other herbs. Common methods of administration include beverages and decoctions (added in near the end of the cooking time), powders, concentrated granules, alcohol extracts, infusions, tablets, and pills. It is in many important formulas such as Yin Qiao San (*Lonicera* and *Forsythia* Powder), Sang Ju Yin (*Morus* and Chrysanthemum Decoction), Xiao Yao San (Free and Easy Wanderer Powder) and all of its derivative formulas, Xiao Feng San (Eliminate Wind Powder), Cang Er Zi San (*Xanthium* Seed Powder), and Chuan Xiong Cha Tiao San (*Ligusticum* Powder to be Taken with Green Tea).

Traditionally, although leaves and stems are usually used together with bò hé, the leaves are considered to have a stronger surface relieving effect while the stems have a stronger effect on regulating the qi.

Momordica charantia (L.)

Common Name: Bitter Melon
Pinyin: Kǔ guā
Family: Cucurbitaceae
Part Used: Fruit

Plant Description

An important edible and medicinal, this curious annual vining gourd grows up to twelve feet and has eight-inch wide, deeply lobed, palmate, dark-green leaves that climb with clasping tendrils. The five-petaled, butter-yellow flowers are 1½ inches across and yield a warty edible fruit. Many varieties have been developed, producing fruits of many shapes and sizes, from long and thin to shorter or more pointed. The five- to eight-inch fruits are roughly ridged lengthwise and are always seriously bumpy. Each one seems to be a variation on a work of art. The immature fruits are either pale or dark green and mature into orange fruit that splits and ejects the brilliant red seed while still hanging on the vine. *Momordica charantia* has a wide geographic distribution, mostly in the tropics as a cultivated vegetable, in China and southeast Asia, Africa, and India. Watch for any invasive qualities, especially in frost-free regions. All USDA hardiness zones.

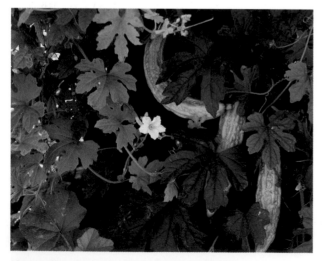

***Momordica charantia* vine in flower and fruit.**

Propagation

Where summers are short or cool, plant the large seed in the greenhouse; direct seed where summers are hot or long. The seed does not store well, so use fresh stock. Warm soil is best for germination, which takes place in a week. Media should be fertile, or supplement with a liquid fertilizer. Pot up if necessary, keeping vines separated.

Garden and Polyculture Planting

Insect-pollinated bitter melon is quite suitable for growing in a vegetable or ornamental garden or hedgerow. Plants, flowers, and fruit are attractive and gardenworthy. Bitter melon prefers warm to hot and humid weather. Take heart—it is possible to get good crops in cooler locations or short-season regions: simply grow cultivars that are either smaller or earlier-maturing, or use season-extending techniques. Strong trellising is a must, as plants are vigorous and fruit production is generally high. Plant two feet apart in full sun in fertile, well-cultivated, draining soils. Bitter melon is monoecious—if seed production is desired, grow several plants to assure getting males and females. When collecting seed, gather as the fruits are turning orange; wait any longer and you'll find the seed expelled on the ground.

Suitable Companions

Achyranthes bidentata, Oxknee, huái niú xī
Allium macrostemon, xiè bái
Andrographis paniculata, Kalmegh, chuān xīn lián
Aster tataricus, Tartar Aster, zǐ wǎn
Belamcanda chinensis, Blackberry Lily, shè gān
Celosia argentea, qīng xiāng zǐ
Celosia cristata, Cockscomb, jī guān huā

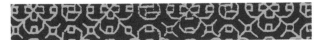

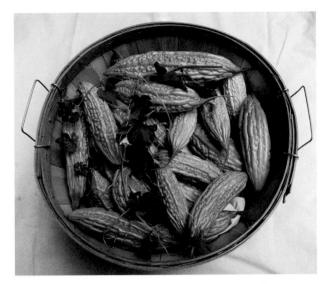

Freshly harvested fruit of *Momordica charantia*–the orange one, though beautiful, is overripe.

Chrysanthemum morifolium, Mum, jú huā
Clerodendrum trichotomum, Glorybower, chòu wú tóng
Crataegus pinnatifida, Chinese Hawthorn, shān zhā
Cyathula officinalis, Hookweed, chuān niú xī
Dianthus superbus, Fringed Pink, qú mài
Dioscorea opposita, Chinese Yam, shān yào
Dolichos lablab, Hyacinth Bean, bái biǎn dòu
Eriobotrya japonica, Loquat, pí pá yè
Forsythia suspensa, lián qiào
Ligusticum jeholense, Chinese Lovage, gǎo běn
Ligustrum lucidum, Chinese Privet, nǔ zhēn zǐ
Lonicera japonica, Honeysuckle, jīn yín huā
Lycium chinense, Chinese Wolfberry, gǒu qǐ zǐ/dì gǔ pí
Magnolia denudata, xīn yí huā
Paeonia lactiflora, Chinese Peony, bái/chì sháo
Platycodon grandiflorus, Balloon Flower, jié gěng
Rehmannia glutinosa, Chinese Foxglove, dì huáng
Saposhnikovia divaricata, Siler, fáng fēng
Sophora flavescens, kǔ shēn

Field Production

Transplant or seed directly on two-foot spacing when soils have warmed in late spring or early summer. Provide a trellis or tripods at least six feet tall. Vigorous and highly productive in most soils, bitter

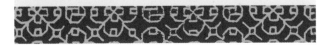

Bitter Melon Recipes

Bitter Melon and Fermented Black Beans

The bitterness of bitter melon is somewhat offset when it is first blanched and then quickly stir-fried in a fermented black bean sauce.

2 bitter melons, about ½ pound each
1 tablespoon salt
1 tablespoon safflower or peanut oil
1 tablespoon fermented black beans, chopped
1 tablespoon ginger, coarsely chopped
1 teaspoon garlic, finely chopped
¼ cup chopped green onions
1 tablespoon soy sauce
1 teaspoon sesame oil
1 teaspoon toasted sesame seeds
Serves four as a side dish

Cut the melons in half lengthwise, and scoop out pith and seeds. Slice the halves across into half-inch pieces. Add water to a medium-size saucepan and set over high heat. Add the salt, and when the water is boiling put in the bitter melon pieces and blanch for three minutes. Drain the melon and set aside.

Place a medium-size saucepan or wok over high heat. When the pan is hot, add the oil, black beans, ginger, garlic, green onions, and soy sauce and cook for one minute, stirring constantly. Add the melon and continue to stir for an additional two minutes, or until the pieces soften. Remove from the heat, add the sesame oil, and stir. Serve immediately with the toasted sesame seeds scattered over the top.

melon prefers warm, fertile, well-drained soils. Bitter melon is not drought tolerant; provide irrigation if rains are not forthcoming. Plants are definitely frost tender and require about one hundred days to reach maturity. In cooler regions the use of row covers or even open-ended hoophouses in the field can boost heat and thus production, though on a larger scale this may not be cost effective.

Pests and Diseases
None.

Harvest and Yield
Collect young fruits before they ripen and turn from green to orange. This stage happens very quickly; to maximize yield, fruits may need to be harvested every few days. Do not peel or deseed the fruits. Simply cut them crosswise in ½-inch-thick slices and put to dry. Drying is quick and easy. Yield for bitter melon is 1¼ pounds per plant fresh. Ratio of fresh to dry for whole fruits is 9:1.

Medicinal Uses of Kǔ guā

Kǔ guā is the fruit (melon) of *Momordica charantia*. Bitter (kǔ guā literally means "bitter melon") and cold, it clears heat, dispels summer heat, and relieves thirst. It is a common medicinal food that is used to help the body deal with environmental heat, heat stroke, elevated thirst, various skin conditions, upper respiratory tract infections, and redness and pain in the eyes. Its modern use has been expanded to improve blood sugar control in adult-onset diabetes.

Kǔ guā is used culinarily and prepared as a vegetable. Other common methods of administration include decoctions, juices, alcohol extracts, and pills.

Ocimum sanctum (L.)
Medicinal Synonyms: *Ocimum tenuiflorum* (L.), *Ocimum gratissimum* (L.)
Common Name: Sacred Basil
Hindi: Tulsi
Family: Lamiaceae
Part Used: Herb

Plant Description
There are two varieties of *Ocimum sanctum* that do best in temperate regions, rama and kapoor. This pleasant, very fragrant herb has stems that are square in cross section, like all in the mint family. It looks similar to and has the same culture as its close relative, culinary basil. A vigorous grower in warm weather, *Ocimum sanctum* has ovate leaves up to two inches long on purple- or green-stemmed, upright, branching plants reaching up to two feet tall and one foot wide. Light blue to purple flowers are borne in racemes or spikes and rise above the soft hairy foliage. Tulsi is an annual, requiring roughly eighty days to maturity. All USDA hardiness zones.

Propagation
Tulsi is a warm season annual; sow by pressing seed into the surface of the soil or medium and barely covering it with soil. It should germinate readily in five to twenty days. Sow early in the greenhouse for a

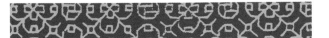

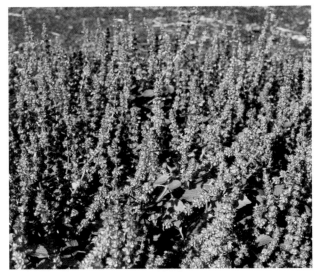

***Ocimum sanctum* growing in the field.**

quick start to the season, or direct seed into the field or garden when soils have warmed. Tulsi grows well in pots but needs to be kept well watered. In the nursery it takes seven weeks from spring sowing to a four-inch transplant or containerized sale.

Garden and Polyculture Planting

Tulsi often reseeds but is not considered invasive. Try transplanting volunteer seedlings to the front of the border on one-foot spacing to organize the planting. Full sun and average water in fertile soils will make tulsi thrive. It is excellent in the garden but a bit small for a hedgerow.

Suitable Companions

Agastache rugosa, Korean Mint, tŭ huò xiāng
Allium macrostemon, xiè bái
Allium tuberosum, Garlic Chives, jiŭ cài zĭ
Angelica dahurica, baí zhĭ
Angelica pubescens, dú huó
Aster tataricus, Tartar Aster, zĭ wǎn
Atractylodes macrocephala, Chinese Thistle Daisy, bái zhú
Belamcanda chinensis, Blackberry Lily, shè gān
Bupleurum chinense, Hare's Ear, chái hú
Carthamus tinctorius, Safflower, hóng huā
Celosia argentea, qīng xiāng zĭ
Celosia cristata, Cockscomb, jī guān huā

Tulsi Recipes

Tulsi is revered in India and is frequently steeped to create a beverage. Pour boiling water over the dried or fresh leaves and steep for two to three minutes. Use a larger quantity of fresh leaves to dried, and adjust the amounts to your taste. If desired, add rose petals or other tealike herbs. Chilled, the tea makes a refreshing hot-weather drink.

Berries with Tulsi Basil Syrup
Tulsi imparts a slight licorice flavor to a simple sugar or honey syrup. This quickly prepared syrup heightens the sweet perfume of berries, particularly strawberries.

½ cup sugar or honey
1 cup water
1 cup fresh tulsi leaves, washed and drained
4 cups of berries, washed, hulled, and drained
Serves four

In a small saucepan, heat together the sugar or honey and water until the mixture just comes to a boil. Remove the syrup from the heat, add the tulsi leaves, and let the tulsi basil syrup cool.

Just before serving, strain off the basil leaves and pour the syrup over the berries.

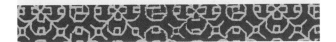

Chrysanthemum morifolium, Mum, jú huā
Clerodendrum trichotomum, Glorybower, chòu wú tóng
Cornus officinalis, Dogwood, shān zhū yú

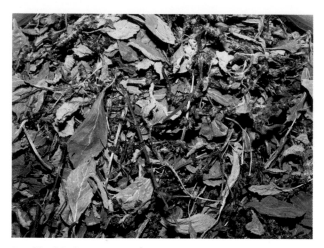

Freshly dried *Ocimum sanctum* leaf, stem, and flower.

Crataegus pinnatifida, Chinese Hawthorn, shān zhā
Cyathula officinalis, Hookweed, chuān niú xī
Dianthus superbus, Fringed Pink, qú mài
Eriobotrya japonica, Loquat, pí pá yè
Eucommia ulmoides, Hardy Rubber Tree, dù zhòng
Ginkgo biloba, Ginkgo, bái guǒ
Lilium lancifolium, L. brownii, Lily, bǎi hé
Magnolia denudata, xīn yí huā
Paeonia lactiflora, Chinese Peony, bái/chì sháo
Paeonia suffruticosa, Tree Peony, mǔ dān pí
Plantago asiatica, Plantain, chē qián zǐ
Platycodon grandiflorus, Balloon Flower, jié gěng
Prunella vulgaris, Heal All, xià kū cǎo
Rehmannia glutinosa, Chinese Foxglove, dì huáng
Rheum palmatum, Chinese Rhubarb, dà huáng
Salvia miltiorrhiza, S. przewalskii, S. bowleyana,
  Red Sage, dān shēn
Saposhnikovia divaricata, Siler, fáng fēng
Schizonepeta tenuifolia, Japanese Catnip, jīng jiè
Scrophularia buergeriana, Figwort, běi xuán shēn
Scutellaria baicalensis, Baikal Skullcap, huáng qín
Scutellaria barbata, Barbat Skullcap, bàn zhī lián
Sophora flavescens, kǔ shēn
Withania somnifera, Ashwagandha

Field Production

Plant or directly seed on one-foot spacing in full sun to part shade in late spring when soils have warmed. Tulsi appreciates a well-drained, fertile soil. It will tolerate some drought conditions, but in areas where

Medicinal Uses of Tulsi

Tulsi is the herb portion of *Ocimum sanctum*. One of the most important Ayurvedic herbs, tulsi in Sanskrit means "Beyond Compare." According to Ayurvedic classification, it is dry, light, acrid, bitter, and hot, with its primary effect on the kapha and pitta humors. It is used to promote longevity; reduce stress and tension; and address issues such as upper respiratory infections, bronchitis, skin disorders, malarial disorders, kidney stones, constipation, mouth ulcers, and insect bites. In modern use it is considered to have strong adaptogenic, antiviral, and anti-inflammatory properties.

Tulsi is used as a single herb and in combination with other herbs. Common methods of administration include tealike infusions, juices, oils, syrups, powders, and chewing or eating the leaves.

In India tulsi is regarded as a sacred plant. It is used in religious rituals, and places where it grows abundantly are considered ideal locations for meditation and spiritual practices.

there are no summer rains, irrigation is necessary; overhead or drip are both suitable. Keep an eye on weeds to facilitate a clean harvest.

Pests and Diseases

Occasional spring aphids are found on tulsi in the nursery. Gophers will occasionally consume all basils.

Harvest and Yield

Tulsi is ready to harvest when it starts to bloom; three harvests per season are possible. For the best quality herb, at first harvest make cuts just above where branching starts. At subsequent harvests, cut immediately above the previous cuts. Harvest early in the day to avoid bee activity and retain cool harvest conditions, because tulsi will discolor if it is picked when warm; refrigerate quickly or put immediately to dry. Drying temperatures should be low, and the dried herb should be green and very fragrant. Yield is one pound per plant per season fresh. Ratio of fresh to dry herb in one-foot bunches is 10:1.

Notes

These basils are revered in the Ayurvedic herbal tradition and are most often used as a caffeine-free tealike beverage. There are several varieties: rama and kapoor (*Ocimum sanctum*), krishna (*Ocimum tenuiflorum*), and vana tulsi (*Ocimum gratissimum*). Krishna and vana tulsi grow well in tropical environs.

Ophiopogon japonicus ([Thunb.] Ker Gawl.)
Common Name: Lilyturf
Pinyin: Mài mén dōng
Family: Convallaricaceae
Part Used: Tuber

Plant Description

Ophiopogon japonicus is a perennial that has been extensively hybridized and is widely available in the nursery trade. Traditionally the species, or more wild form, is used in Chinese medicine; floristically speaking, it is less ornamental. This evergreen, grasslike groundcover blooms in summer with modest panicles that produce bright blue, basally situated fruits. The thin linear-shaped leaves are dark green and lightly serrate, producing a tufted six-inch-tall plant. *Flora of China* notes that this native Asian plant can be found growing in "forests, dense scrub in ravines, moist and shady places on slopes and along streams . . . [and] cliffs."[130] *Ophiopogon japonicus* prefers a moist soil that is somewhat well drained and is in a shady location. Cold hardy to at least zero degrees. USDA hardiness zones 6–10.

Propagation

To increase planting stock, take divisions spring through fall. Slow-growing, they need at least a season to bulk up; consequently they keep well in pots. You can also sow seed in spring and fall; separate the seed from the psychedelic blue-colored fruit before sowing. Lilyturf is not a cool-soil germinator, so use bottom heat or a heated greenhouse. Fertilizer needs are low.

Garden and Polyculture Planting

Lilyturf is useful in the shade or semishade ornamental garden; it fills the niche of an understated

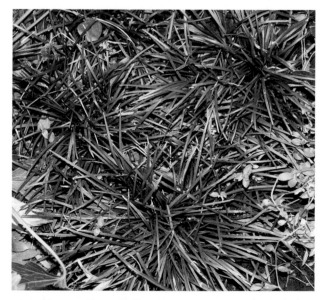

Cultivating *Ophiopogon japonicus*.

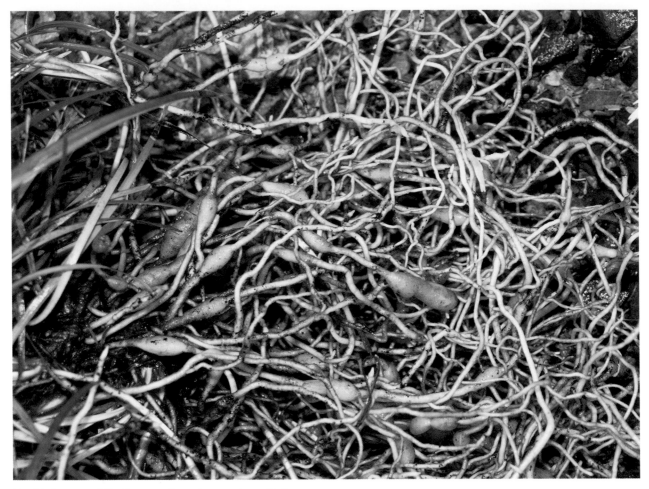

Freshly harvested *Ophiopogon japonicus* roots and tubers.

evergreen mounding groundcover. Mass them in the front of the border or use them as an edging for planting beds; their dark green color will set off many a specimen. Plant six to eight inches on center and they will fill in within a year or so. Beyond weeding no pruning or upkeep is necessary.

Suitable Companions
Acanthopanax gracilistylus, wǔ jiā pí
Albizia julibrissin, Mimosa, hé huān pí/huā
Angelica sinensis, Dang Gui, dāng guī
Asparagus cochinchinensis, tiān mén dōng
Bacopa monnieri, Brahmi
Centella asiatica, Gotu Kola, jī xuě cǎo
Codonopsis pilosula, Poor Man's Ginseng, dǎng shēn

Coix lacryma-jobi, Job's Tears, yì yǐ rén
Cornus officinalis, Dogwood, shān zhū yú
Crataegus pinnatifida, Chinese Hawthorn, shān zhā
Eclipta prostrata, Eclipta, mò hàn lián
Eucommia ulmoides, Hardy Rubber Tree, dù zhòng
Gentiana scabra, lóng dǎn cǎo
Gentiana straminea, qín jīao
Ginkgo biloba, Ginkgo, bái guǒ
Gynostemma pentaphyllum, Sweet Tea Vine, jiǎo gǔ lán
Houttuynia cordata, yú xīng cǎo
Magnolia denudata, xīn yí huā
Pinellia ternata, bàn xià
Schisandra chinensis, Five Flavored Fruit, wǔ wèi zǐ
Scutellaria barbata, Barbat Skullcap, bàn zhī lián

Medicinal Uses of Mài mén dōng

Mài mén dōng is the tuber of *Ophiopogon japonicus*. Sweet, slightly bitter, and cool, it nourishes the yin, moistens the lungs, nourishes the stomach, generates fluids, clears the heart, and moistens the intestines. It is used to address a range of disorders that involve dryness, including acute or chronic dry cough, postviral cough, sore throat, loss of voice, dry throat, nosebleed, stomach pain with thirst, nausea and vomiting, excessive thirst, irritability, insomnia, and constipation.

Mài mén dōng is usually used in combination with other herbs. Common methods of administration include decoctions, powders, concentrated granules, tablets, and pills. It is used in many important formulas, including Mai Men Dong Tang (*Ophiopogon* Combination), Qing Zao Jiu Fei Tang (Clear Dryness and Rescue the Lungs Decoction), Sheng Mai San (Generate the Pulse Powder), Zeng Ye Tang (Increase Fluids Decoction), Yu Nu Jian (Jade Woman Combination), and Ba Xian Chang Shou Wan (Eight Immortals Pill for Longevity).

Field Production

After one season in the nursery, situate in a shady or semishady location six to eight inches on center. Keep watered—lilyturf is not at all drought tolerant and prefers moist soil that is not boggy. Otherwise, it is an undemanding and durable—albeit slow growing—shallowly rooted herb.

Pests and Diseases

Occasionally gophers will consume the roots.

Harvest and Yield

Dig whole plants in the summer of the third year (or more) and remove the one-inch-long fleshy tubers from the tops and other connecting root material. Repot crowns that have small tubers attached for future stock. Wash and use the tasty, crunchy tubers fresh or dry. The tubers should be separated from the thin connecting root, which is considered undesirable. The tubers seem to dry easily enough, and turn a bit translucent, but it appears that the herb is hydroscopic and attracts moisture—be sure to monitor stored material. Two-season-old yield is a quarter-pound per plant fresh. Ratio of fresh to dry herb is 4:1.

Paeonia lactiflora (Pall.)
Common Name: Chinese Peony
Pinyin: Bái/chì sháo
Family: Paeoniaceae
Part Used: Root

Plant Description

Cultivated for over 2,000 years in China and Siberia, this medicinal herb made its Western debut roughly 200 years ago as a beautiful horticultural introduction and now graces many gardens throughout cold winter regions. Growing from two to four feet tall, *Paeonia lactiflora* is a long-lived herbaceous perennial that has dark green leaves that are twice divided into three lanceolate to obovate leaflets. Flowers with showy yellow stamens are three to four inches across and are usually single and white, sometimes pink or red, and are alluringly fragrant. Brown-skinned roots cover a white interior. In the Russian far east and central to northeast China, *Paeonia lactiflora* is endemic in woods and grasslands from roughly 1,200–7,000 feet in elevation.[131] These beautiful peonies do best in areas that receive a good long winter chill and summer heat. USDA hardiness zones 3–8.

Propagation

Sowing the black half-inch roundish seed requires patience. Nick the hard seed coat and sow in fall in deep flats and expose to winter's chill; do not allow the soil to dry out or become waterlogged. It can take a year for seeds to germinate. Grow in the nursery for at least a season before planting out. Seed-grown plants will bloom in three years. Chinese peonies make excellent permanent potted specimens; keep fertilized and repot every third year with fresh medium. Anhui province in Central China is considered one of the premiere growing regions for bái/chì sháo. I was fortunate enough to visit a farm there during harvest. They propagated the Chinese peonies by removing the crowns and replanting them at the same time as harvesting the roots. The usual time to divide the clumps is in late summer or fall, retaining several buds on each division.

Garden and Polyculture Planting

Coarsely handsome and possessing a graceful habit, Chinese peonies lend beauty to the garden or hedgerow. Transplant two-year-old nursery-grown containers or bareroot plants in fall; place in full sun where summers are mild and part shade in regions with pronounced summer heat. Plant in soils that are friable, fertile or well-amended and well-drained. Plant spacing is three to four feet; irrigate and top-dress with compost, and mulch yearly for even moisture. As a cut flower the quality of Chinese peonies is

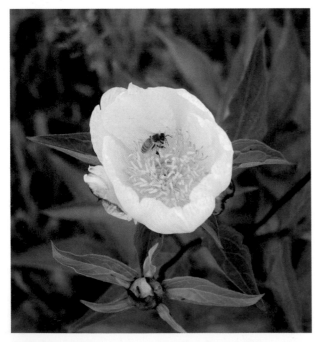

Honeybee working a *Paeonia lactiflora* flower. Photo courtesy of Jean Giblette.

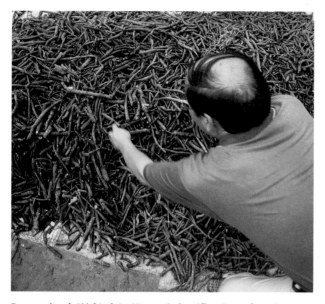

Processing bái/chì sháo (*Paeonia lactiflora*) at a farm in Anhui Province, China.

unsurpassed. In autumn cut and remove spent foliage to avoid any potential disease issues.

Suitable Companions

Anemarrhena asphodeloides, zhī mǔ
Angelica dahurica, bái zhǐ
Angelica pubescens, dú huó
Asparagus cochinchinensis, tiān mén dōng
Aster tataricus, Tartar Aster, zǐ wǎn
Belamcanda chinensis, Blackberry Lily, shè gān
Chrysanthemum morifolium, Mum, jú huā
Codonopsis pilosula, Poor Man's Ginseng, dǎng shēn
Cornus officinalis, Dogwood, shān zhū yú
Crataegus pinnatifida, Chinese Hawthorn, shān zhā
Dianthus superbus, Fringed Pink, qú mài
Eucommia ulmoides, Hardy Rubber Tree, dù zhòng

Medicinal Uses of Bái/chì sháo

Bái sháo, also called bái sháo yao, is the root of *Paeonia lactiflora*. Bitter, sour, and cool, it nourishes the yin, preserves the blood, nourishes the liver, calms liver yang, softens the liver, and relieves spasms. It is one of the most commonly used herbs in TCM for addressing liver patterns of disharmony. It is used to address a wide range of health issues, including muscle spasms, twitches, tremors, numbness and tingling of the extremities, headache, vertigo, abdominal cramping, leg cramping, dizziness, fatigue, dry hair and nails, premenstrual syndrome, menstrual cramping, abnormal uterine bleeding, night sweats, spontaneous sweating, diarrhea with cramping, and dysentery.

Bái sháo is usually used in combination with other herbs. Common methods of administration include decoctions, powders, concentrated granules, alcohol extracts, tablets, and pills. It is in close to one hundred important formulas, including formulas such as Si Wu Tang (Four Substances Decoction), Xiao Yao San (Free and Easy Wanderer), Gui Zhi Tang (Cinnamon Twig Decoction), Shao Yao Gan Cao Tang (Peony and Licorice Decoction), Dang Gui Shao Yao San (*Angelica sinensis* and Peony Powder), Chai Hu Shu Gan San (*Bupleurum* Powder to Spread the Liver), and Si Ni San (Frigid Extremities Powder).

Although unprocessed (dried) bái sháo is commonly used for all of its applications, unprocessed or fresh bái sháo is best for calming the liver and addressing headaches, dizziness, and similar issues. Dry-frying bái sháo enhances its effect on nourishing the blood and preserving the yin, while alcohol-frying increases its ability to treat spasms and cramping.

Paeonia lactiflora is sometimes also used as the source for chì sháo, an important herb for clearing heat, cooling the blood, dispelling blood stagnation, and relieving pain.

Gentiana scabra, lóng dǎn cǎo
Gentiana straminea, qín jiāo
Ginkgo biloba, Ginkgo, bái guǒ
Lilium lancifolium, L. brownii, Lily, bǎi hé
Magnolia denudata, xīn yí huā
Momordica charantia, Bitter Melon, kǔ guā
Ocimum sanctum, Sacred Basil, Tulsi
Ophiopogon japonicus, Lilyturf, mài mén dōng
Paeonia suffruticosa, Tree Peony, mǔ dān pí
Platycodon grandiflorus, Balloon Flower, jié gěng
Prunella vulgaris, Heal All, xià kū cǎo
Rehmannia glutinosa, Chinese Foxglove, dì huáng
Rheum palmatum, Chinese Rhubarb, dà huáng
Salvia miltiorrhiza, S. przewalskii, S. bowleyana,
    Red Sage, dān shēn
Saposhnikovia divaricata, Siler, fáng fēng
Schizonepeta tenuifolia, Japanese Catnip, jīng jiè
Scrophularia buergeriana, Figwort, běi xuán shēn
Scutellaria baicalensis, Baikal Skullcap, huáng qín
Scutellaria barbata, Barbat Skullcap, bàn zhī lián
Sophora flavescens, kǔ shēn
Trichosanthes kirilowii, Chinese Cucumber, guā
    lóu/tiān huā fěn

Field Production

Plant out two-year nursery-grown stock on three-foot spacing, in full sun where summers are mild and part shade in regions with pronounced heat. Amend the soil well with compost and fertilizer before planting. Provide drip irrigation where needed and mulch to maintain even moisture levels. Cultivate to keep weed and resource competition low.

Pests and Diseases

In humid regions botrytis, a fungal disease, can be problematic. At the Anhui province farm the harvesters exposed a grub that ate the roots of Chinese peony; they called it "earth tiger" and mentioned it was usually only a problem with Chinese peonies grown longer than three years in one location. Unfortunately I do not know the name or if we have the pest in North America.

Harvest and Yield

Lift roots from three- to four-year-old plants in summer or fall.[132] First remove the upper material from the crown and dig up the root system. Cut off the roots and remove the bark. The farm in Anhui uses a machine that circulates water and rocks and roots to remove the root bark. The cylindrical roots are then cut on a diagonal of no more than a quarter inch and then dried. "Good quality consists of thick, solid, and heavy roots with a white cross section without clefts and hollow parts."[133] I have not harvested this herb at the Chinese Medicinal Herb Farm and thus don't have any yield data for it.

Notes

- There are many ornamental cultivars of Chinese peony, and you may have to look to specialty peony growers for the species form used in Chinese medicine.
- Chì sháo, or red peony root, is the same plant as bái sháo but is wild-harvested in spring and processed differently.
- I think there is potential for wild-cultivating Chinese peonies, and I hope to hear from growers in the future who are trying it in areas and habitats that are suitable for this hands-off technique.

Paeonia suffruticosa (Andr.)

Common Name: Tree Peony
Pinyin: Mǔ dān pí
Family: Paeoniaceae
Part Used: Root Bark

Plant Description

One of the most admired and prized of medicinal and horticultural specimens, *Paeonia suffruticosa* is also one of the most beautiful and often-depicted Chinese plants. It is a multistemmed deciduous shrub, eventually growing three to five feet tall and just as wide. Spring flowers bloom at the terminus of gray-brown stems. In the species form, flowers are single, from four inches across when young to almost a foot across when older. I grow a medicinal cultivar called 'White Phoenix'; at six years, these plants threw a dozen white, seven-inch, pink-blushed flowers with showy yellow stamens around hot pink pistils. Green leaves often show purple coloration in response to winter's chill and are thrice divided. Each leaflet is deeply lobed or dissected; petioles

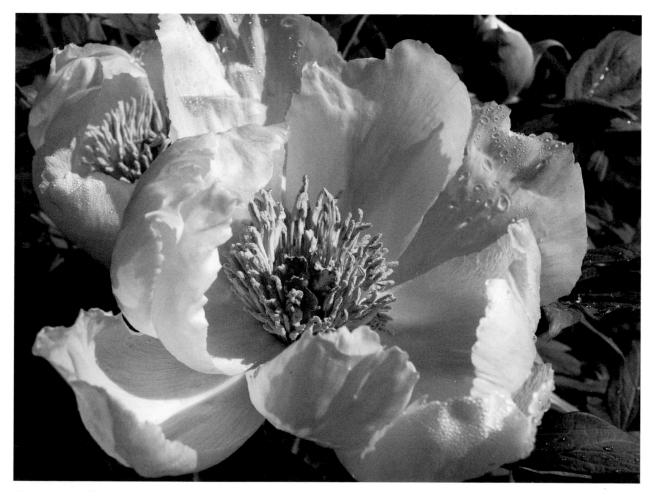

The gorgeous flower of *Paeonia suffruticosa*.

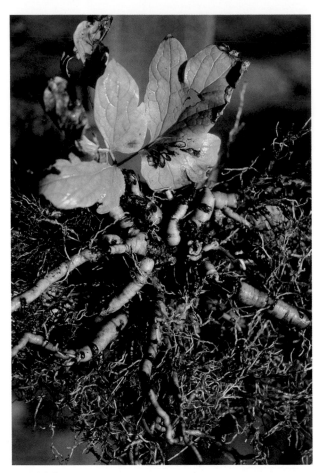

Freshly unearthed *Paeonia suffruticosa* plant. Photo by Nina Zhito.

are strong and rigid. Thickened tuberous roots are tannish. *Paeonia suffruticosa* requires fewer chill hours than *P. lactiflora*. It is native to Anhui and Henan provinces in central China.[134] Cultivation is now widespread and suitable in USDA hardiness zones 5–9 or 10.

Propagation

As with Chinese peony, one needs patience to grow tree peonies from seed. The seed is about the size of a marble with a hard seed coat you should scarify (one method is to rub the seed against sandpaper just until the brown barely yields to white). Sow the seeds one inch deep in a large flat that is five to eight inches deep. Keep moist but not wet (cold is fine, but protect from excessive rain) for at least a year, possibly more, until mass germination surprises the doubtful grower. Grow in the flat for a year and transplant

when dormant (one per gallon pot), grow for a year, and plant out or sell. Division of root clumps in autumn or semihardwood cuttings in spring are other methods of increasing stock. Peonies have a long history of (and do well) growing permanently in large containers. Treat with a balanced fertilizer in spring, and repot every three to four years with new media.

Garden and Polyculture Planting

These gracefully stout plants make excellent garden or border additions, preferring afternoon shade and soils that are fertile, well amended, and freely draining. Prune out any dead wood in late winter, when they are admittedly not much to look at. The flowers are a delight when they appear; it is roughly three years from germination to bloom. Tree peony makes a wonderfully fragrant cut flower.

Suitable Companions

Agastache rugosa, Korean Mint, tǔ huò xiang
Anemarrhena asphodeloides, zhī mǔ
Angelica dahurica, baí zhǐ
Angelica pubescens, dú huó
Asparagus cochinchinensis, tiān mén dōng
Aster tataricus, Tartar Aster, zǐ wǎn
Belamcanda chinensis, Blackberry Lily, shè gān
Chrysanthemum morifolium, Mum, jú huā
Codonopsis pilosula, Poor Man's Ginseng, dǎng shēn
Cornus officinalis, Dogwood, shān zhū yú
Dianthus superbus, Fringed Pink, qú mài
Eclipta prostrata, Eclipta, mò hàn lián
Eriobotrya japonica, Loquat, pí pá yè
Eucommia ulmoides, Hardy Rubber Tree, dù zhòng
Gentiana scabra, lóng dǎn cǎo
Gentiana straminea, qín jiāo
Ginkgo biloba, Ginkgo, bái guǒ
Ligustrum lucidum, Chinese Privet, nǔ zhēn zǐ
Lilium lancifolium, *L. brownii*, Lily, bǎi hé
Magnolia denudata, xīn yí huā
Ophiopogon japonicus, Lilyturf, mài mén dōng
Paeonia lactiflora, Chinese Peony, bái/chì sháo
Plantago asiatica, Plantain, chē qián zǐ

Medicinal Uses of Mǔ dān pí

Mǔ dān pí is the root bark of *Paeonia suffruticosa*. Acrid, bitter, and cool, it clears heat, cools the blood, invigorates the blood, and dispels blood stasis. It is used to address issues such as excessive menstruation, early menstruation, painful menstruation, menopausal symptoms such as nighttime heat and thirst, skin disorders, hypertension, abdominal masses such as fibroids, intestinal abscess, early stage appendicitis—and musculoskeletal injuries with inflammation, bruising, and swelling.

Mǔ dān pí is usually used in combination with other herbs. Common methods of administration include decoctions, powders, concentrated granules, alcohol extracts, tablets, and pills. Mǔ dān pí plays a supportive role in many important formulas including Liu Wei Di Huang Wan (Six Flavor *Rehmannia* Pills) and all of its derivatives, Jia Wei Xiao Yao San (Augmented Free and Easy Wanderer), Gui Zhi Fu Ling Wan (Cinnamon and *Poria* Pill), and Qing Wei San (Clear the Stomach Powder).

Unprocessed (dried) mǔ dān pí is usually used for clearing heat and cooling the blood, while alcohol-frying enhances its ability to move the blood and treat blood stagnation. Charring increases its ability to stop abnormal bleeding.

Mǔ dān yè, the leaf of *Paeonia suffruticosa*, is sometimes used to clear damp heat from the intestines and treat dysentery.

Prunella vulgaris, Heal All, xià kū cǎo
Rehmannia glutinosa, Chinese Foxglove, dì huáng
Rheum palmatum, Chinese Rhubarb, dà huáng
Salvia miltiorrhiza, *S. przewalskii*, *S. bowleyana*, Red Sage, dān shēn
Saposhnikovia divaricata, Siler, fáng fēng
Schisandra chinensis, Five Flavored Fruit, wǔ wèi zǐ
Scrophularia buergeriana, Figwort, běi xuán shēn
Scutellaria barbata, Barbat Skullcap, bàn zhī lián

Field Production
To avoid transplant shock gently plant out two-year-old plants on three-foot spacing. Grow in amended, well-draining soil and fertilize yearly in springtime. Afternoon shade with the root area consistently shaded is the ideal siting. Mulch and provide even water.

Pests and Diseases
Gophers occasionally relieve the grower of in-ground stock.

Harvest and Yield
Harvest roots in the fall (October or November) from three- to five-year-old plants.[135] Cut away all aboveground plant material, separate the roots from the crown, and wash well. Score the root lengthwise and excise the cortex. Cut into three-quarter- to one-inch cross sections and dry. Good bark quality is described as having a strong aroma and being thick, white, and without xylem.[136] To date I have harvested from only one tree peony plant. It was a seed-grown plant, and I waited to harvest until it was nine years old. The yield was three-quarters of a pound fresh. Ratio of fresh to dry is unknown.

Notes
There are many ornamental cultivars, and one may have to look to specialty peony growers for the species form used in Chinese medicine.

Panax ginseng (C.A. Mey.)

Common Name: Asian Ginseng
Pinyin: Rén shēn
Family: Araliaceae
Part Used: Root

Plant Description

This herb, which stands up to 2½ feet tall, has palmately compound leaves arranged in whorls and divided into five leaflets with toothed margins. Small yellow-green, umbrella-shaped inflorescences bloom in spring and mature into bright red, globe-shaped fruits in fall. The thick, aromatic white roots have a history of use dating back several thousands of years. Like *Panax quinquefolius* (American ginseng), this Asian species ginseng is herbaceous and prefers predominantly shady, mixed coniferous and broad-leaved cold temperate forests with moist but well-drained, deep soils rich in organic matter. Wild stands of *Panax ginseng* are rare or extinct in ginseng's historic native habitat in China and Korea; only in Russia are there some intact remnant natural stands. There are some people growing *Panax ginseng* domestically in natural habitats similarly suitable for *Panax quinquefolius* mostly in the mountainous northeastern to southeastern United States. USDA hardiness zones 3–8.

![Panax ginseng plant]

***Panax ginseng*, the plant source of rén shēn. Photo by Steven Foster ©2011.**

Propagation

Sow fresh or stratified seed a half inch deep in the fall in large, deep flats in nursery mix that is high in organic matter; leave exposed to the winter elements. Seeds can take two seasons to germinate. Sow thinly so the resulting seedlings will not touch one another in the flat. Grow for one to three years before transplanting into a hardwood forest site. Another option

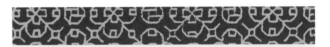

Asian Ginseng Recipes

Ginseng is a well-known tonic for many different ills, but combined with other tea herbs, it enhances its medicinal use with culinary pleasure.

Licorice-Flavored Ginseng Tea

　　1 cup ginseng roots, preferably small tendrils
　　1 cup fresh Korean mint (*Agastache rugosa*) leaves, or a half-cup dried

　　Place the roots and the leaves in a teapot, and fill with boiling water. Let steep for eight to ten minutes. You can continue to refresh the pot with boiling water until the tea seems too weak. If desired, stir a teaspoon of honey into each individual cup.

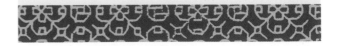

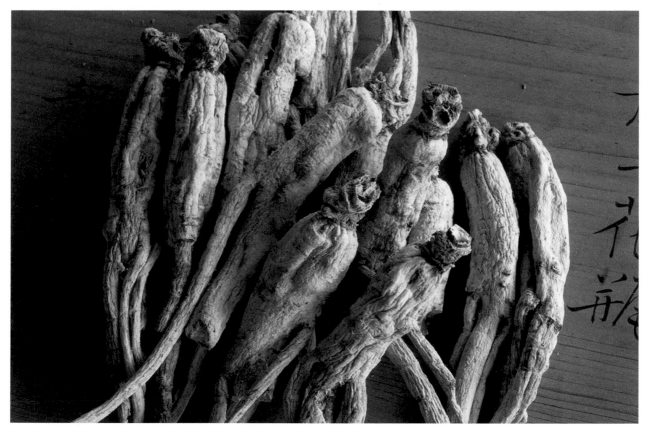

Dried roots of *Panax ginseng,* rén shēn. Photo by Steven Foster ©2011.

is to direct sow the seed by pulling back the forest duff, sowing half an inch deep, and replacing the natural forest dressing. Asian ginseng holds a traditional position in Asia as a homegrown porch plant.

Garden and Polyculture Planting

Asian ginseng and American ginseng share the same understory hardwood forest niche habitat (see the *Panax quinquefolius* entry after this one). A good bet might be to trial an interplanting of Asian ginseng with related species that are known companions in its indigenous habitat. These species include *Abies* spp. (Fir), *Betula* spp. (Birch), *Carpinus* spp. (Hornbeam), *Picea* spp. (Spruce), *Pinus* spp. (Pine), *Quercus* spp. (Oak), and *Tilia* spp. (Linden, Basswood).[137] Give plants plenty of room in order to lessen competition.

Suitable Companions

Angelica sinensis, Dang Gui, dāng guī
Asparagus cochinchinensis, tiān mén dōng

Gentiana scabra, lóng dǎn cǎo
Gentiana straminea, qín jīao
Ophiopogon japonicus, Lilyturf, mài mén dōng
Pinellia ternata, bàn xià
Schisandra chinensis, Five Flavored Fruit, wǔ wèi zǐ

Field Production

The Chinese Medicinal Herb Farm does not have any suitable sites for growing Asian ginseng. But if you are fortunate enough to have the right conditions on your property, I encourage you to try growing this plant. As with American ginseng, plant fresh or stratified Asian ginseng seed directly into the forest duff, sowing half an inch deep and replacing the natural forest dressing. Space one foot apart, in areas that poachers are unlikely to find. Use of transplants will yield a quicker crop. Collect and use forest duff as a mulch to conserve and moderate water, as well as a nutrient source. The use of fertilizer is not recommended. Keep weeded, taking care not to disturb the plants. It is difficult to bring a successful crop to harvest; trial plots mitigate potential financial losses. From every source I've consulted crop rotation is recommended for all *Panax* species; areas where ginseng has been grown and harvested should not be used again for a number of years to rid soils of pathogens. Field production is not recommended, as many deleterious inputs are needed to yield a harvestable crop (and the market price is much lower).

Pests and Diseases

Slugs, rodents, and other mammals enjoy ginseng plants. Numerous diseases affect ginseng crops, particularly when crops are not grown in a natural forest setting.

Harvest and Yield

According to one materia medica, six- to seven-year-old cultivated plants are harvested in September or October and wild material is collected in August through September.[138] Good quality dried root should be thick and long with a yellowish white cortex.[139]

Notes

- There is almost no wild *Panax ginseng* in China or Korea, and wild *Panax ginseng* is considered "at risk." It should be cultivated, not harvested from wild stands; it is currently listed in Appendix II of the Convention on International Trade in Endangered Species of Wild Fauna and Flora (CITES) list. Because "natural populations of ginseng are currently in a state of extreme depletion"[140] we should simulate wild-cultivated material for botanical medicine and allow natural (if not aided) regeneration of wild stands.

- The high value of the roots encourages poaching and will be problematic for forest-grown *Panax ginseng*, just as it is for *Panax quinquefolius*.

Medicinal Uses of Rén shēn

Rén shēn is the root of *Panax ginseng*. It is probably the most well-known Chinese medicinal herb throughout the world. Bitter, sweet, and warm, it tonifies the source qi, strengthens the spleen and lung, generates fluids, calms the shen, enhances the production of blood, and is used to tonify the correct qi in deficient patients with an external condition. It is used to address conditions such as weakness, fatigue, lack of appetite, loose stools, diarrhea, organ prolapse, chronic cough, wheezing, shortness of breath, blood loss, excessive loss of fluids, insomnia, forgetfulness, depression, excessive worrying, and impotence.

Rén shēn is used as a single herb and in combination with other herbs. Common methods of administration include decoctions, powders, alcohol extracts, concentrated granules, tablets, and pills. It is also added to many food and beauty products. It is in well over a hundred commonly used herb formulas, including combinations such as Si Junzi Tang (Four Gentlemen) and its many derivatives, all of the Chai Hu Tang (*Bupleurum* Decoction) variations, Bu Zhong Yi Qi Tang (Tonify the Center and Benefit the Qi Decoction), Gui Pi Tang (Restore the Spleen Decoction), Bu Fei Tang (Tonify the Lungs Decoction), Qing Xin Lian Zi Yin (Lotus Seed Decoction to Clear the Heart), and Sheng Mai San (Generate the Pulse Powder).

Rén shēn yè, the leaf of *Panax ginseng*, is a rarely used herb that relieves summer heat and generates fluids.

Panax quinquefolius (L.)

Common Name: American Ginseng
Pinyin: Xī yáng shēn
Family: Araliaceae
Part Used: Root

Plant Description

One of the most revered Asian medicinal herbs turns out to be none other than *Panax quinquefolius* root—indigenous to eastern North America from southern Canada down to Georgia. Used by Native Americans at least as early as the beginning of the 1700s, *Panax quinquefolius* was recognized as being very similar to *Panax ginseng* (Asian ginseng) by a Jesuit missionary, Joseph Francois Lafitau, in 1715—after reading a description of *Panax ginseng* by another missionary, Petrus Jartoux, who was on a mapping expedition in northern China. Samples were sent to China and the trade of *Panax quinquefolius* began around 1720.[141] It grows one to two feet tall with three to five palmately compound, coarsely toothed leaflets on long petioles and a half-inch umbel of white- to green-colored flowers in spring, followed by red-berried fruits containing two seeds. *Panax quinquefolius* is an herbaceous medicinal with aromatic white forked roots. Every time ginseng goes dormant, the process leaves a mark on the neck of the root, and the years can be counted out by the scars. USDA hardiness zones 3–8.

Propagation

Sow fresh or stratified seed a half-inch deep in the fall in large, deep flats in nursery mix that is high in organic matter; leave exposed to the winter elements. Seeds can take two seasons to germinate. Sow thinly so the resulting seedlings will not touch one another in the flat. Grow for one to three years before transplanting into a hardwood forest site, or direct sow the seed by pulling back the forest duff, sowing half an inch deep, and replacing the natural forest dressing.

Garden and Polyculture Planting

Plant American ginseng in a forest community on the northern side of a slope, providing 50 percent or more shade and plenty of space—do not crowd. Suitable forest companions in eastern areas include *Acer saccharum* (sugar maple), *Actaea racemosa* (black cohosh), *Hydrastis canadensis* (goldenseal), *Podophyllum peltatum* (mayapple), *Polygonatum biflorum* (Solomon's seal), *Sanguinaria canadensis*

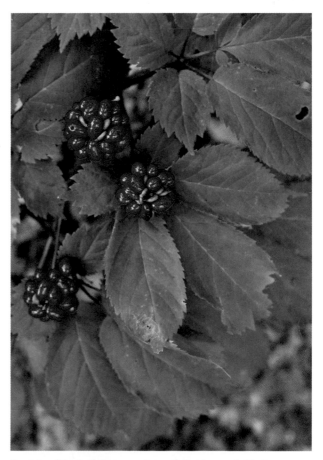

Forest cultivated *Panax quinquefolius* in seed. Photo courtesy of Eric P. Burkhart.

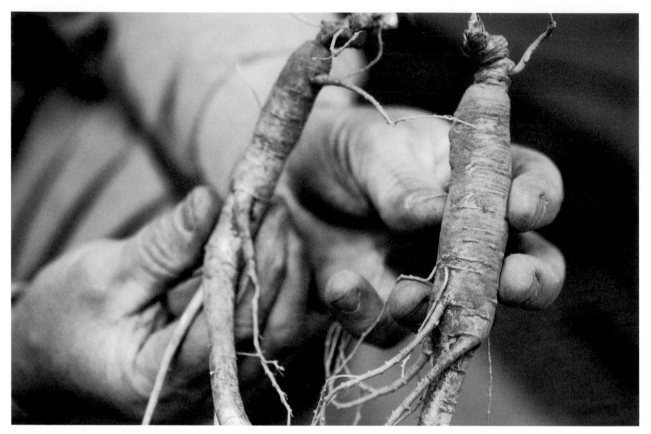

Forest cultivated fresh roots of *Panax quinquefolius*. Photo courtesy of Eric P. Burkhart.

(bloodroot), and *Trillium* spp. (Trillium). (Additionally, some Eastern tree genera associated with American ginseng include *Juglans* (walnut), *Populus* (poplar), *Quercus* (oak), and *Tilia* (basswood).[142]) Western companions include *Maianthemum racemosum* (false Solomon's seal), *Mahonia nervosa* (Oregon grape), *Trillium* spp. (Trillium), and *Asarum canadense* (wild ginger).[143] "Avoid planting under conifers or other shallow-rooted trees as they compete with ginseng for soil moisture and nutrients."[144] No fertilizers are necessary; mulch is recommended.

Suitable Companions
Angelica sinensis, Dang Gui, dāng guī
Asparagus cochinchinensis, tiān mén dōng
Gentiana scabra, lóng dǎn cǎo
Gentiana straminea, qín jiāo
Ophiopogon japonicus, Lilyturf, mài mén dōng
Pinellia ternata, bàn xià
Schisandra chinensis, Five Flavored Fruit, wǔ wèi zǐ

Field Production
American ginseng requires a very specific habitat: hardwood forest with 50–75 percent shade, ample moisture, and well-drained deep soils. Provide supplemental irrigation if rainfall is below twenty inches annually.[145] There are many considerations that make growing ginseng a high-risk venture. Highly modified environments, including raised beds and shade cloth, are often input intensive. It requires cold winter temperatures and is not a suitable crop for warm winter regions. For the best success and best price point, wild-cultivate American ginseng within its native forest habitat and geographic range. There is much in-depth and well-researched information available on growing this plant. Use fresh or stratified seed and sow directly into prepared forest soils one foot apart in areas that poachers are unlikely to find. Transplants will yield a quicker crop than seed. Use mulch to conserve and moderate water as well as a nutrient source. The use of fertilizer is

Medicinal Uses of Xī yáng shēn

Xī yáng shēn is the root of *Panax quinquefolius*. Sweet, bitter, and cold, it tonifes the qi, nourishes the yin, clears fire, and generates fluids. It is used to address issues such as weakness, fatigue, coughing, wheezing, dry throat and mouth, and excessive thirst. In modern China it is often used to address side effects of chemotherapy and radiation and to treat diabetes.

Xī yáng shēn is commonly used as a single herb and is also used in combination with other herbs. Common methods of administration include decoctions, powders, concentrated granules, and pills. It is the chief herb in the formula Qing Shu Yi Qi Tang (Clear Summer Heat and Augment the Qi Decoction).

not recommended. Keep weeded, taking care not to disturb the plants. It is difficult to bring a successful crop to fruition; trial plots mitigate potential financial losses.

Pests and Diseases

Slugs, rodents, and other mammals enjoy ginseng plants. Numerous diseases affect ginseng crops, particularly when they are not grown in the woods.

Harvest and Yield

Harvest the roots in the fall of their fifth year, taking care not to damage any rootlets. Wash gently, and dry whole—gently and slowly—starting with lower temperatures and increasing the heat to ninety degrees.[146] The best quality roots are yellowish white (not a bleached white), deeply aromatic, heavy for their size, showing lateral lines, and powdery when cut.[147] "Yields of dried roots from a well-managed planting average about 1 ton/acre, although greater yields are often reported."[148] Ratio of fresh to dry is 3½:1.[149]

Notes

- Wild *Panax quinquefolius* is considered "at risk" and should be cultivated, not harvested from wild stands; it is currently listed in Appendix II of the Convention on International Trade in Endangered Species of Wild Fauna and Flora (CITES) list. This regulation attempts to monitor the trade and protect the species from extinction by overharvesting (however, the designation does not apply to artificially cultivated American ginseng material).
- Interestingly enough, this US native is now being extensively cultivated in northeast China, corresponding to USDA hardiness zone 4, as well as two more southern interior provinces near the 25th and 30th parallels (Guizhou, Jiangxi) and coastal Jiangsu corresponding to USDA hardiness zones 8 and 9.[150]
- As with other high-value crops, growing American ginseng under the cloak of forest cover brings the risk of theft.

Pinellia ternata ([Thunb.] Makino)
Common Name: None
Pinyin: Bàn xià
Family: Araceae
Part Used: Tuber

Plant Description

Pinellia ternata is an herbaceous tuber-forming perennial with bright green, thrice-divided palmate leaves. Air bulbils are white with papery tan-brown coverings and are frequently found on the petioles, while larger tubers are subterranean. Under favorable conditions *Pinellia ternata* exhibits invasive qualities and spreads by the underground tubers. The striking flowers are borne in summer and are green spathes with black spadices that sit above the foliage at a height of one to two feet. Endemic to China, Japan, and Korea, *Pinellia ternata* grows at lower elevations in "grasslands, secondary forests, and wastelands . . . [and] cultivated lands."[151] USDA hardiness zones 5–9; however, temperatures over 95–100 degrees can drive this plant into summer dormancy.

Propagation

It is easy to increase stock in the spring or fall by taking divisions of underground tubers or potting up the pea-sized bulbils. Slow growing, the plants hold well in pots. It takes a season of growth (or more) to size up for containerized sale. Do not allow potted stock of *Pinellia ternata* to dry out. Fertilizer needs are low.

Garden and Polyculture Planting

Pinellia ternata is a curious looking plant that would grow well in a shady and moist but well-drained, front-of-the-border location. The plantings expand slowly, but they are persistent; watch for invasive qualities. It appears in the U.S. nursery trade as a landscape ornamental. This plant has toxic attributes in raw form, so do not plant it where it may be eaten by mistake. Processing is necessary before ingestion.

Suitable Companions

Asparagus cochinchinensis, tiān mén dōng
Bacopa monnieri, Brahmi
Centella asiatica, Gotu Kola, jī xuě cǎo
Clerodendrum trichotomum, Glorybower, chòu wú tóng
Codonopsis pilosula, Poor Man's Ginseng, dǎng shēn
Coix lacryma-jobi, Job's Tears, yì yǐ rén
Cornus officinalis, Dogwood, shān zhū yú
Crataegus pinnatifida, Chinese Hawthorn, shān zhā
Eclipta prostrata, Eclipta, mò hàn lián

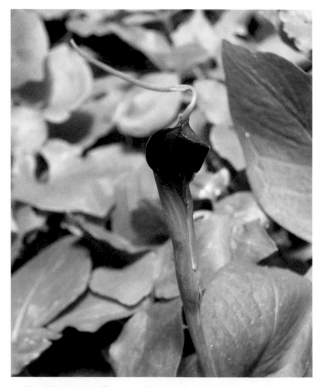

In *Pinellia ternata* flowers the green sheathlike spathe encircles the projecting spadix on which the plant's flowers are borne.

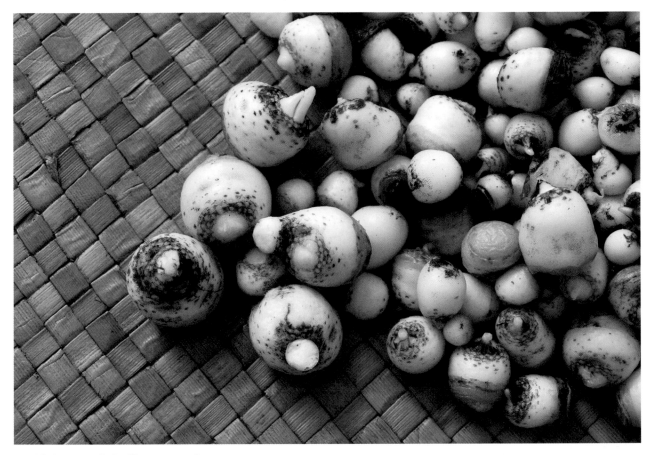

Freshly harvested *Pinellia ternata* tubers.

Eriobotrya japonica, Loquat, pí pá yè
Eucommia ulmoides, Hardy Rubber Tree, dù zhòng
Gentiana scabra, lóng dǎn cǎo
Gentiana straminea, qín jiāo
Ginkgo biloba, Ginkgo, bái guǒ
Gynostemma pentaphyllum, Sweet Tea Vine, jiǎo gǔ lán
Houttuynia cordata, yú xīng cǎo
Lilium lancifolium, L. brownii, Lily, bǎi hé
Lonicera japonica, Honeysuckle, jīn yín huā
Magnolia denudata, xīn yí huā
Ophiopogon japonicus, Lilyturf, mài mén dōng
Plantago asiatica, Plantain, chē qián zǐ
Scutellaria barbata, Barbat Skullcap, bàn zhī lián

Field Production

Pinellia ternata is shade- and moisture-loving and does not tolerate drought; soils should be somewhat well-drained and of average fertility. Where it is happy it can be invasive. Transplant six-month to one-year-old plants on eight-inch centers in the shade to semi-shade. Keep moist—drip or overhead irrigation works equally well. This medicinal is grown two to three years before harvesting. Small tubers have a tendency to persist in the soil even after thorough harvesting, making this plant a good candidate for planting in a permanent location. To control its invasive tendencies, and if only small amounts are needed, try growing it in large containers filled with a mixture of half nursery medium and half native soil.

Pests and Diseases

Occasionally gophers will eat this herb.

Harvest and Yield

Harvest half-inch and larger roundish tubers in late summer after two to three years of growth. Due to the plant's toxic qualities, it's a good idea to wear

Medicinal Uses of Bàn xià

Bàn xià is the tuber of *Pinellia ternata*. Acrid and warm, it is one of the most important herbs in TCM for treating phlegm and damp patterns. It dries dampness, transforms phlegm, redirects qi downward, and dissipates nodules. It is used to address problems such as cough with profuse sputum, shortness of breath, nausea and vomiting due to many causes, dizziness, headache, chest congestion and pressure, thyroid nodules, and some skin disorders.

Bàn xià is usually used in combination with other herbs. Common methods of administration include decoctions, powders, concentrated granules, alcohol extracts, tablets, and pills. It is in a large number of important formulas, including Er Chen Tang (Two-Cured Decoction), Ban Xia Hou Po Tang (*Pinellia* and *Magnolia* Bark Decoction), Liu Junzi Tang (Six Gentlemen Decoction), Wen Dan Tang (Warm Gallbladder Decoction), Dao Tan Tang (Guide Out the Phlegm Decoction), Ding Chuan Tang (Arrest Wheezing Decoction), and all of the Chai Hu Tang (*Bupleurum* Decoction) variations.

Bàn xià is processed before use, as unprocessed bàn xià has some toxicity. There are various methods of processing to eliminate toxicity, with each method slightly changing the function. Qing bàn xià is processed by soaking in water and then cooking with alumen, which produces the most mild and gentle form of bàn xià. Fa bàn xià is processed in water, alumen, calcium oxide, and gān cǎo (*Glycyrrhiza uralensis*), which is one of the most common methods of processing. Jiang bàn xià is processed with ginger juice, which increases its warming functions and ability to treat nausea and vomiting.

gloves when handling this herb. To harvest, dig eight inches deep below the crop, transfer by shovelful into a box with a hardware cloth bottom, and sift the tubers from the soil. Rinse the harvest by hosing off the larger-than-half-inch material that's collected on the screen to reveal the white tubers. Tubers that are smaller than half an inch are too small for medicinal purposes and should be used for future planting stock. To remove the baggy tuber skin, roll the tubers over the screen numerous times and rinse off once more. Drying bàn xià is easy; leave tubers whole. It is fully dry when centers have a powdery feel; cut open to check for doneness. The yield is 0.6 pounds per square foot fresh for a three-year-old crop. Ratio of fresh to dry herb is 3:1.

NOTES

This herb should only be sold to licensed practitioners of Chinese medicine.

Plantago asiatica (L.)

Common Name: Plantain
Pinyin: Chē qián zǐ
Family: Plantaginaceae
Part Used: Seed

Plant Description

Looking very much like the ubiquitous Western weed commonly called broad-leaved plantain (*Plantago major*), this Asian species has bright green, parallel, seven-veined, broadly ovate leaves. Leaf margins have small teeth that can be felt more than seen. A perennial with exclusively basal leaves and petioles eight to ten inches long, the whole leaf reaches 1¼

feet tall. Rigid flowering stalks rise above the foliage to a total height of 2½ feet. These stalks are densely packed with small white flowers ascending the flowering stem to 1½ feet. Flowering takes place over a long summer season, maturing on the stem from the bottom up. Each fruiting capsule contains many brown seeds, which reseed readily in moist to wet areas in gardens and nurseries; in fact this plant may

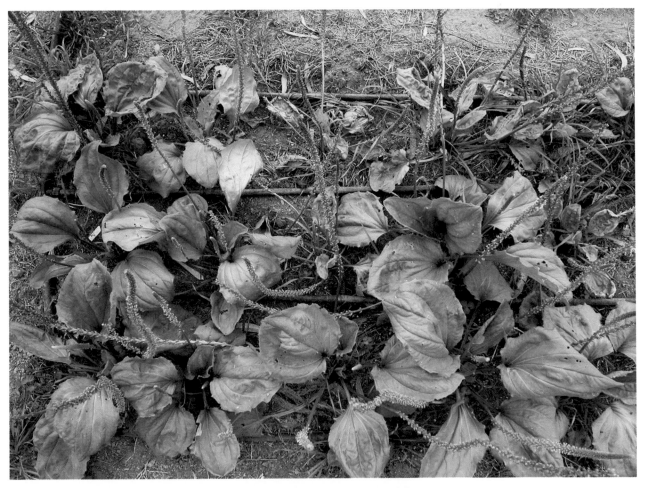

These three-foot-tall row cropped plants of *Plantago asiatica* are moving from flower into seed.

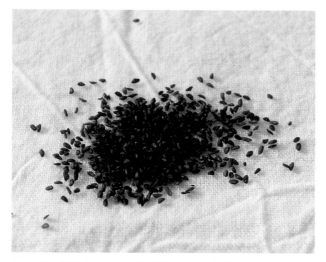

Chē qián zǐ is the dry seed of *Plantago asiatica*.

be weedy in regions with summer rainfall. *Plantago asiatica* is hardy in all USDA zones.

Propagation

The small seeds are light-dependent germinators; sow on the surface of the soil in situ or in nursery medium. Germination is at twenty-eight days and ongoing in cool soils. Plants hold very well in pots and make a surprisingly handsome, if informal, potted winter specimen in mild winter regions.

Garden and Polyculture Planting

Plaintain prefers full sun to part shade in average soils that are not well drained; moist to wet soils are favored. Transplant or directly surface sow toward the front of the garden or border. Due to plantain's invasive inclinations, do not plant in naturally occurring wetlands or riparian areas.

Suitable Companions

Alisma plantago-aquatica subsp. *orientale*, zé xiè
Bacopa monnieri, Brahmi
Coix lacryma-jobi, Job's Tears, yì yǐ rén
Eclipta prostrata, Eclipta, mò hàn lián
Gynostemma pentaphyllum, Sweet Tea Vine, jiǎo gǔ lán
Houttuynia cordata, yú xīng cǎo
Mentha haplocalyx, Field Mint, bò hé

Medicinal Uses of Chē qián zǐ

Chē qián zǐ is the seed of *Plantago asiatica*. Sweet and cold, it clears damp heat, drains dampness, stops diarrhea, clears liver heat, benefits the eyes, clears the lung, and transforms phlegm. It is used to address issues such as painful urination, burning urination, urgency with inability to urinate, diarrhea, eye redness and swelling, headache, dizziness, blurred vision, and cough.

Chē qián zǐ is used by itself and in combination with other herbs. Common methods of administration include powders, decoctions, concentrated granules, tablets, and pills. It is in important formulas including Ba Zheng San (Eight Rectifications Powder), Qing Xin Lian Zi Yin (Heart Clearing Lotus Seed Decoction), and Long Dan Xie Gan Tang (*Gentiana* Decoction to Drain the Liver).

Pinellia ternata, bàn xià
Prunella vulgaris, Heal All, xià kū cǎo
Scrophularia buergeriana, Figwort, běi xuán shēn

Field Production

Transplant on one-foot spacing in beds that are well irrigated. For best growth and yields, keep well watered. These plants are durable and can manage some drought stress.

Pests and Diseases

Slugs, snails, and earwigs riddle the leaves with holes. If damage becomes too great use baits, traps, or exclusionary techniques such as iron phosphate baits for snails or wet, rolled-up newspapers. A few holes are acceptable; shredded leaves indicate action is needed.

Harvest and Yield

Plantain will bloom in the first season if sown in early spring; chē qián zǐ is the ripe seed. The summer and fall seed ripens to a loose rattle in the fruiting capsule; collect several times per season by stripping just the mature seed capsules off the standing fruiting stem. Or if you've grown a sufficient quantity to collect enough seed in just one harvest, cut the stems off completely (for a harvest of roughly a third of the plant's potential seed production capacity). Invert the seed capsules over a clean vessel and the ripe seed will tumble out easily. Blow off the chaff or any extraneous matter, and use or sell the seed fresh or dry. Good quality is said to be "full, hard, brownish black seeds."[152] Seed yield for first season plants is 0.08 pounds per plant. Seed when harvested is almost dry, so the difference between the fresh to dry weight is negligible.

Notes

- In addition to the market for *Plantago asiatica* seed, there is an active Western market for the leaf; conduct a trial for economic feasibility.
- *Plantago depressa* is also a standard species in the Chinese materia medica; however, it is a much smaller plant and seed production is minimal.

Platycodon grandiflorus ([Jacq.] A. DC.)
Common Name: Balloon Flower
Pinyin: Jié gěng
Family: Campanulaceae
Part Used: Root

Plant Description

Platycodon grandiflorus has bright blue-purple, two-inch, terminal blooming flowers exhibiting the characteristic bell shape of the Campanulaceae family. The buds swell before opening, giving the plant its common name of balloon flower. The species form of this popular garden flower grows up to two feet tall and is a prolific summer bloomer. Perennial and herbaceous, erect plants form clumps of foliage with simple, two-inch, ovate, serrate, alternately arranged leaves. When bruised, the stems exude a white sticky latex. The range of *Platycodon grandiflorus* is "Siberia (southern and western regions, the Far East), northeastern China, Korea and Japan. Dry meadows, rocky places among shrubs or in forest clearings."[153] Balloon flower is cold hardy to at least minus thirty degrees. USDA hardiness zones 3–10.

Propagation

Sow seeds in the nursery or indoors very early in the spring, or in the fall for planting out the following summer. Germination is two to three weeks in the heated greenhouse. Seed is small but reliably easy to propagate; there are no special requirements for

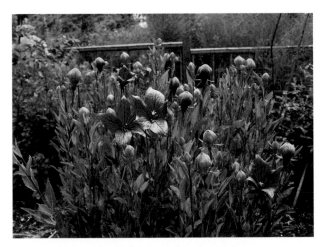

The very gardenworthy *Platycodon grandiflorus*.

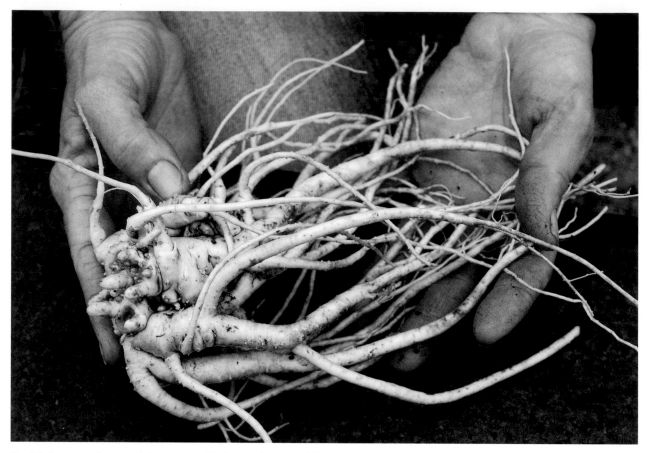

Freshly harvested roots of three-year-old *Platycodon grandiflorus*. Photo by Nina Zhito.

germination. Balloon flower holds very well in pots and makes a good ornamental container plant as well.

Garden and Polyculture Planting

Showy balloon flower has a long history of cultivation and is very gardenworthy. Plant in masses one foot apart in average soil in full sun. For the most ornamental value, the summer flowers will need staking. As the seasons progress the root mass will increase in size and the number of flowers will multiply. It makes a fair cut flower.

Suitable Companions

Agastache rugosa, Korean Mint, tǔ huò xiāng
Allium macrostemon, xiè bái
Allium tuberosum, Garlic Chives, jiǔ cài zǐ
Anemarrhena asphodeloides, zhī mǔ
Angelica dahurica, baí zhǐ

Aster tataricus, Tartar Aster, zǐ wǎn
Belamcanda chinensis, Blackberry Lily, shè gān
Carthamus tinctorius, Safflower, hóng huā
Celosia argentea, qīng xiāng zǐ
Celosia cristata, Cockscomb, jī guān huā
Chrysanthemum morifolium, Mum, jú huā
Codonopsis pilosula, Poor Man's Ginseng, dǎng shēn
Dianthus superbus, Fringed Pink, qú mài
Dolichos lablab, Hyacinth Bean, bái biǎn dòu
Ligusticum jeholense, Chinese Lovage, gǎo běn
Ligustrum lucidum, Chinese Privet, nǚ zhēn zǐ
Lilium lancifolium, *L. brownii*, Lily, bǎi hé
Momordica charantia, Bitter Melon, kǔ guā
Ocimum sanctum, Sacred Basil, Tulsi
Paeonia lactiflora, Chinese Peony, bái/chì sháo
Paeonia suffruticosa, Tree Peony, mǔ dān pí
Prunella vulgaris, Heal All, xià kū cǎo
Rehmannia glutinosa, Chinese Foxglove, dì huáng

Salvia miltiorrhiza, S. przewalskii, S. bowleyana,
  Red Sage, dān shēn
Saposhnikovia divaricata, Siler, fáng fēng
Schizonepeta tenuifolia, Japanese Catnip, jīng jiè
Scutellaria baicalensis, Baikal Skullcap, huáng qín
Scutellaria barbata, Barbat Skullcap, bàn zhī lián
Trichosanthes kirilowii, Chinese Cucumber, guā
  lóu/tiān huā fěn

Field Production

Balloon flower grows best in full sun in moist but
well-drained sandy loam soil. It has average fertilizer
and compost needs. Transplant seedlings one foot
apart in rows one foot apart. Supplement with water
if needed; drip irrigation is ideal as it provides water
without pulling the flowers earthward. Though
balloon flower grows in grasslands in its native Asia,
weeding is recommended to keep nutrient competition low.

Pests and Diseases

Gophers are quite fond of the roots.

Harvest and Yield

Dig the bulbous taproots while dormant in the spring
or fall after at least two years of growth. The shallowly rooted, soft, white, branching taproots grow
about eight inches long. Washing is easy as there is
little root bark; slice roots lengthwise. They dry easily
to a yellow-tan color. "Good quality consists of thick,
white, heavy roots with a bitter taste."[154] The yield is a
half pound per plant fresh for three-year roots. Ratio
of fresh to dry herb is 3½:1.

Notes

- Much work has been done in the nursery
  trade to modify the height, flower, and so
  on of this plant for ornamental purposes—
  potentially at the expense of the medicinal
  properties. When sourcing seed or planting stock, choose unselected species—not
  cultivars or named varieties.

Medicinal Uses of Jié gĕng

Jié gĕng is the root of *Platycodon grandiflorus.* Bitter, acrid, and neutral, it opens the lungs, transforms phlegm, benefits the throat, dispels pus, and raises the qi. It is used to address cough, phlegm, sore throat, hoarse voice, chest discomfort, lung abscess, diarrhea, and water retention. It is one of the most commonly used herbs for treating lung disorders and its influence on the chest makes it a common envoy to guide the functions of a formula to that region.

Jié gĕng is usually used in combination with other herbs. Common methods of administration include decoctions, powders, concentrated granules, alcohol extracts, tablets, and pills. It is in formulas such as Sang Ju Yin (Mulberry and Chrysanthemum Decoction), Yin Qiao San (*Lonicera* and *Forsythia* Decoction), Zhi Sou San (Stop Cough Powder), Xue Fu Zhu Yu Tang (Eliminate Stasis in the Mansion of Blood Decoction), Huo Xiang Zheng Qi San (*Agastache* Powder to Rectify Qi), and Shen Ling Bai Zhu San (Ginseng, *Poria,* and *Atractylodes* Powder).

Jié gĕng is sometimes honey-baked to enhance its ability to moisten the lung and transform phlegm.

- Occasionally there will be a genetic kick-
  back and a white flower form will bloom
  in a field of blue.

Prunella vulgaris (Greene)
Common Name: Heal All
Pinyin: Xià kū cǎo
Family: Lamiaceae
Part Used: Herb

Plant Description
This creeping perennial groundcover has attractive two- to four-inch spikes of purple flowers that bloom in a few short months after sowing, from summer into fall. The plants sport lance-shaped one- to two-inch leaves and grow one foot tall, spreading to form a thick mat. *Prunella vulgaris* grows indigenously on several continents and can reseed or spread by runners readily in many environments—thus it is often labeled as invasive. *Prunella vulgaris* can be winter deciduous; it is widely grown and hardy to at least minus ten degrees. USDA hardiness zones 4–9.

Propagation
Seeds are small but easy to start in the spring, or plants can be divided. Start seed indoors or outside after the danger of frost has passed. Germination occurs in about two weeks, and heat is not necessary. Due to their quick growing habit these plants do not hold well in pots—they need to be repotted often as they easily become pot-bound.

Garden and Polyculture Planting
Heal all is useful and attractive in the garden or front of the border or in a hedgerow where it can move around. Plant on eight-inch to one-foot spacing en masse as a groundcover and give room for it to travel without smothering nearby delicate plants. Water in summer as needed to keep it looking its best; it will survive with scant water, but will become rather scraggly. Prune after blooming (or harvest) to keep it looking neat. Heal all is a durable plant.

Suitable Companions
Acanthopanax gracilistylus, wǔ jiā shēn/pí
Agastache rugosa, Korean Mint, tǔ huò xiāng
Albizia julibrissin, Mimosa, hé huān pí/huā
Angelica dahurica, baí zhǐ
Angelica pubescens, dú huó
Aster tataricus, Tartar Aster, zǐ wǎn
Belamcanda chinensis, Blackberry Lily, shè gān
Carthamus tinctorius, Safflower, hóng huā
Chrysanthemum morifolium, Mum, jú huā
Clerodendrum trichotomum, Glorybower, chòu wú tóng
Coix lacryma-jobi, Job's Tears, yì yǐ rén
Cornus officinalis, Dogwood, shān zhū yú
Crataegus pinnatifida, Chinese Hawthorn, shān zhā
Cyathula officinalis, Hookweed, chuān niú xī
Dolichos lablab, Hyacinth Bean, bái biǎn dòu
Eriobotrya japonica, Loquat, pí pá yè
Eucommia ulmoides, Hardy Rubber Tree, dù zhòng
Forsythia suspensa, lián qiào
Lilium lancifolium, L. brownii, Lily, bǎi hé

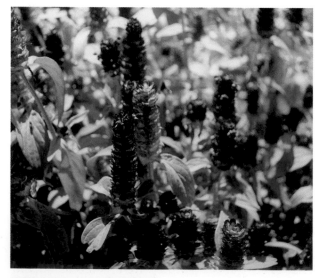

Field-grown *Prunella vulgaris*.

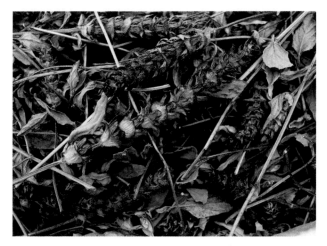

Xià kū cǎo is the dried flower spike and some leaves of *Prunella vulgaris*.

Lonicera japonica, Honeysuckle, jīn yín huā
Magnolia denudata, xīn yí huā
Rheum palmatum, Chinese Rhubarb, dà huáng
Sophora flavescens, kǔ shēn
Trichosanthes kirilowii, Chinese Cucumber, guā lóu/tiān huā fěn

Field Production

Direct seed or transplant easy-to-grow heal all in full sun to part shade on one-foot centers and it will fill in by midsummer. It tolerates soils that are fairly wet to dry, rich to lean, but it prefers moist soils. To keep it healthy as a semipermanent crop, foliar feed it or top-dress with compost in winter. Before spring growth resumes, use hedge shears, a string trimmer, or another tool to prune back hard-to-remove old flower spikes in preparation for summer harvests. Keep weeded to facilitate quick and clean harvests.

Pests and Diseases

Gophers occasionally consume, deer and rabbits browse the flowers, and mites can cause light leaf damage.

Harvest and Yield

For the traditional Chinese herb market the crop is ready to harvest when a majority of the flowers are starting to turn brown. However, for the Western herb market, you'll need to harvest when the flowers

Medicinal Uses of Xià kū cǎo

Xià kū cǎo is the flower spike herb of *Prunella vulgaris*. Bitter, spicy, and cold, xià kū cǎo clears heat and liver fire, clears hot phlegm, and disperses stagnation. It is used to address issues such as redness and swelling of the eyes, headaches, high blood pressure, enlargement of the liver, hyperthyroidism, and swellings and nodules.

Xià kū cǎo is commonly used as an individual herb as well as in herbal formulas. Common methods of administration include decoctions, powders, concentrated granules, alcohol extracts, and pills.

When treating hypertension, it is common in modern China to use the entire plant rather than just the flower spike.

are in full bloom. This is one of the quickest herbs from transplant to first harvest; it can be just nine weeks. Two or possibly three harvests are possible per season, with the second being smaller for both Eastern and Western types. Harvest early in the day to avoid bee activity. If only harvesting a small amount, long-handled scissors yield much more faster than hand pruners. A gas hedge trimmer makes quick work of cutting the top six or eight inches; put it to dry on bench screens or racks. The dry crop doesn't require further handling unless a "cut and sift" specific size is desired. For the ideal result with secondary harvests, cut the herb above where the first cut of the previous harvest was made. The best quality Chinese product consists of two-inch-long mature brown flower spikes and short stalks without leaves,[155] and for the Western herb market it will be young flower spikes with the purple flowers still colorful when the crop is dry. Yield is 0.3 pounds per plant fresh. Ratio of fresh to dry is 4½:1.

Notes

- There are many cultivated varieties created for ornamental and not medicinal purposes—use species, or unselected varieties, found in the medicinal herb trade.
- Potential diversification of sales is possible by servicing both the Eastern and Western herb markets. I will often take the first harvest when immature for the Western trade and dry it if I do not have a contract for fresh herb. Then I will grow the subsequent harvests until they are more mature and harvest them for the Chinese market.

Rehmannia glutinosa ([Gaertn.] DC.)

Common Name: Chinese Foxglove
Pinyin: Dì huáng
Family: Scrophulariaceae
Part Used: Root

Plant Description

Rehmannia glutinosa is an important Chinese botanical, but it is not commonly grown in the United States. This creeping herbaceous perennial has attractive, muted pink, tubular flowers come spring on spikes to 1½ feet tall. The hairy, textured or crenate, softly toothed leaves are arranged in a basal rosette. These are many natural varieties and variations in the species; some bear flowers that are more orange in color than pink, some only grow eight inches tall, and some have roots that are more brittle than others. Some plants exhibit more overall purple tones than others. They spread by pale, orange-skinned, fleshy rhizomes. This herb is widely cultivated in China and occurs naturally from sea level to 3,500 feet and as far north as Mongolia.[156] USDA hardiness zones 4–9.

Propagation

Chinese foxglove is easy to propagate by root division. Seed is very small, and I have found production to be scant, but if you wish to use seed sow it in early spring and use bottom heat to ensure that seedlings will be ready to plant by summer. The plants have adventitious roots; rhizomes that are one year old or with several eyes can also be sectioned off and replanted from March through November. I've found that fungal disease can destroy a planting of Chinese foxglove in a very short time; to guard against loss keep stock in several locations, as well as nursery stock held back. We've also learned that it's critical to supply bottom heat for newly divided nursery stock or the entire crop may be lost. Different landraces are variable in terms of their susceptibility to disease. Chinese foxglove holds fairly well as container stock. Take care not to overwater, especially while winter dormant.

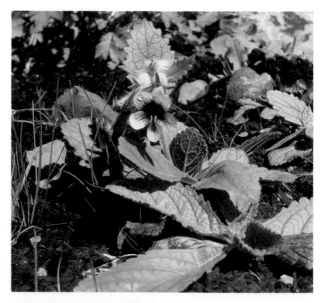

Rehmannia glutinosa **in flower.**

Garden and Polyculture Planting

Chinese foxglove makes an attractive addition for the front of the border or hedgerow. Preferring full sun and very well-drained, average to rich soil, it will do well in an elevated planting or placed where soil drains very well. Grow away from herbs that prefer more irrigation. There will be die-off in times of excess rain, especially when dormant. However, some rhizomes will most likely remain to repopulate the bed. They tend to travel around but are never invasive. Plant en masse, encourage a colony, and enjoy numerous beautiful foxglovelike flowers.

Suitable Companions

Agastache rugosa, Korean Mint, tǔ huò xiāng
Angelica dahurica, baí zhǐ
Angelica pubescens, dú huó
Aster tataricus, Tartar Aster, zǐ wǎn
Belamcanda chinensis, Blackberry Lily, shè gān
Carthamus tinctorius, Safflower, hóng huā
Chrysanthemum morifolium, Mum, jú huā
Cyathula officinalis, Hookweed, chuān niú xī
Dolichos lablab, Hyacinth Bean, bái biǎn dòu
Lilium lancifolium, *L. brownii*, Lily, bǎi hé
Lonicera japonica, Honeysuckle, jīn yín huā
Momordica charantia, Bitter Melon, kǔ guā
Prunella vulgaris, Heal All, xià kū cǎo
Rheum palmatum, Chinese Rhubarb, dà huáng
Salvia miltiorrhiza, *S. przewalskii*, *S. bowleyana*, Red Sage, dān shēn
Saposhnikovia divaricata, Siler, fáng fēng
Scutellaria baicalensis, Baikal Skullcap, huáng qín
Withania somnifera, Ashwagandha

Field Production

Chinese foxglove will appreciate full sun in cooler climates or part shade where there is summer heat. Transplant in spring from nursery pots to one foot on center, being careful not to damage the rhizomes. They will spread into a groundcover by fall. Extremely well-draining soil is necessary, especially while dormant; while in the growth phase, irrigate plants regularly—they are not drought tolerant. Drip or overhead irrigation works equally well. On the other hand, cultivation

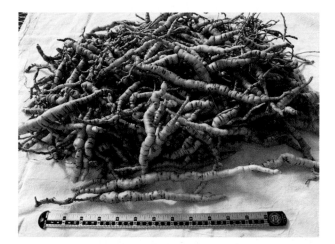

Freshly harvested roots of *Rehmannia glutinosa*; these were cooked with rice wine to become sticky black shú dì huáng.

of this valuable crop is not suitable in areas with high rainfall. Chinese foxglove grows naturally in waste areas and does not require much fertilizer. When growing well, they return in late spring and seem to thrive until the next winter season, when they frequently tend to suffer die-off due to fungal diseases.

Pests and Diseases

In the nursery thrips and spider mites can be problematic, and the previously mentioned fungal disease is a distinct threat. Deer occasionally browse the foliage.

Harvest and Yield

The rather brittle, orange, thin-skinned rhizomes with white interiors can be harvested in the late fall if planted out the previous spring; however, two seasons yield larger and more plentiful roots. If growing in a wet winter area, harvest just after the plants go dormant to avoid crop loss to rot. Save the rootlets and pot them up at this time to increase next season's stock. Rhizomes darken as they dry. The best quality is described as being large, thick, and heavy with thin outer bark and a soft texture, producing roughly eight roots per pound (domestic yields are more in the range of twenty per pound). But it is curious to note that the best roots are said to be black and shiny in cross section. I can only imagine that the reference is to processed and not raw or freshly

Medicinal Uses of Dì huáng

Dì huáng is the root of *Rehmannia glutinosa*. It has significantly different properties depending on whether it is processed or not. When processed it is called shú dì huáng and is one of the most important tonic herbs for nourishing the blood and yin in TCM. When dried it is called sheng dì huáng, and when fresh it is xian dì huáng.

Shú dì huáng is sweet and slightly warm. It nourishes the blood, tonifies the liver and kidney yin, restores the jing (essences), and stops cough and wheezing. It is one of the most frequently used tonics and is used to address anemia, fatigue, weakness, dizziness, palpitations, insomnia, irregular menstruation, infertility, night sweats, many menopausal symptoms, ringing in the ears, developmental delay in children, premature aging, and certain types of respiratory disorders.

Shú dì huáng is usually used in combination with other herbs. Common methods of administration include decoctions, alcohol extracts, powders, concentrated granules, tablets, and pills. It is in many important formulas, including Si Wu Tang (Four Substances Decoction), Ba Zhen Tang (Eight Treasures Decoction), Liu Wei Di Huang Wan (Six Ingredient Pill with *Rehmannia*) and its many derivative formulas, Zuo Gui Yin (Restore the Left Kidney Decoction), and You Gui Wan (Restore the Right Kidney Pills).

Sheng dì huáng (dried, unprocessed *Rehmannia glutinosa*) is sweet, bitter, and cold. It clears heat, cools the blood, nourishes the yin, and promotes the generation of body fluids. It is used to address issues such as excessive menstruation, gastrointestinal bleeding, nose bleeds, rashes, hives, high thirst, night sweats, dry throat, constipation, and painful urination.

Xian dì huáng (fresh *Rehmannia glutinosa*) is bitter, sweet, and very cold. It primarily clears heat and cools the blood and does not have a pronounced nourishing effect. It is less commonly used than the other forms of dì huáng.

dried material,[157] because I have dried many Chinese foxglove roots and they are never black in their raw form (upon processing with wine they do turn black and shiny). The yield is 0.5 pounds per plant fresh for one season and 0.8 pounds per plant fresh for two years old. Ratio of fresh to dry herb is 4:1.

Notes

Do not confuse this plant with *Rehmannia elata*, which is taller and has bright pink flowers; it is a common landscaping plant.

Rheum palmatum (L.)

Common Name: Chinese Rhubarb
Pinyin: Dà huáng
Family: Polygonaceae
Part Used: Root

Plant Description

Rheum palmatum is a commonly used herb in the Chinese materia medica, with a long history of use and trade. It is a large, coarse, and unassuming plant with cordate to rounded, two-foot wide, red-petioled, basally arranged leaves that are deeply lobed to palmate. This three-foot-wide herbaceous perennial grows for a few years before shooting a summer flowering stalk six feet high. The clustered insignificant flowers form small, flat, green-blushed-with-red seed on the typical *Rheum palmatum* hollow flowering stem. The dark orange roots are thick, stout, and fragrant. It is found growing in mountains from 4,500–13,000 feet in China, in the arid western region as well as in northern and central China.[158] USDA hardiness zones 4–9.

Propagation

Large seeds sown in the nursery or indoors in spring will germinate in two weeks without benefit of heat. Provide fertile media and average water. Grow for two months for four-inch potted transplant or sale. Root division is another method, but seed is easy and offers genetic diversity without the effort of digging up a large, heavy plant. Chinese rhubarb is not a good candidate as a permanently potted specimen because the roots are so stout that they outgrow pots rapidly.

Garden and Polyculture Planting

All rhubarbs are considered to be northern plants, enjoying cold weather and mild summers. Plant in groups in the midsection of the garden border or hedgerow on three-foot spacing in full sun to part shade in fertile, well-drained soil. These are large mounding plants that share garden or border space with other plants well.

Suitable Companions

Achyranthes bidentata, Oxknee, huái niú xī
Agastache rugosa, Korean Mint, tǔ huò xiāng
Allium tuberosum, Garlic Chives, jiǔ cài zǐ
Anemarrhena asphodeloides, zhī mǔ
Angelica dahurica, bái zhǐ
Angelica pubescens, dú huó
Aster tataricus, Tartar Aster, zǐ wǎn

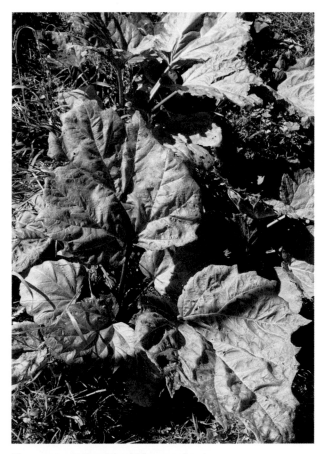

First season's growth of *Rheum palmatum*.

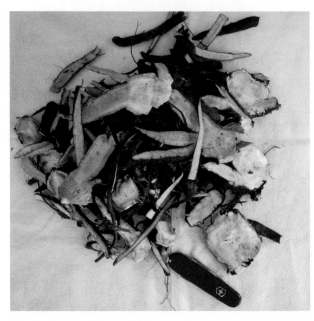

Freshly harvested root of *Rheum palmatum*.

Atractylodes macrocephala, Chinese Thistle Daisy, bái zhú

Belamcanda chinensis, Blackberry Lily, shè gān

Bupleurum chinense, Hare's Ear, chái hú

Carthamus tinctorius, Safflower, hóng huā

Chrysanthemum morifolium, Mum, jú huā

Codonopsis pilosula, Poor Man's Ginseng, dǎng shēn

Cornus officinalis, Dogwood, shān zhū yú

Crataegus pinnatifida, Chinese Hawthorn, shān zhā

Eucommia ulmoides, Hardy Rubber Tree, dù zhòng

Forsythia suspensa, lián qiào

Gentiana scabra, lóng dǎn cǎo

Gentiana straminea, qín jiāo

Ginkgo biloba, Ginkgo, bái guǒ

Lilium lancifolium, *L. brownii*, Lily, bǎi hé

Magnolia denudata, xīn yí huā

Paeonia lactiflora, Chinese Peony, bái/chì sháo

Paeonia suffruticosa, Tree Peony, mǔ dān pí

Platycodon grandiflorus, Balloon Flower, jié gěng

Prunella vulgaris, Heal All, xià kū cǎo

Rehmannia glutinosa, Chinese Foxglove, dì huáng

Salvia miltiorrhiza, *S. przewalskii*, *S. bowleyana*, Red Sage, dān shēn

Saposhnikovia divaricata, Siler, fáng fēng

Scrophularia buergeriana, Figwort, běi xuán shēn

Chinese Rhubarb Recipes

Culinarily Chinese rhubarb is very similar to European rhubarb. Rhubarb is valued for its tart flavor, used alone or in harmonious combinations in sweet desserts and preserves.

Chinese Rhubarb Crumble

Crumbles are quick to assemble for an easy dessert. Use only the rhubarb stalks; the leaves are poisonous. Older stalks may need to be peeled, but earlier in the summer the tender fresh stalks need only be chopped.

> 4 cups Chinese rhubarb stalks, coarsely chopped
> ¾ cup dark brown sugar
> ½ cup olive or safflower or camellia oil
> 1 cup uncooked oatmeal
> 1 teaspoon cinnamon
> 1 cup walnuts, coarsely chopped
> Serves four to six

Preheat oven to 350 degrees. Place the chopped rhubarb in a nine-inch pie pan. Mix together the brown sugar, oil, oatmeal, cinnamon, and walnuts, and sprinkle evenly over the rhubarb. Bake for thirty to forty minutes, or until the rhubarb softens and the topping browns.

Serve warm.

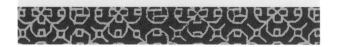

Scutellaria baicalensis, Baikal Skullcap, huáng qín

Scutellaria barbata, Barbat Skullcap, bàn zhī lián

Sophora flavescens, kǔ shēn

Trichosanthes kirilowii, Chinese Cucumber, guā lóu/tiān huā fěn

Field Production

Transplant or directly sow pregerminated seed on three-foot spacing in full sun or part shade in regions with summer heat. This crop does not tolerate hot, humid conditions well; plants will go dormant early in response. Soil should be fertile, loose, and well-drained. Strong winds break the sail-like leaves, making it difficult for the crop to grow due to loss of leaf material.

Pests and Diseases

None.

Harvest and Yield

Harvest Chinese rhubarb after three years or more, while it is dormant. Wear gloves when coming in contact with the root for long periods of time; this is an action-prone herb, and its laxative properties will be absorbed through the skin. Use a pruning saw to cut off the crown. Using a power washer, clean the roots well, removing any flaking bark or old tissue. Saw through the roots from the crown down in even slabs no more than a quarter-inch thick. Drying is easy and should be uneventful; as usual, check carefully for doneness before storing. Good quality roots are said to be dense and heavy "with oily content, a yellowish brown surface, fresh aromatic fragrance, and a bitter but not astringent taste. When chewed, it should stick to the teeth."[159] Yield is three pounds per plant fresh. Ratio of fresh to dry is 3:1.

Notes

- Be careful—the leaves of Chinese rhubarb are toxic.
- *Rheum tanguticum* var. *tanguticum* and *R. officinale* are also utilized as dà huáng.

Medicinal Uses of Dà huáng

Dà huáng is the root of *Rheum palmatum*. It is one of the most important herbs for addressing constipation due to many causes. Bitter and cold, it purges downward, clears heat, purges fire, eliminates toxins, activates the blood, removes blood stasis, clears damp heat, and drains dampness. It addresses issues such as constipation, late-stage dysentery, headache, red eyes, sore throat, swollen gums, mouth ulcers, gastrointestinal bleeding, intestinal abscess, lack of menstruation, abdominal masses, water retention, and painful urination.

Dà huáng is usually used in combination with other herbs. Common methods of administration include decoctions, powders, concentrated granules, tablets, and pills. It is in many important formulas, such as all of the Cheng Qi Tang (Order the Qi Decoction) formulas, Run Chang Tang (Moisten the Intestines Decoction), Ma Zi Ren Tang (Hemp Seed Decoction), and Ba Zheng San (Eight Rectifications Powder).

Salvia miltiorrhiza (Bge.)
Alternate Species: *Salvia przewalskii* (Maxi., Bull.), *S. bowleyana* (Dunn)
Common Name: Red Sage
Pinyin: Dān shēn
Family: Lamiaceae
Part Used: Root

Plant Description
This attractive and gardenworthy sage grows up to two feet tall and almost as wide. The attractive foliage is dark green and has slightly crenate, pinnate leaves with purple highlights. The flowers are purple and are held on spikes above the foliage, blooming in spring and summer. The taproots, as one can imagine from the common name, are red. *Salvia miltiorrhiza* is long-lived and can be found in its native China on hillsides, on stream banks, and in forests—from roughly 300–4,000 feet in elevation.[160] *Salvia miltiorrhiza* is reliably cold hardy in USDA hardiness zones 6–9.

Propagation
If kept properly, fresh seed has good viability for at least three years. Germination generally occurs in ten to twenty-one days. Bottom heat is not necessary, but it will speed up plant emergence. It is possible to propagate red sage by root suckers, but the seed is vigorous, best for genetic diversity, and will more reliably create a good stand. This herb holds well in pots and makes dependable transplants for containerized sale. Sow in fall or very early spring; it takes fourteen weeks to produce a four-inch plant for spring containerized sale.

Garden and Polyculture Planting
This long-blooming sage makes a fine addition to the front or middle of a border in an ornamental garden or section of a hedgerow. Honeybees and other pollinating insects frequently visit red sage flowers. Beautiful, low maintenance, and a valuable habitat plant—who could ask for more? The beautiful purple flower spikes make nice cut flowers, but they have only average longevity. In an ornamental setting remove the spent foliage after the tops have gone fully dormant. To give added winter cold protection in cold winter areas, however, wait to prune until spring—just before new growth emerges.

Suitable Companions
Achyranthes bidentata, Oxknee, huái niú xī
Agastache rugosa, Korean Mint, tǔ huò xiāng

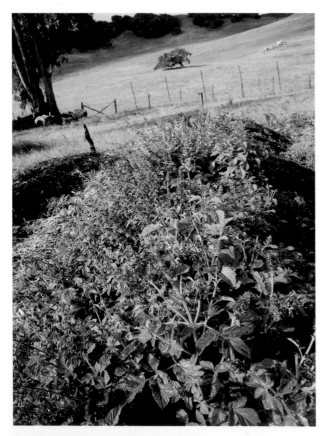

Two-year-old *Salvia miltiorrhiza* plants.

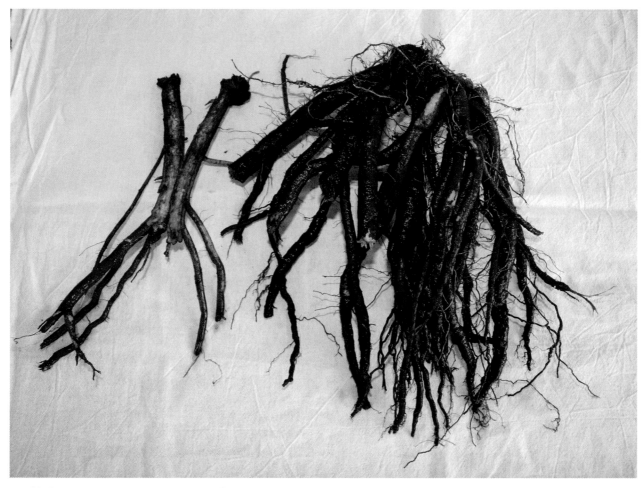

Freshly harvested *Salvia miltiorrhiza* root from 1 three-year-old plant.

Allium macrostemon, xiè bái
Allium tuberosum, Garlic Chives, jiǔ cài zǐ
Angelica dahurica, bái zhǐ
Angelica pubescens, dú huó
Aster tataricus, Tartar Aster, zǐ wǎn
Atractylodes macrocephala, Chinese Thistle Daisy, bái zhú
Belamcanda chinensis, Blackberry Lily, shè gān
Carthamus tinctorius, Safflower, hóng huā
Celosia argentea, qīng xiāng zǐ
Celosia cristata, Cockscomb, jī guān huā
Chrysanthemum morifolium, Mum, jú huā
Cornus officinalis, Dogwood, shān zhū yú
Crataegus pinnatifida, Chinese Hawthorn, shān zhā
Cyathula officinalis, Hookweed, chuān niú xī
Dianthus superbus, Fringed Pink, qú mài
Dolichos lablab, Hyacinth Bean, bái biǎn dòu

Eriobotrya japonica, Loquat, pí pá yè
Eucommia ulmoides, Hardy Rubber Tree, dù zhòng
Ginkgo biloba, Ginkgo, bái guǒ
Ligusticum jeholense, Chinese Lovage, gǎo běn
Lilium lancifolium, *L. brownii*, Lily, bǎi hé
Lonicera japonica, Honeysuckle, jīn yín huā
Ocimum sanctum, Sacred Basil, Tulsi
Platycodon grandiflorus, Balloon Flower, jié gěng
Rehmannia glutinosa, Chinese Foxglove, dì huáng
Saposhnikovia divaricata, Siler, fáng fēng
Schizonepeta tenuifolia, Japanese Catnip, jīng jiè
Scutellaria baicalensis, Baikal Skullcap, huáng qín
Withania somnifera, Ashwagandha

Field Production

Red sage is easy to grow in a full sun site. Soil should be at least fairly well drained, of average fertility, and kept weeded to produce a good root crop. Set out the transplants on one- to two-foot centers. Although the plants are somewhat drought tolerant, an average amount of water makes for the best growth. In arid regions, drip is preferable to overhead irrigation. In the field during the second or successive seasons, the plants may look like they could benefit from some maintenance pruning, but this is an unnecessary labor expenditure (and contradictory if the farming practice is to mimic wild cultivation).

Pests and Diseases

Gophers will occasionally consume the roots but red sage is not their first choice. Occasionally deer will browse the flowers. Prolonged wet periods may cause roots to rot.

Harvest and Yield

Collect or dig one-year or older roots in the late fall to early spring, while the plants are dormant. (Slower to express dormancy than most herbs, red sage does not lose its leaves until temperatures hit twenty or twenty-five degrees.) Good quality roots have bright, brick-red bark and a white interior; they are thick, straight, fleshy, and slightly brittle, with little root bark appearing. Remove the crown and small rootlets prior to cleaning. The easiest method to clean the roots is by power washing; however, take care not to wash too vigorously or the red will wash off! Slice the roots from the crown end down into no more than quarter-inch slices before drying. To facilitate even drying, take care to make cuts of equal thickness. "Good quality consists of large, purplish red,

Medicinal Uses of Dān shēn

Dān shēn is the root of *Salvia miltiorrhiza*. Cool and bitter, it is one of the most important herbs in Chinese medicine for activating and moving the blood and dispelling blood stagnation. Other functions include cooling the blood and calming the shen (spirits). It is used to address cardiovascular and circulatory disorders, many types of pain, traumatic injury, lack of menstruation, painful menstruation, abdominal masses, skin sores, abscesses, mental agitation, and insomnia.

Dān shēn is commonly used as a single herb as well as in herbal formulas. Common methods of administration include decoctions, alcohol extracts, powders, concentrated granules, tablets, and pills. It is in formulas such as Dān Shēn Yin (*Salvia* Decoction), Huo Luo Xiao Ling Dan (Wonderfully Effective Pill to Invigorate the Collateral Channels), and Tian Wang Bu Xin Dan (Emperor of Heaven's Special Pill to Tonify the Heart).

unfragmented roots with thin root bark and without root heads or fine hairy roots."[161] Two-season-old roots yield an average of a quarter- to a half-pound per plant fresh. Ratio of fresh to dry herb is 4:1.

Saposhnikovia divaricata ([Turcz.] Schisck.)

Common Name: Siler
Pinyin: Fáng fēng
Family: Apiaceae
Part Used: Root

Plant Description

Saposhnikovia divaricata is an attractive herbaceous perennial that grows to 2½ feet tall. Its glaucous blue-green flattened leaves are long and deeply cut. The foliage is basally situated, and at first glance the plants look a lot like *Eschscholzia californica* (California poppies). After several seasons a mass of three-inch white flowers appears in summer in the typical umbel fashion. Roots are whitish-yellow, ropy, two-foot-long taproots with no bark. When broken the roots exude a small amount of white, sticky latex. Persistent leaf fibers from years past surround the crown. Endemic to stony hillsides and grasslands of central and northern China as well as Korea, Mongolia, and Eastern Siberia,[162] *Saposhnikovia divaricata* is hardy in USDA hardiness zones 3–9.

Propagation

If seed is sown in the fall, plants should be seven or eight inches tall by midspring and ready for transplant. Fall cool-soil germination time without heat is twenty-five days and about three weeks in early spring with bottom heat; both seeding times are easily successful. Seed that has been stored well remains viable for at least four years. Root cuttings work for propagation too but offer little genetic diversity. Siler holds extremely well in pots, but take care not to overwater during the winter dormant period.

Garden and Polyculture Planting

Siler prefers a sunny site in soils that are well drained and of medium fertility. With somewhat coarse foliage and a rounded form, this perennial works well in the front of the garden or border. Space one foot apart in groupings to enhance their coloration and rounded effect. For a more ornamental showing, stake the floral stalks.

Suitable Companions

Acanthopanax gracilistylus, wǔ jiā pí
Achyranthes bidentata, Oxknee, huái niú xī
Agastache rugosa, Korean Mint, tǔ huò xiāng
Allium macrostemon, xiè bái
Allium tuberosum, Garlic Chives, jiǔ cài zǐ
Anemarrhena asphodeloides, zhī mǔ
Angelica dahurica, baí zhǐ

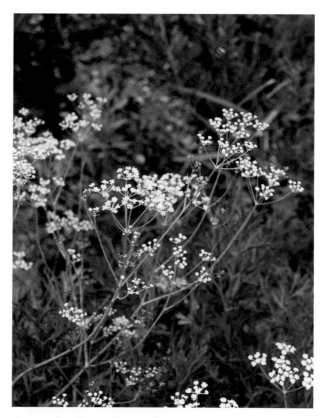

Saposhnikovia divaricata **in flower.**

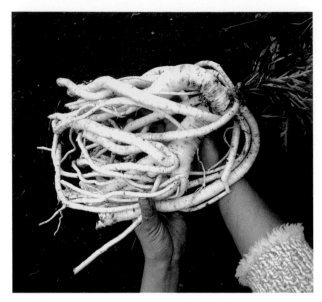

Sample of a whole *Saposhnikovia divaricata* plant.

Aster tataricus, Tartar Aster, zǐ wǎn

Atractylodes macrocephala, Chinese Thistle Daisy, bái zhú

Belamcanda chinensis, Blackberry Lily, shè gān

Bupleurum chinense, Hare's Ear, chái hú

Carthamus tinctorius, Safflower, hóng huā

Celosia argentea, qīng xiāng zǐ

Celosia cristata, Cockscomb, jī guān huā

Chrysanthemum morifolium, Mum, jú huā

Cyathula officinalis, Hookweed, chuān niú xī

Dianthus superbus, Fringed Pink, qú mài

Dioscorea opposita, Chinese Yam, shān yào

Dolichos lablab, Hyacinth Bean, bái biǎn dòu

Ligusticum jeholense, Chinese Lovage, gǎo běn

Lilium lancifolium, *L. brownii*, Lily, bǎi hé

Momordica charantia, Bitter Melon, kǔ guā

Ocimum sanctum, Sacred Basil, Tulsi

Paeonia lactiflora, Chinese Peony, bái/chì sháo

Paeonia suffruticosa, Tree Peony, mǔ dān pí

Platycodon grandiflorus, Balloon Flower, jié gěng

Prunella vulgaris, Heal All, xià kū cǎo

Rehmannia glutinosa, Chinese Foxglove, dì huáng

Rheum palmatum, Chinese Rhubarb, dà huáng

Salvia miltiorrhiza, *S. przewalskii*, *S. bowleyana*, Red Sage, dān shēn

Schizonepeta tenuifolia, Japanese Catnip, jīng jiè

Medicinal Uses of Fáng fēng

Fáng fēng is the root of *Saposhnikovia divaricata*. Acrid, sweet, and slightly warm, it dispels wind; releases the exterior; clears wind, cold, and dampness; dispels internal liver wind; relieves diarrhea; and stops bleeding. It is used to address fever, headache, muscle aches, red eyes, sore throat, skin disorders with itching, arthritic pain, muscle spasms, diarrhea with abdominal pain, and excessive menstrual bleeding.

Fáng fēng is usually used with other herbs in herbal formulas. Common methods of administration include decoctions, alcohol extracts, powders, concentrated granules, tablets, and pills. It is in formulas such as Jing Fang Bai Du San (*Schizonepeta* and *Saposhnikovia* Powder to Overcome Pathogenic Influences), Yu Ping Feng San (Jade Windscreen Powder), Xiao Feng San (Eliminate Wind Powder), and Tong Xie Yao Fang (Important Formula for Painful Diarrhea).

Fáng fēng is generally used unprocessed and also charred to stop bleeding.

Scutellaria baicalensis, Baikal Skullcap, huáng qín

Sophora flavescens, kǔ shēn

Trichosanthes kirilowii, Chinese Cucumber, guā lóu/tiān huā fěn

Field Production

Plant one foot on center, with one to two feet between rows in full sun. A well-drained, moist soil is best. Irrigate where summers are dry and provide adequate, but not too much, nutrition. Siler is a persistently tough but slow grower. Weed to keep competition in check.

Pests and Diseases

This may be the favorite food of gophers; the rodents can eat entire plantings in a very short time. Trapping can be effective—if one keeps with it daily. Rabbits and deer eat foliage. Siler may suffer from the virus-like disease called aster yellows, which shows as distorted, yellow leaves and loss of plant vigor.

Harvest and Yield

The best fáng fēng is said to be long, thick, and unbranched (roots)—with annulations, or ring sections, near the crown. A cross section shows faint radiating marks that look somewhat like chrysanthemum flowers.[163] Fall and spring are both traditional harvest times. Generally, harvestable plants are several seasons old. If gophers are a problem in your area, harvest in the fall immediately after the leaves have died back. The gophers are so problematic at our farm that I grow only a small amount of plants in beds lined with hardware cloth (and the gophers will just eat the root portions that protrude through the mesh), but this is often not cost effective on a large scale. Washing the straight white roots is easy with a power washer or direct flow nozzle. Cut across the root into quarter- to half-inch sections and dry. Cross sections dry rapidly and without fuss to a ruddy yellow color. The yields for three-year plants are one pound per plant fresh (that's accounting for gopher damage). Ratio of fresh to dry herb is 5:1.

Notes

Practitioners occasionally use the outdated names of *Ledebouriella seseloides* and *Siler divaricatum*.

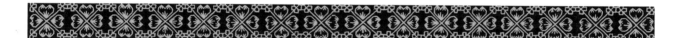

Schisandra chinensis ([Turcz.] Baill.)
Common Name: Five Flavored Fruit
Pinyin: Wǔ wèi zǐ
Family: Schisandraceae
Part Used: Fruit

Plant Description

Featuring a deliciously tart fruit of much report, *Schisandra chinensis* has the rare distinction of possessing all five flavors in Chinese medicine—and thus is considered to be perfectly balanced. Also referred to as northern *Schisandra,* it is a hardy woody vine climbing to at least twenty feet, often clambering in and through trees. It is perennial and deciduous with alternately arranged, tough, green, three-inch-long elliptically shaped leaves with red petioles. White, one-inch, magnolialike, lightly fragrant flowers bloom in springtime. Plants are dioecious; male and female flowers are borne on separate plants, so both sexes must be present for fruiting to occur. Fall fruit is ovoid and red and borne in hanging clusters. Geographically distributed in hills (from roughly 3,500–5,000 feet in elevation) and along riverbanks and wooded regions of northeastern

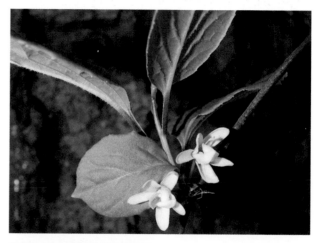

***Schisandra chinensis* in flower.**

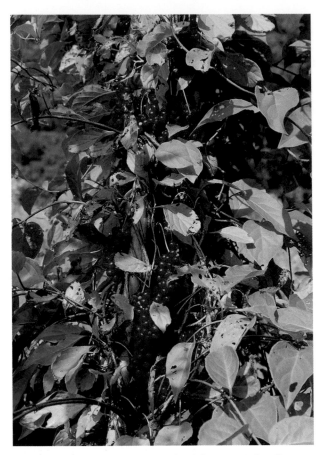

Schisandra chinensis **vine full of fresh fruit at High Falls Gardens, New York. Photo courtesy of Regina Serkin.**

Medicinal Uses of Wǔ wèi zǐ

Wǔ wèi zǐ is the fruit of *Schisandra chinensis*. Sour and warm, it stabilizes lung qi, stops cough, generates fluids, stabilizes the exterior, nourishes the kidneys, binds the jing (essences), nourishes the heart, and calms the shen (spirits). It is used to address issues such as chronic cough, asthma, spontaneous sweats, night sweats, chronic diarrhea, spermatorrhea, urinary incontinence, insomnia, and anxiety. Its use has been expanded in recent times to include addressing liver disease such as hepatitis, as well as being used as an adaptogen (increasing the body's ability to adapt to stress).

Wǔ wèi zǐ is used as a single herb and in combination with other herbs. Common methods of administration include decoctions, powders, alcohol extracts, concentrated powders, and pills. It is in formulas such as Ba Xian Chang Shou Wan (Eight Immortal Pill for Longevity), Sheng Mai San (Generate the Pulse Powder), Shi Bu Wan (Ten Tonics Pill), Ming Mu Di Huang Wan (Brighten the Eyes Pill with *Rehmannia*), and Tian Wang Bu Xin Dan (Emperor of Heaven's Special Pill to Tonify the Heart).

China and in Korea, northern Japan, and eastern Russia.[164] USDA hardiness zones 4 or 5–9.

Propagation

Five flavored fruit is propagated by fall-sown seed, stem cuttings, layering, or root suckers. Soak overnight to remove the smooth kidney-shaped seed from the fruit, plant an eighth- or quarter-inch deep in tall nursery flats, and expose to the winter elements (except in heavy rainfall areas, where the flats need to be protected from excess moisture); expect germination in spring. Alternately, cold stratify in the refrigerator for three months and then sow in the spring. When true leaves appear, transplant these starts into their own pots and grow for another year or two before planting in the ground. Potting media should be well drained; do not overwater.

Garden and Polyculture Planting

This ornamental vine requires a trellis—or in its native forest habitat, trees to grow on. Ideal sites are those with winter-cold, shady, moist but very well-drained, deep, rich soils. Clay soils are not suitable. Remember to grow male and female plants if your goal is to harvest fruit. If you start with unsexed nursery stock, grow at least three plants to hedge the bets. Try permanent potted culture where soils are heavy and drain poorly.

Suitable Companions

Asparagus cochinchinensis, tiān mén dōng
Codonopsis pilosula, Poor Man's Ginseng, dǎng shēn
Gentiana scabra, lóng dǎn cǎo
Gentiana straminea, qín jiāo
Gynostemma pentaphyllum, Sweet Tea Vine, jiǎo gǔ lán
Panax ginseng, Asian Ginseng, rén shēn
Panax quinquefolius, American Ginseng, xī yáng shēn
Pinellia ternata, bàn xià

Field Production

Given a suitable siting, five flavored fruit is an ideal candidate for forest farming. Soils must be very well-drained, much amended, and friable. Light to deep shade is recommended. Vines can get to be heavy, so provide a sturdy trellis or strong tree as a good armature. Plant with roughly ten-foot spacing.

Pests and Diseases

None.

Harvest and Yield

Harvest the fruits in fall after several years' growth and after the frost; remove the stems and any other extraneous matter and dry.[165] Good quality is said to be a "large fruit with thick, purplish red, fleshy, and oily pulp, and an intense aroma."[166] Yields will vary depending on the crop's age. Mature vines will yield many pounds of fruit per plant. Although I grow five flavored fruit plants, they have not yet fruited, so I am not able to provide information on ratio of fresh to dry weights at this time.

Notes

- Freshly dried fruits have an amazing flavor that unfortunately diminishes quickly with age; store no longer than one year.
- *Schisandra sphenanthera*, or southern Schisandra, is also used as wǔ wèi zǐ.

Schizonepeta tenuifolia (Briq.)
Botanical Synonym: *Nepeta tenuifolia* (Benth.)
Common Name: Japanese Catnip
Pinyin: Jīng jiè
Family: Lamiaceae
Part Used: Herb

Plant Description

Schizonepeta tenuifolia is a quick-growing annual extending up to three feet tall by two feet wide. The whole plant has a strong, pleasant, heady, menthol-like fragrance. Many upright red branches are oppositely arranged with rather sparse, grey-green, lanceolate, pointed 1½-inch-long-by-¾-inch-wide leaves, each thrice divided. Small lavender flowers are borne in profusion in two- to six-inch spikes, three per terminus. When in seed the red-blushed fruiting spikes resemble those of *Vitex agnus-castus* (chaste tree). *Schizonepeta tenuifolia* grows throughout China. All USDA hardiness zones.

Propagation

The dark brown seeds of Japanese catnip are long-lived; I've had seed stored (properly) for eight years that yielded 100 percent germination. Sowing by seed is easy, but the seedlings don't transplant well, so I recommend direct seeding or transplanting carefully when seedlings are young. If transplanting, do not allow the plants to linger and become pot-bound.

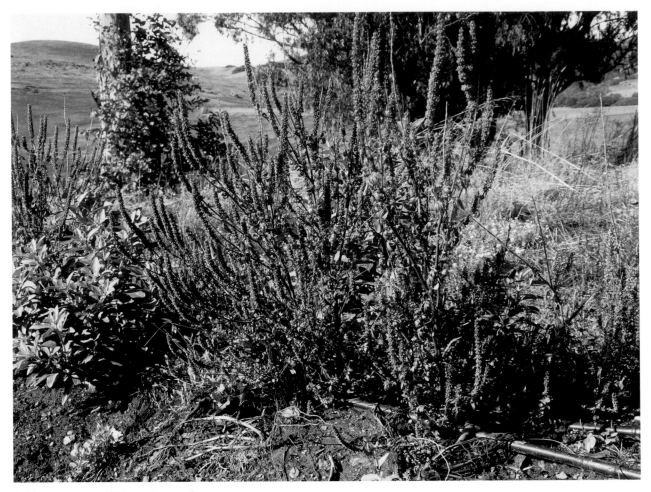

***Schizonepeta tenuifolia* setting seed.**

Sow in spring, barely beneath the soil surface; germination with heat is four to nine days. If Japanese catnip is unhappy, in the interests of fulfilling its genetic destiny it will bloom prematurely—then die.

Garden and Polyculture Planting

Plant this attractive annual a few feet into the border with other sun-loving plants. Toss some seed in the hedgerow; the plants are a good source of nectar for pollinators. You'll need to water it if there is scant summer rain. Upright plants need no staking and are carefree growers. Occasionally they will reseed but it gives no sign on our farm of being invasive.

Suitable Companions

Agastache rugosa, Korean Mint, tǔ huò xiāng

Albizia julibrissin, Mimosa, hé huān pí/huā

Allium macrostemon, xiè bái

Allium tuberosum, Garlic Chives, jiǔ cài zǐ

Anemarrhena asphodeloides, zhī mǔ

Angelica dahurica, bái zhǐ

Angelica pubescens, dú huó

Aster tataricus, Tartar Aster, zǐ wǎn

Atractylodes macrocephala, Chinese Thistle Daisy, bái zhú

Belamcanda chinensis, Blackberry Lily, shè gān

Bupleurum chinense, Hare's Ear, chái hú

Carthamus tinctorius, Safflower, hóng huā

Celosia argentea, qīng xiāng zǐ

Celosia cristata, Cockscomb, jī guān huā

Chrysanthemum morifolium, Mum, jú huā

Clerodendrum trichotomum, Glorybower, chòu wú tóng

Cornus officinalis, Dogwood, shān zhū yú

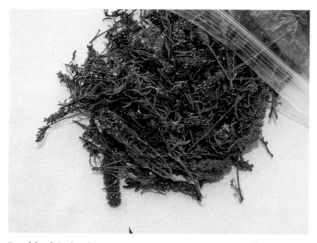

Freshly dried *Schizonepeta tenuifolia* flower, leaf, and stem—the source of jīng jiè.

Crataegus pinnatifida, Chinese Hawthorn, shān zhā
Cyathula officinalis, Hookweed, chuān niú xī
Dianthus superbus, Fringed Pink, qú mài
Eriobotrya japonica, Loquat, pí pá yè
Eucommia ulmoides, Hardy Rubber Tree, dù zhòng
Ginkgo biloba, Ginkgo, bái guǒ
Ligusticum jeholense, Chinese Lovage, gǎo běn
Ligustrum lucidum, Chinese Privet, nǚ zhēn zǐ
Lilium lancifolium, *L. brownii*, Lily, bǎi hé
Magnolia denudata, xīn yí huā
Ocimum sanctum, Sacred Basil, Tulsi
Paeonia lactiflora, Chinese Peony, bái/chì sháo
Paeonia suffruticosa, Tree Peony, mǔ dān pí
Platycodon grandiflorus, Balloon Flower, jié gěng
Prunella vulgaris, Heal All, xià kū cǎo
Rehmannia glutinosa, Chinese Foxglove, dì huáng
Rheum palmatum, Chinese Rhubarb, dà huáng
Salvia miltiorrhiza, *S. przewalskii*, *S. bowleyana*,
  Red Sage, dān shēn
Saposhnikovia divaricata, Siler, fáng fēng
Scutellaria baicalensis, Baikal Skullcap, huáng qín
Scutellaria barbata, Barbat Skullcap, bàn zhī lián
Sophora flavescens, kǔ shēn

Medicinal Uses of Jīng jiè

Jīng jiè is the flowering herb or aerial portion of *Schizonepeta tenuifolia*. Acrid and slightly warm, it is a commonly used herb for releasing the exterior and dispelling wind cold and wind heat. It also stops bleeding and dispels wind to relieve spasms, vent rashes, and alleviate itching. It is used for upper respiratory tract infection with fever, headache, and sore throat; muscle spasms following exposure to wind; unerupted measles, eczema, rashes, and skin sores; excessive menstruation; nosebleeds; blood in the urine; and bleeding hemorrhoids.

Jīng jiè is used as a single herb and in combination with other herbs. Common methods of administration include decoctions (added at the end), powders, concentrated granules, alcohol extracts, tablets, and pills. It is in well-known formulas such as Yin Qiao San (*Lonicera* and *Forsythia* Powder), Jing Fang Bai Du San (*Schizonepeta* and *Saposhnikovia* Powder to Overcome Pathogenic Influences), Xiao Feng San (Eliminate Wind Powder), Chuan Xiong Cha Tiao Wan (*Ligusticum* Powder to Be Taken with Green Tea), and Zhi Sou San (Stop Cough Powder).

Jīng jiè is used unprocessed to release the exterior, charred to stop bleeding, and often powdered and used topically for skin disorders.

Field Production

Direct sow after danger of frost has passed; place three to five seeds per emitter or on one-foot spacing. Grow Japanese catnip in full sun to part shade in soils that have average fertility and are well drained. If the soil is too lean the leaves will be very sparse and crop yield will be poor. It is moderately drought and frost tolerant. Cultivate out weeds to facilitate harvesting of the low branches.

Pests and Diseases

None—the grey-green foliage and strong smell repel insect as well as herbivorous animal pests.

Harvest and Yield

All aerial parts of the plants are regularly used, but sometimes practitioners call for them separately; the flower spikes are considered to be top quality.[167] The top six inches or so of the floral tips are harvested when in full bloom. The herb is easy and quick to bench dry. The best quality herb is very aromatic; the volatile oils should be present, giving the herb an ascending quality similar to menthol. Yield is a quarter pound per plant fresh. Ratio of fresh to dry is 4:1.

Notes

Although Japanese catnip is in the same family as the Western herb called *Nepeta cataria* (catnip or catmint), cats do not have the same affinity for rolling in, eating, or otherwise destroying Japanese catnip.

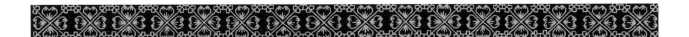

Scrophularia buergeriana (Miq.)
Medicinal Synonym: *Scrophularia ningpoensis* (Hemsl.)
Common Name: Figwort
Pinyin: Běi xuán shēn
Family: Scrophulariaceae
Part Used: Root

Plant Description

Growing to three feet tall, *Scrophularia buergeriana* has an upright to relaxed branching habit spreading up to three feet wide. This Scrophulariaceae family member has lanceolate, bright green, oppositely arranged leaves, and the undersides have prominent veining and finely serrate margins. The foliage is extremely odiferous, smelling strongly of burning tires—much more so than either *S. ningpoensis* or the Western native *S. californica*, all of which look similar. The short bilabiate or two-lipped roundish flowers are green with dark red markings on the upper portion of the floret and ascend up the last foot of the flower spike. These summer flowers develop by fall into small brown seed capsules with numerous tiny dark brown seeds. *Scrophularia buergeriana* can reseed to the point of being potentially invasive in moist regions. The slightly bulbous rhizomes have a light brown (almost barkless) exterior and a white interior. The *Flora of China* mentions that *Scrophularia buergeriana* natively grows on hilly slopes and in moist grasslands in a swath across the northern median of China.[168] USDA hardiness zones 4–9.

Propagation

Press the very small seeds into nursery medium in a nursery flat and water gently from below or with a watering wand fitted with a misting nozzle. Sow in early spring and place the flat outside. Germination occurs in approximately four weeks; times will vary depending on growing geography and local temperatures. Seed can be sown directly as well. Keep well watered. Plants can be set out in the first season; they hold well in pots.

Garden and Polyculture Planting

Try planting figwort at the front or in the middle of a garden bed or border. It will do best in moist soils that are well drained, loose, and of average fertility. Although figwort prefers a moist site, it can manage with some summer drought.

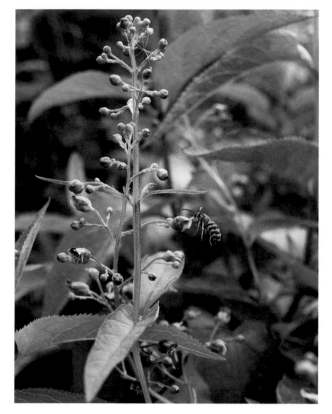

Wasp visiting a flower of *Scrophularia buergeriana*.

Suitable Companions

Acanthopanax gracilistylus, wǔ jiā shēn/pí
Agastache rugosa, Korean Mint, tǔ huò xiāng
Allium macrostemon, xiè bái
Allium tuberosum, Garlic Chives, jiǔ cài zǐ
Anemarrhena asphodeloides, zhī mǔ
Angelica dahurica, bái zhǐ
Angelica pubescens, dú huó
Asparagus cochinchinensis, tiān mén dōng
Aster tataricus, Tartar Aster, zǐ wǎn
Belamcanda chinensis, Blackberry Lily, shè gān
Bupleurum chinense, Hare's Ear, chái hú
Chrysanthemum morifolium, Mum, jú huā
Clerodendrum trichotomum, Glorybower, chòu
  wú tóng
Codonopsis pilosula, Poor Man's Ginseng,
  dǎng shēn
Cornus officinalis, Dogwood, shān zhū yú
Crataegus pinnatifida, Chinese Hawthorn, shān zhā
Cyathula officinalis, Hookweed, chuān niú xī

Medicinal Uses of Běi xuán shēn

Běi xuán shēn is the root of *Scrophularia buergeriana* and is a regional variant and substitute (with identical properties) for *Scrophularia ningpoensis*. Bitter, sweet, salty, and cold, it clears heat, nourishes the yin, cools the blood, eliminates toxins, and disperses nodules. It is a common herb to use when excess heat has damaged the fluids. It is used to address issues such as elevated thirst, dry mouth and throat, sore throat, dry cough, certain skin disorders characterized by dark purple blotches, goiter, and skin lesions with abscesses or ulcerations.

Běi xuán shēn is most often used in combination with other herbs. Common methods of administration include decoctions, powders, concentrated granules, tablets, and pills. It is in formulas such as Zeng Ye Tang (Increase the Fluids Decoction), Xiao Luo Wan (Reduce Scrofula Pill), and Bai He Gu Jing Tang (Lily Bulb Decoction to Preserve Metal).

Dianthus superbus, Fringed Pink, qú mài
Eriobotrya japonica, Loquat, pí pá yè
Eucommia ulmoides, Hardy Rubber Tree, dù zhòng
Forsythia suspensa, lián qiào
Ginkgo biloba, Ginkgo, bái guǒ
Ligusticum jeholense, Chinese Lovage, gǎo běn
Ligustrum lucidum, Chinese Privet, nǔ zhēn zǐ
Lilium lancifolium, *L. brownii*, Lily, bǎi hé
Lonicera japonica, Honeysuckle, jīn yín huā
Magnolia denudata, xīn yí huā
Ocimum sanctum, Sacred Basil, Tulsi
Paeonia lactiflora, Chinese Peony, bái/chì sháo

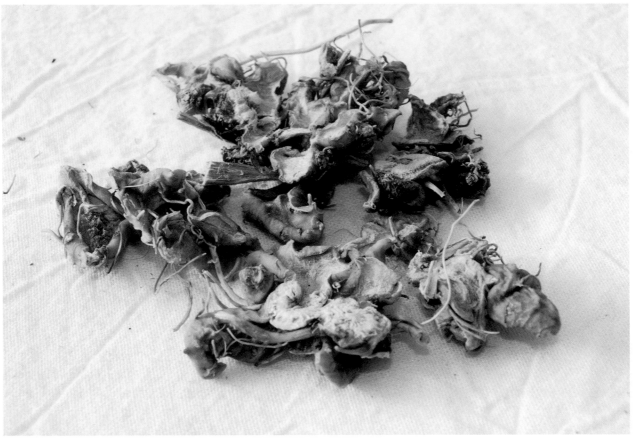

Dried roots of *Scrophularia buergeriana*, běi xuán shēn.

Paeonia suffruticosa, Tree Peony, mǔ dān pí
Plantago asiatica, Plantain, chē qián zǐ
Platycodon grandiflorus, Balloon Flower, jié gěng
Prunella vulgaris, Heal All, xià kū cǎo
Rheum palmatum, Chinese Rhubarb, dà huáng
Salvia miltiorrhiza, *S. przewalskii*, *S. bowleyana*, Red Sage, dān shēn
Saposhnikovia divaricata, Siler, fáng fēng
Schizonepeta tenuifolia, Japanese Catnip, jīng jiè
Scutellaria barbata, Barbat Skullcap, bàn zhī lián
Sophora flavescens, kǔ shēn

Field Production
Grow on one-foot spacing in amended or loose soils; provide summer irrigation where rains are scarce. Plant in full sun to part shade; *Scrophularia buergeriana* prefers a sunnier siting than *S. ningpoensis*. As with some other roots, if grown in heavy soil they may become distorted—it really is amazing how determined they are to grow!

Pests and Diseases
Despite figwort's strong smell, deer are quite willing to eat its foliage.

Harvest and Yield
Lift roots in the third year (or beyond) in the winter while they are dormant. Remove any small roots from the rhizomes, then wash the rhizomes and cut for drying by slicing in quarter-inch slabs from the crown down. Yield for three-year fresh root is one pound per plant. Ratio of fresh to dry is 4:1.

Notes
Scrophularia buergeriana, the source of běi xuán shēn, is both cultivated and wild-collected in China.

Scutellaria baicalensis (Georgi)
Common Name: Baikal Skullcap
Pinyin: Huáng qín
Family: Lamiaceae
Part Used: Root

Plant Description

Scutellaria baicalensis is but one of many medicinal herbs in the *Scutellaria* genus. This one is a gardenworthy deciduous perennial subshrub growing up to 1½ feet tall by 2 feet wide. Simple lanceolate leaves ascend the many branching stems, which terminate in truly beautiful purple-blue flowers that arrive in summer and are followed by a heavy crop of black seed in the fall. The stems, like all mint family species, are square; the branching roots are a saturated yellow color. Although plants in this genus are insect pollinated, I have not seen any outcrossing with other skullcaps. Widely distributed across northern and northeastern China, Japan, Korea, Mongolia, and Russia,[169] *Scutellaria baicalensis* is hardy in USDA zones from at least 4 to at least 9. It is a tough plant and can survive partly due to its adventitious roots but does not reseed or become weedy.

Propagation

Transplants that are nursery sown in March will be ready for the field in late spring or early summer—or you can direct sow seed in the field in late spring. Good quality seed will germinate in one to two weeks. Easy-to-grow baikal skullcap holds well in containers—take care not to overwater. Plants do not tolerate saline conditions; the indication of too much salt is that the foliage turns a bright turquoise blue— and death ensues.

Garden and Polyculture Planting

With its strikingly attractive and very floriferous blue flowers, baikal skullcap is every bit as ornamental as any garden center perennial. It also makes a good rock garden specimen. Place this sun-loving plant in well-drained soil of low to average fertility; space plants one to two feet apart. In keeping with the concepts of wild quality, winter woody material does not need to be "cleaned up" unless perhaps in an ornamental setting where the need for a neat appearance may prevail.

Suitable Companions

Achyranthes bidentata, Oxknee, huái niú xī
Agastache rugosa, Korean Mint, tǔ huò xiāng
Allium macrostemon, xiè bái
Allium tuberosum, Garlic Chives, jiǔ cài zǐ
Aster tataricus, Tartar Aster, zǐ wǎn

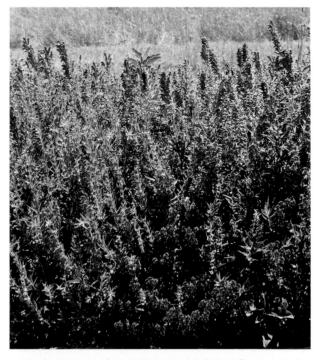

Second-year crop of *Scutellaria baicalensis*—it flowers in the first year as well.

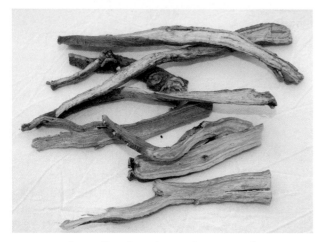

Dry roots of *Scutellaria baicalensis*, the source of huáng qín.

Atractylodes macrocephala, Chinese Thistle Daisy, bái zhú
Belamcanda chinensis, Blackberry Lily, shè gān
Bupleurum chinense, Hare's Ear, chái hú
Carthamus tinctorius, Safflower, hóng huā
Chrysanthemum morifolium, Mum, jú huā
Dolichos lablab, Hyacinth Bean, bái biǎn dòu
Ligusticum jeholense, Chinese Lovage, gǎo běn
Lilium lancifolium, *L. brownii*, Lily, bǎi hé
Prunella vulgaris, Heal All, xià kū cǎo
Salvia miltiorrhiza, *S. przewalskii*, *S. bowleyana*, Red Sage, dān shēn
Saposhnikovia divaricata, Siler, fáng fēng
Schizonepeta tenuifolia, Japanese Catnip, jīng jiè
Withania somnifera, Ashwagandha

Field Production

This species of *Scutellaria* prefers full sun and a low-to-average amount of water in soils that are at least somewhat well drained. Set seed or plants on one-foot centers its cultural requirements are easy to fulfill. If directly seeded into the field, thin to just one plant per spot or emitter to maximize the root size. If directly sown, be watchful of field moisture and do not let seeds dry out—or use a row crop cover to protect emerging seedlings from the drying effects of wind and sun, late frost, and footfalls from clueless visitors. Its late-season drought tolerance is unexpected in this genus of water-loving herbs. Indeed this *Scutellaria* can manage well in heavy clay, as

Medicinal Uses of Huáng qín

Huáng qín is the root of *Scutellaria baicalensis*. Bitter and cold, it is an important herb for clearing heat. It clears heat, dries dampness, sedates fire, eliminates toxins, cools the blood and stops bleeding, and calms the fetus. It is used to address issues such as hepatitis, dysentery, jaundice, epigastric burning, constipation, oral ulcers, cough with yellow sputum, sore throat, fever, skin lesions, eye disorders, excessive menstruation, blood in the stool, and blood in the urine.

Huáng qín is usually used in combination with other herbs. Common methods of administration include decoctions, powders, concentrated granules, alcohol extracts, tablets, and pills. It is in approximately eighty of the primary, commonly used formulas of TCM, including all of the Chai Hu Tang (*Bupleurum* Decoction) formulas, Ding Chuan Tang (Arrest Wheezing Decoction), Qing Xin Lian Zi Yin (Lotus Seed Decoction to Clear the Heart), Huang Lian Jie Du Tang (*Coptis* Decoction to Relieve Toxicity), Huang Lian E Jiao Tang (*Coptis* and Gelatin Decoction), and Long Dan Xie Gan Tang (*Gentiana* Decoction to Drain the Liver).

Huáng qín is usually charred to stop bleeding, steamed with liquor to clear lung heat, and used dried and unprocessed to clear heat and eliminate toxins. It can be used fresh to clear damp heat from the intestines and treat dysentery.

long as there is not standing water, as well as alkaline and acid soils (however, growers in the eastern U.S. have reported root rot due to wet soils). Fertilizer needs are low.

Pests and Diseases

Occasionally gophers will eat the roots. Excess water can lead to root rot.

Harvest and Yield

Harvest the bright yellow roots (with even more brilliantly yellow interiors) while winter dormant, in fall or early spring, after at least two full seasons of growth. This is one of the first Chinese root botanicals to go dormant in the fall. Expect roots to be about one inch thick, branched, and about a foot or more long. Power wash down to the yellow root surfaces to remove extraneous material. Slice the roots lengthwise; they will occasionally develop light green streaks upon slicing. Drying is easy, especially if not cut too thick, but be sure to test for doneness. The yield is 0.4 pounds per two-year plant fresh. Ratio of fresh to dry root is 3:1.

Notes

- This is one of the more commonly used herbs in the Chinese pharmacopeia and is eminently marketable.
- The green coloration that frequently presents on the root after slicing is often a source of confusion; there are varying differences of opinion about the origin of the coloration and its effect on the medicinal quality. One authority states that "bluish green roots reflect improper processing, which can result in low content of glycosides"[170]; however, since the greenish blue color appears right after root slicing of freshly harvested material, it seems unlikely to be improper processing. Yet agreement can certainly be found in the statement that "Good quality consists of big, golden yellow, full roots with few if any withered areas in the center."[171]

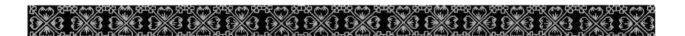

Scutellaria barbata (D. Don)
Common Name: Barbat Scullcap
Pinyin: Bàn zhī lián
Family: Lamiaceae
Part Used: Herb

Plant Description

Profusely branching and with an upright habit, *Scutellaria barbata* grows to a maximum of 1½ feet tall, slowly spreads by runners, and has leaves that are 1 inch long by ½ inch wide with margins that are softly dentate. Bright blue flowers are ¾ of an inch long and borne in leaf axils ascending up the pliant stems. Plants produce copious, tiny, dark-brown seed in fall. An herbaceous perennial dormancy is initiated around twenty-three degrees. *Scutellaria barbata* grows under 6,000 feet in central, southern, and the east coast of China—as well as areas in India, Japan, Korea, Laos, Nepal, Thailand, and Vietnam.[172] USDA hardiness zones 7–10.

Propagation

Spring-sown seed is easy and reliable. Due to the small size of the seed, sow just below the medium surface and water gently; germination occurs in two weeks without the aid of heat. If sown in fall or early enough in spring, transplants will be ready for the field in twelve weeks, plenty of time for one (if not two) harvests.

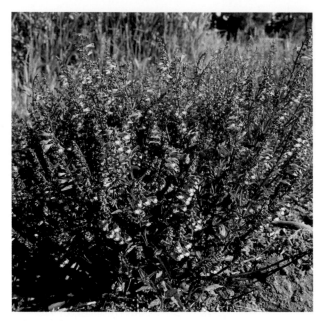

One *Scutellaria barbata* specimen in full bloom.

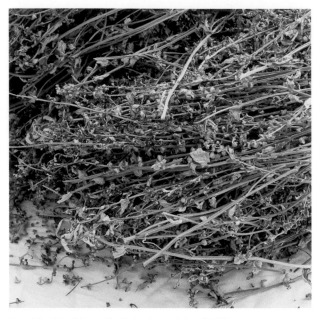

Freshly dried *Scutellaria barbata*, bàn zhī lián.

Garden and Polyculture Planting

Uncommon in cultivation, this attractive blue flowering perennial is definitely gardenworthy. Mass it as a ground cover in the front of the border or garden. Barbat skullcap prefers a moist, well-drained, average fertility soil. Plant one foot apart in a full sun location or part shade where summers are hot.

Suitable Companions

Agastache rugosa, Korean Mint, tǔ huò xiang
Albizia julibrissin, Mimosa, hé huān pí/huā
Allium macrostemon, xiè bái
Allium tuberosum, Garlic Chives, jiǔ cài zǐ
Andrographis paniculata, Kalmegh, chuān xīn lián
Anemarrhena asphodeloides, zhī mǔ
Angelica dahurica, baí zhǐ
Angelica pubescens, dú huó
Asparagus cochinchinensis, tiān mén dōng
Aster tataricus, Tartar Aster, zǐ wǎn
Bacopa monnieri, Brahmi
Belamcanda chinensis, Blackberry Lily, shè gān
Centella asiatica, Gotu Kola, jī xuě cǎo
Chrysanthemum morifolium, Mum, jú huā
Clerodendrum trichotomum, Glorybower, chòu wú tóng

Codonopsis pilosula, Poor Man's Ginseng, dǎng shen
Coix lacryma-jobi, Job's Tears, yì yǐ rén
Cornus officinalis, Dogwood, shān zhū yú
Crataegus pinnatifida, Chinese Hawthorn, shān zhā
Dianthus superbus, Fringed Pink, qú mài
Eclipta prostrata, Eclipta, mò hàn lián
Eriobotrya japonica, Loquat, pí pá yè
Eucommia ulmoides, Hardy Rubber Tree, dù zhòng
Gentiana scabra, lóng dǎn cǎo
Gentiana straminea, qín jiāo
Ginkgo biloba, Ginkgo, bái guǒ
Gynostemma pentaphyllum, Sweet Tea Vine, jiāo gǔ lán
Houttuynia cordata, yú xīng cǎo
Ligustrum lucidum, Chinese Privet, nǔ zhēn zǐ
Magnolia denudata, xīn yí huā
Mentha haplocalyx, Field Mint, bò hé
Ocimum sanctum, Sacred Basil, Tulsi
Ophiopogon japonicus, Lilyturf, mài mén dōng
Paeonia lactiflora, Chinese Peony, bái/chì sháo
Paeonia suffruticosa, Tree Peony, mǔ dān pí
Pinellia ternata, bàn xià
Plantago asiatica, Plantain, chē qián zǐ
Prunella vulgaris, Heal All, xià kū cǎo

Schizonepeta tenuifolia, Japanese Catnip, jīng jiè
Scrophularia buergeriana, Figwort, běi xuán shēn

Field Production

Transplant one foot apart in moist soils. Drought severely impacts production: plants grow to only a few inches high, yield is low, and harvesting is difficult. If you plan to grow barbat skullcap for more than a few years in the same location, top-dress with compost to maintain fertility and soil tilth. Early in the second and successive seasons cut the crop very low to even out errant stems and facilitate clean future harvests. Temperatures over one hundred degrees can initiate summer dormancy.

Pests and Diseases

I've noticed spider mites on these plants in late summer, but the infestation hasn't been too severe.

Harvest and Yield

In many regions barbat skullcap can be harvested three times per season. The traditional time is when plants are in full flower; the first cut will be the largest and subsequent ones will be smaller. For a superior product make the first harvest low, about three or four inches from the ground, and subsequent harvests just above the previous cut. Remember to spray the crop with water one or two days before harvest to clean off dust and other impurities. Drying is easy and properly dried herb should still show blue flowers and green stems. Yield is 0.4 pounds per plant per year, with three harvests per plant per year. Ratio of fresh to dry is 4:1.

Medicinal Uses of Bàn zhī lián

Bàn zhī lián is the herb or aerial portion of *Scutellaria barbata*. Acrid, slightly bitter, and cool, it has primary functions of clearing heat, eliminating toxins, and reducing swelling—and secondary functions of draining dampness and stopping bleeding. In modern China this is one of the most important anticancer herbs, most commonly used for tumors of the digestive tract and carcinoma of the liver, lung, cervix, and breast. It is also used for upper respiratory tract infections, skin disorders characterized by swelling, painful urination, chronic hepatitis, and liver disease leading to ascites.

Bàn zhī lián is usually used in combination with other herbs. Common methods of administration include decoctions, powders, concentrated granules, alcohol extracts, tablets, and pills.

Bàn zhī lián can be used fresh or dried, although the dosage is usually doubled when used fresh.

Sophora flavescens (Ait.)
Common Name: None
Pinyin: Kǔ shēn
Family: Fabaceae
Part Used: Root

Plant Description
Sophora flavescens is an herbaceous, multibranched shrub growing up to seven feet tall and five to six feet wide. Pinnate leaves are up to ten inches long with many individual lanceolate leaflets, each growing one to two inches long. Graceful, pale yellow, terminal blooming racemes are comprised of pealike flowers and grow ten to twelve inches long. By fall they mature into five-inch-long, skinny green bean pods that turn brown. This species is a sometimes opportunistic shrub that grows on slopes and hillsides in all provinces in China as well as in areas within India, Japan, Korea, and Russia.[173] It reseeds in some, but not all, settings. USDA hardiness zones 6–10.

Propagation
Reddish-brown, eighth-inch roundish seeds are easy to sow and more reliable than cuttings for creating new plants. The seed coat is hard but doesn't require scarification or other pretreatment. Sow seed in the spring or fall: nothing fancy, just straight-on sowing a quarter-inch deep with average water in average media. Germination will take about four weeks. Transplant to individual pots and grow for a season before planting out or selling. Plants hold well as potted stock.

Garden and Polyculture Planting
Sophora flavescens is a rather ungainly large deciduous shrub; stems stick out from the base in all directions. Plant it near the back of an informal garden or in a hedgerow. Late summer is when they look their best, all decked out in arching yellow flowers or big green seedpods. Plant six feet apart and water during times of drought.

Suitable Companions
Achyranthes bidentata, Oxknee, huái niú xī
Agastache rugosa, Korean Mint, tǔ huò xiāng
Albizia julibrissin, Mimosa, hé huān pí/huā
Allium macrostemon, xiè bái
Allium tuberosum, Garlic Chives, jiǔ cài zǐ
Andrographis paniculata, Kalmegh, chuān xīn lián
Anemarrhena asphodeloides, zhī mǔ
Angelica dahurica, bái zhǐ
Angelica pubescens, dú huó
Aster tataricus, Tartar Aster, zǐ wǎn
Atractylodes macrocephala, Chinese Thistle Daisy, bái zhú
Belamcanda chinensis, Blackberry Lily, shè gān
Bupleurum chinense, Hare's Ear, chái hú
Carthamus tinctorius, Safflower, hóng huā
Celosia argentea, qīng xiāng zǐ
Celosia cristata, Cockscomb, jī guān huā
Chrysanthemum morifolium, Mum, jú huā

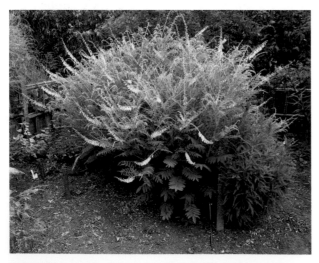
Pale yellow pealike blossoms adorn *Sophora flavescens*.

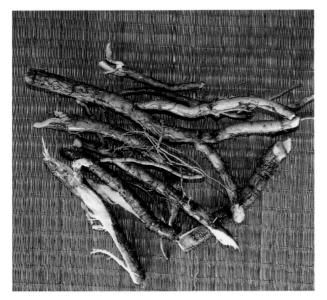

Freshly harvested root of *Sophora flavescens*.

Clerodendrum trichotomum, Glorybower, chòu wú tóng

Codonopsis pilosula, Poor Man's Ginseng, dǎng shēn

Cornus officinalis, Dogwood, shān zhū yú

Crataegus pinnatifida, Chinese Hawthorn, shān zhā

Cyathula officinalis, Hookweed, chuān niú xī

Dianthus superbus, Fringed Pink, qú mài

Dolichos lablab, Hyacinth Bean, bái biǎn dòu

Eriobotrya japonica, Loquat, pí pá yè

Eucommia ulmoides, Hardy Rubber Tree, dù zhòng

Forsythia suspensa, lián qiào

Ginkgo biloba, Ginkgo, bái guǒ

Ligusticum jeholense, Chinese Lovage, gǎo běn

Ligustrum lucidum, Chinese Privet, nǚ zhēn zǐ

Lilium lancifolium, *L. brownii*, Lily, bǎi hé

Lonicera japonica, Honeysuckle, jīn yín huā

Lycium chinense, Chinese Wolfberry, gǒu qǐ zǐ/dì gǔ pí

Magnolia denudata, xīn yí huā

Mentha haplocalyx, Field Mint, bò hé

Momordica charantia, Bitter Melon, kǔ guā

Ocimum sanctum, Sacred Basil, Tulsi

Platycodon grandiflorus, Balloon Flower, jié gěng

Prunella vulgaris, Heal All, xià kū cǎo

Rehmannia glutinosa, Chinese Foxglove, dì huáng

Rheum palmatum, Chinese Rhubarb, dà huáng

Medicinal Uses of Kǔ shēn

Kǔ shēn is the root of *Sophora flavescens*. Bitter and cold, it clears heat, dries dampness, dispels wind, kills parasites, relieves itching, and promotes urination. It is used to address issues such as diarrhea, dysentery, yellow vaginal discharge, genital itching, bleeding hemorrhoids, skin itching, skin lesions, and painful urination.

Kǔ shēn is usually used in combination with other herbs, although it is sometimes used alone to make a topical wash. Common methods of administration include decoctions, powders, concentrated granules, tablets, and pills. It is in formulas such as She Chuang Zi San (*Cnidium* Powder) and Xiao Feng San (Eliminate Wind Powder).

Salvia miltiorrhiza, *S. przewalskii*, *S. bowleyana*, Red Sage, dān shēn

Saposhnikovia divaricata, Siler, fáng fēng

Schizonepeta tenuifolia, Japanese Catnip, jīng jiè

Scutellaria baicalensis, Baikal Skullcap, huáng qín

Trichosanthes kirilowii, Chinese Cucumber, guā lóu/tiān huā fěn

Field Production

Plant in full sun to part shade, six to eight feet apart, in rows or in an orchard, set up with irrigation. *Sophora flavescens* prefers sandy soils but is tolerant and adaptable to other types; good drainage is recommended. As new growth starts to emerge in spring, remove old woody stems back to the crown. Mulch with compost to maintain even moisture and provide nutrients. Fertilizer needs are low.

Pests and Diseases

Gophers eat the roots.

Harvest and Yield

Harvest roots in the fall of the third year or beyond when the plants are dormant. Cut down the leafless stems to the ground and dig, starting two feet away from the plant (the roots grow laterally outward from the crown). Roots have a yellowish brown bark and should be cylindrical and thick. The interior of the bark is white. Cut into manageable lengths and power wash. Make quarter-inch slices diagonally with a sharp knife and dry. Good quality kǔ shēn is said to be "a uniform root with a yellowish white cross section and an extremely bitter taste."[174] Yield for a four-year-old plant is five pounds per plant fresh. Ratio of fresh to dry is 2:1.

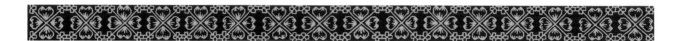

Trichosanthes kirilowii (Maxim.)

Common Name: Chinese Cucumber
Pinyin: Guā lóu/Tiān huā fěn
Family: Cucurbitaceae
Part Used: Fruit, root

Plant Description

Trichosanthes kirilowii is an attractive, herbaceous, perennial, climbing vine with six-inch broadly ovate lobed leaves. Vigorous plants emerge in late spring and grow rapidly up to fifteen feet. Pure white tubular flowers are deeply dissected and borne on either male or female plants; there is no fruit production without at least two plants present, representing both sexes. You can tell flower sex by looking at the base of the blossom to see whether or not there is a fruit initiate—similar to garden cucumbers. A swelling (very small immature fruit) indicates the plant is a female. Round fruits are green when young and orange when mature. *Trichosanthes kirilowii* is cold hardy to at least minus twenty degrees, and like most cucurbits it enjoys hot summers. USDA hardiness zones 5–9.

Propagation

Seeds sown in the heated greenhouse give a long season of growth; however, they will germinate in cool soils as well. Seed emergence takes place in three to four weeks in both warm and cool soils. In the nursery it takes eight weeks from spring sowing to four-inch transplant or containerized sale. Chinese cucumber develops a significant root; repot seedlings as needed to keep plants from becoming pot-bound.

Garden and Polyculture Planting

Plants thrive in warm soils in sunny, warm regions. The showy white flowers and the large, dark-green leaves make Chinese cucumber very ornamental;

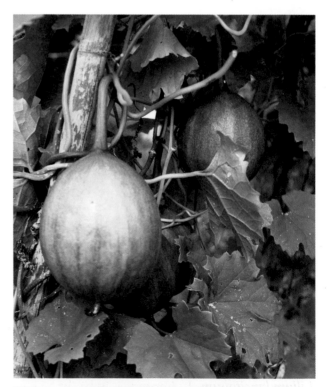

Trichosanthes kirilowii **fruit grown at High Falls Gardens, New York. Photo courtesy of Jean Giblette.**

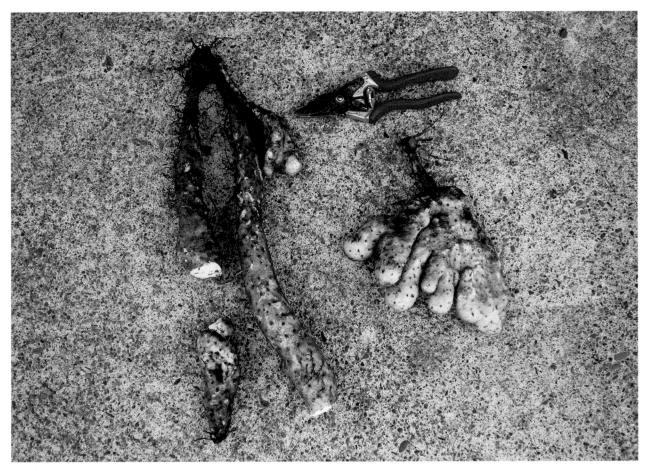

Two fresh root harvests of *Trichosanthes kirilowii* showing two different root forms.

its large fruits certainly add visual interest. Provide a sturdy trellis to accommodate the fifteen-foot-long vines and heavy fruit. Flower production is high, but flowers last only a day or wilt in hot afternoons and have poor vase value.

Suitable Companions

Agastache rugosa, Korean Mint, tǔ huò xiāng
Allium tuberosum, Garlic Chives, jiǔ cài zǐ
Angelica dahurica, baí zhǐ
Angelica pubescens, dú huó
Aster tataricus, Tartar Aster, zǐ wǎn
Belamcanda chinensis, Blackberry Lily, shè gān
Carthamus tinctorius, Safflower, hóng huā
Chrysanthemum morifolium, Mum, jú huā
Cyathula officinalis, Hookweed, chuān niú xī
Lilium lancifolium, *L. brownii*, Lily, bǎi hé
Prunella vulgaris, Heal All, xià kū cǎo

Rheum palmatum, Chinese Rhubarb, dà huáng
Salvia miltiorrhiza, *S. przewalskii*, *S. bowleyana* Red Sage, dān shēn
Saposhnikovia divaricata, Siler, fáng fēng
Schizonepeta tenuifolia, Japanese Catnip, jīng jiè
Scutellaria baicalensis, Baikal Skullcap, huáng qín
Sophora flavescens, kǔ shēn
Withania somnifera, Ashwagandha

Field Production

Grow Chinese cucumber in a sunny location in well-drained, average soil with medium fertility. Plant one foot apart and provide stout support for the climbing tendrils. Soil should drain well; if not, vines and roots will show evidence of dieback. Chinese cucumber is not considered drought tolerant. First-year roots grow one or two feet deep and are shaped like a baseball bat; in subsequent years they grow to three

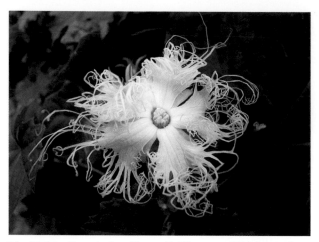

The highly dissected and beautiful flowers of *Trichosanthes kirilowii* last only one day.

feet deep. The plants break dormancy rather late in the spring.

Pests and Diseases
Soils that are excessively wet enable root rot.

Harvest and Yield
Dig roots while plants are dormant in the late fall or early winter after at least two years of growth. The brittle, white roots grow three feet straight down, making hand harvesting the norm as a machine harvest will miss much of the root. Wash thoroughly, cut roots a little less than a quarter-inch thick on a slight diagonal, and dry. Harvest fruit in the fall when red and ripe, slice a quarter-inch thick, and dry. The best fruit is considered to be large pieces with an orange wrinkled surface.[175] In considering the root, the best quality is said to be "large, heavy, white, and powdery."[176] The yield for roots is 0.3–0.5 pounds per plant fresh for first season root. Ratio of fresh to dry herb is 3:1. The ten plants in my permanent planting of this crop all appear to be males; harvest data on fruit is not currently available.

Notes
- The seeds (guā lóu rén) and fruit peel (guā lóu pí) of Chinese cucumber are also sometimes used separately in Chinese medicine.
- The roots of this plant look very much

Medicinal Uses of Guā lóu/ Tiān huā fěn

Guā lóu is the fruit of *Trichosanthes kirilowii*. Sweet and cold, it clears the lungs, transforms phlegm, regulates the qi, expands the chest, dissipates nodules, and eliminates pus. It is used to address productive cough with phlegm, wheezing, chest congestion and pain, and intestinal abscesses. It is used as a single herb and in combination with other herbs. It is most commonly administered in decoctions, powders, concentrated granules, tablets, and pills—as are guā lóu pí and guā lóu rén.

Guā lóu pí is the peel of the fruit of *Trichosanthes kirilowii*. It has similar properties and functions to the fruit, although it has a stronger effect on addressing cough and phlegm.

Guā lóu rén is the seed of *Trichosanthes kirilowii* and has similar functions to the fruit, except with a stronger moistening and lubricating effect. It is used to address dry cough with sticky phlegm and for constipation. It is usually dry-fried before administration.

Tiān huā fěn is the root of *Trichosanthes kirilowii*. Bitter, slightly sweet, and cold, it clears heat, generates body fluids, and dispels pus. It is most commonly used to address Xiao Ke syndrome, which often corresponds to diabetes, and to address breast abscesses.

like *Dioscorea opposita* (Chinese yam, shān yào) roots. Do not confuse them; it is important to label all herbs well. They have very different effects and are quite different medicines.

Withania somnifera ([L.] Dunal)

Common Name: Ashwagandha
Sanskrit: Ashwagandha
Family: Solanaceae
Part Used: Root

Plant Description

Withania somnifera is a strong-smelling tender perennial. Leaves are bright green, obovate, and lightly pubescent on green-stemmed plants up to three feet tall and three feet wide. Small, clustered, light green flowers yield bright orange fruits, each of which holds many tan, flattened seeds encased in a dry, papery, lantern-shaped calyx. This plant tends to cast its seed about quite successfully, giving it invasive tendencies. Although it is endemic not only to India and other Asian countries as well as some areas in Africa, currently the extent of *Withania somnifera* is reported to be Gansu and Yunnan (Afghanistan, India, Pakistan; SW Asia, Europe).[177] USDA hardiness zones 7 or 8 to 10 or 11.

Propagation

To give the longest growing season possible for first-year harvest, sow seed in very early spring in a heated greenhouse. The seed is a light-dependent germinator; cover lightly with sand or medium. Emergence takes place in two to four weeks. Well-kept seed retains its viability for three years. It is quick and easy to grow and may need to be potted up before planting out (roughly ten weeks after sowing). Alternately, sow in deep wooden flats and transplant directly into the field. The plants do not hold well in pots.

Garden and Polyculture Planting

Ashwagandha resides easily alongside many other drought-tolerant plants that also prefer a sunny, hot location. Birds are fond of the ripe fruit and may facilitate the spread of the plants in irrigated areas

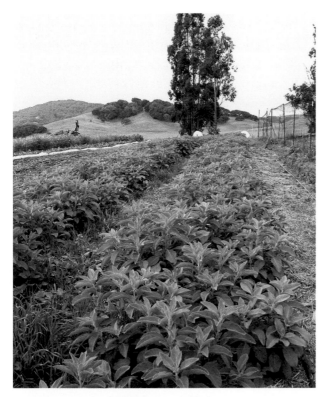

Young row cropped *Withania somnifera*.

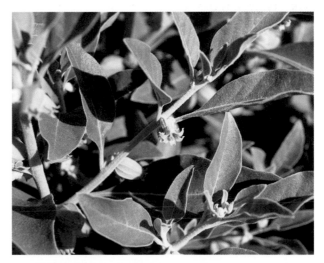

The diminutive green inflorescence of *Withania somnifera*.

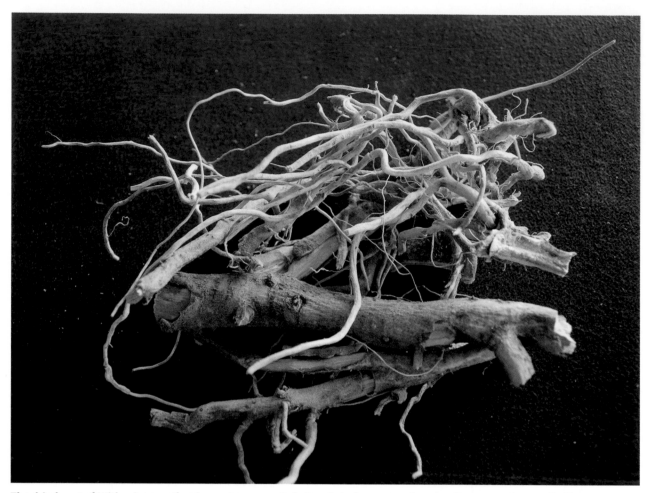

The dried root of *Withania somnifera* has a strong smell—in Sanskrit the name ashwagandha means the smell of horses.

or in regions with summer rain. Plant ashwagandha on two- or three-foot centers and it will develop into large, rounded, green-foliaged mounds.

Suitable Companions

Aster tataricus, Tartar Aster, zǐ wǎn
Astragalus membranaceus, Milk Vetch, huáng qí
Belamcanda chinensis, Blackberry Lily, shè gān
Carthamus tinctorius, Safflower, hóng huā
Ephedra sinica, Ephedra, má huáng/má huáng gēn
Lycium chinense, Chinese Wolfberry, gǒu qǐ zǐ/dì gǔ pí
Salvia miltiorrhiza, S. przewalskii, S. bowleyana, Red Sage, dān shēn
Ziziphus jujuba, Chinese Date, dà zǎo
Ziziphus jujuba var. *spinosa*, suān zǎo rén

Field Production

Grow ashwagandha two feet apart in warm, well-drained, sandy soil; sunny, hot, dry conditions are ideal. If soil is heavy, or in areas of high rainfall, plant in raised beds. The roots tend to rot and fail to overwinter in cold wet soils; in areas of high rainfall or where winters go below twenty degrees, treat it as an annual. Apply fertilizers and compost sparingly. Growing ashwagandha lean (low water, low fertilizer) makes superior medicine. If grown for several seasons with irrigation, these semiwoody plants can grow 3–4 feet tall and 3 feet wide; without supplemental water, expect plants closer to 1½ feet tall and 1½ feet wide. Dryland-farmed ashwagandha produce smaller but potent roots and may be a good choice for areas without the benefit of irrigation. This is a low-maintenance crop.

Pests and Diseases

Small outbreaks of aphids in springtime are common in the greenhouse. Roots rot in cold, wet soils.

Harvest and Yield

Dig the woody roots late in the fall, after one to three seasons' growth; roots will be larger if they grow more than one season. The whitish-yellow branching root system grows from one foot to more than two feet deep. The roots should smell deeply pungent. To process, cut or saw off the crowns, wash thoroughly with a power washer, make a cut with pruners down from the top, split by pulling the roots apart lengthwise, and dry. If the roots are large, utilize large pruners or a saw to reduce the size for drying. The fresh yield for dryland cultivated roots is a quarter pound per plant and a half pound per plant for first-season irrigated crops. Ratio of fresh to dry herb is 3:1.

Notes

- The market for this herb is expanding; many Chinese as well as Western herbalists are finding ashwagandha to be a useful herb.
- Occasionally Ayurvedic practitioners will request berry or leaf harvests; it is difficult to find a price agreement with buyers, as these two crops are labor-intensive to harvest.

Medicinal Uses of Ashwagandha

Ashwagandha is the root of *Withania somnifera*. It is probably the most famous Ayurvedic herb and is sometimes called "Indian ginseng." According to Ayurvedic classification, it is light, bitter, acrid and sweet, sweet post-digestive, and hot. It balances vata and pacifies kapha. It is used to strengthen the body and promote longevity as well as address issues such as fatigue, mental and physical exhaustion, infertility, impotence, anxiety, insomnia, high blood pressure, arthritis, low body weight, low appetite, frequent colds and flu, skin disorders, cough, wheezing, chronic urinary tract infections, kidney stones, and constipation.

Ashwagandha is used as a single herb and in combination with other herbs. It is used topically and internally. Common methods of administration include alcohol extracts, juices, decoctions, powders, ghee preparations, milk preparations, syrups, pastes, capsules, and pills.

Although the root is most commonly used, the whole plant is sometimes used—particularly when preparing medicinal oils and other topical applications.

Ashwa means "horse" and gandha means "smell." Many traditional Ayurvedic practitioners consider this to refer not only to the pungent scent of the herb but also as a reference to the character or essence of the horse and its associated qualities (strength, stamina, virility, and so on).

Ziziphus jujuba (Mill.)
Common Name: Chinese Date
Pinyin: Dà zǎo
Family: Rhamnaceae
Part Used: Fruit

Plant Description

Highly adaptable, *Ziziphus jujuba* can grow well in warm and cold climates from southern Canada, through the United States, and down into South America—and of course Asia! These small trees are deciduous, thorny to less-thorny (depending on variety), and grow about thirty feet tall. Leaves are glossy and bright green with margins that are lightly serrate. Small, sweet-smelling yellow flowers bloom in leaf axils in summer. *Ziziphus jujuba* endemically grows in central, eastern, and southeastern China on sunny and dry mountain slopes under 5,000 feet[178] and generally tolerates temperatures from -20 to 115 degrees. USDA hardiness zones 5 or 6–11.

Propagation

Choosing a variety suited to the locale can be the key to good harvests. Many cultivars of Chinese date have been commercially introduced, with 'Li' and 'Lang' being two of the most popular. Tree starts are available in the nursery trade. Seeds, grafts, or suckers are also commonly used. Fruit grower Roger Meyer wrote that one could stratify the seed and wait for up to two years for germination, or one could take a seed and cut it along the natural suture, presprout, and then sow for immediate germination. Sunstar Herbs in New Mexico has reported more than a 75 percent germination rate with cold stratification methods.

Garden and Polyculture Planting

Although Chinese date trees really do enjoy a good summer heat, there are varieties that are adapted to many different environments. Good for the home garden, or in a mixed orchard, place trees away from paths due to thorns. Chinese date ripens over a two-month period in warm climates, making for ongoing harvests.

Suitable Companions

Astragalus membranaceus, Milk Vetch, huáng qí
Carthamus tinctorius, Safflower, hóng huā
Ephedra sinica, Ephedra, má huáng/má huáng gēn
Lycium chinense, Chinese Wolfberry, gǒu qǐ zǐ/dì gǔ pí
Salvia miltiorrhiza, S. przewalskii, S. bowleyana, Red Sage, dān shēn
Withania somnifera, Ashwagandha
Ziziphus jujuba var. *spinosa*, suān zǎo rén

Field Production

For large-scale production the arid Southwest may be the best orchard siting. Chinese date is tolerant of hot, semiarid conditions as well as poor soils. The

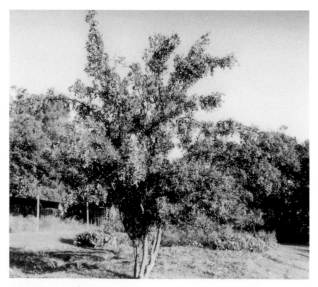
Ziziphus jujuba **tree at Elixir Farm Botanicals, Missouri.**

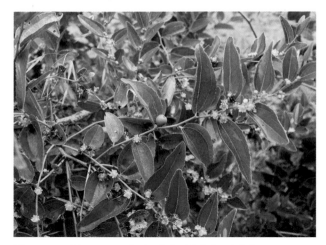

Flowers and immature fruit of the *Ziziphus jujuba* tree.

trees have a low winter-chill requirement. It grows productively in a variety of soils, including slightly acid, strongly alkaline, and saline.[179] Although well-drained soils are ideal, it is tolerant of wet soils as long as they are elevated in a berm; in fact, they may send out more suckers in wet areas. Supplement with irrigation for best fruit production. To modify the size or shape, prune in winter. It breaks dormancy and sets fruit late, often avoiding damage from late frosts. Plant nursery-grown trees on fifteen- to twenty-foot centers in full sun. In severe drought it will abort fruit, and in areas with short seasons or low heat the fruit may not ripen. Where the seasons are short or cool summers prevail, keeping fruit from maturing, hedge your bets and plant in the sunniest location or against a south-facing wall.

Pests and Diseases

Gophers occasionally eat the roots; where they are present plant in a large root basket made of aviary wire or hardware cloth. Rabbits may browse on the trunk; use a protectant made for this purpose (it will double as a trunk protector from wayward string trimmers).

Harvest and Yield

Nursery-grown trees start bearing fruit when they are as young as three years old. For fresh harvest, pick fruit when it is in the early stages of turning from light green to red-brown. Harvest fruits for drying

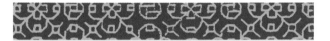

Chinese Date Recipes

Chinese date fruits may be eaten fresh, dried, or cooked. To use them in a braised meat dish, soak them for an hour first. Try this dessert of cooked fruit topped with bits of crystallized ginger.

> 2 cups Chinese date fruit, pitted and coarsely chopped
> 4 cups water
> half cup sugar
> 2 tablespoons lemon juice
> 2 tablespoons crystallized ginger, chopped
> Serves four

In a medium saucepan, add the fruit, water, and sugar and cook over low heat for thirty minutes, or until fruit softens. Check to make sure the syrup doesn't completely boil away—if the pan begins to sizzle, add an additional quarter-cup more water. Remove the pan from the heat and stir in lemon juice. Add the chopped ginger to the top of each portion just before serving. Serve warm or at room temperature.

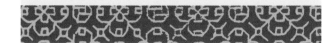

when they are completely brown. Depending on the variety; fruit can be small and shaped like a cherry or long and rounded (or oblong) and up to two inches long. For the best flavor, sweetness, and texture, experiment with harvest times from green to red-brown. Also try an early morning harvest. Smaller fruit may not have any seeds, but it is still perfectly good. When fruit is in the ripening phase rain can cause it to split. The best quality red fruits are sweet tasting, full and thick, and light red in color.[180] Many

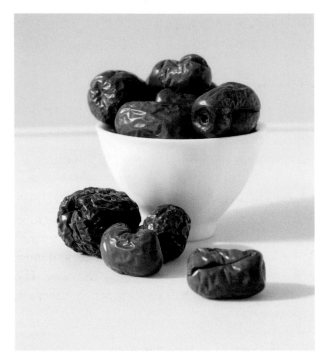

Dà zǎo; the sweet tasty Chinese date from the *Ziziphus jujuba* tree. Photo by Nina Zhito.

varieties were developed for fresh or dry fruit. For varieties that produce best in your area, contact the local county agricultural commissioner, nurseries, or the California Rare Fruit Growers Association. Yields vary according to variety and location.

Notes
"Red dates" are merely dried *Ziziphus jujuba* fruit and "black dates" are the same, but parboiled before drying.[181]

Medicinal Uses of Dà zǎo

Dà zǎo is the fruit of *Ziziphus jujuba*. Sweet and warm, it tonifies the spleen and stomach, benefits the qi, nourishes the blood, calms the shen, and harmonizes other herbs. It is frequently used in combination with gān cǎo (*Glycyrrhiza uralensis*) and shēng jiāng (*Zingiber officinale*) to harmonize the middle jiao and support the overall functions of the formula. It is used to address issues such as fatigue, low body weight, loose stools or diarrhea, scanty menstruation, dry skin and hair, irritability, and insomnia.

Dà zǎo is used as a single herb as well as in combination with other formulas. Common methods of administration include decoctions, powders, concentrated granules, alcohol extracts, tablets, and pills. It is also commonly used as a medicinal food and included in congees, soups, and other dishes. It is in many important formulas such as Ba Zhen Tang (Eight Treasures Decoction), all of the Gui Zhi Tang (Cinnamon Twig Decoction) derivatives, all of the Chai Hu Tang (*Bupleurum* Decoction) variations, Huo Xiang Zheng Qi San (*Agastache* Powder to Rectify the Qi), Ping Wei San (Calm the Stomach Powder), Zhi Gan Cao Tang (Licorice Decoction), and Su Zi Jiang Qi Tang (*Perilla* Decoction to Direct Qi Downward).

Ziziphus jujuba var. *spinosa* ([Bunge] Hu ex F. H. Chen)
Common Name: None
Pinyin: Suān zǎo rén
Family: Rhamnaceae
Part Used: Seed

Plant Description
Ziziphus jujuba var. *spinosa* is an uncommon but durable, deciduous shrubby tree, with many fine spines along the length of the branches. The glossy leaves are simple with slightly toothed margins. Insignificant, sweet-smelling yellow flowers bloom in leaf axils in summer and yield a round, sour fruit in fall. The *Flora of China* mentions its wide distribution from Tibet to northeast of Beijing and from southern to central China, with habitats to be on "hills, sunny dry slopes and plains."[182] I have seen these trees growing prolifically in the wild just north of Beijing. They were rather weedy and scrubby-looking but were up to ten feet tall. USDA hardiness zones 3–9.

Propagation
Scarify or crack the hard seed coat enough to allow water to reach the seed within. Germination takes a minimum of two months and is ongoing. Sow seed in large deep flats and leave it outside to receive nature's winterization. These seeds would probably respond well to an artificial stratification via the refrigerator. There is a high transplant mortality rate, and more work needs to be done to determine the cause. The plants hold well in pots if undisturbed, but they are slow growers.

Garden and Polyculture Planting
This scraggly small tree is not necessarily of specimen quality, but it will fit into the home landscape or hedgerow and offer nectar and serviceable fruit. Place with other drought-tolerant plants in full sun. It is thorny, so give it a respectable amount of space—about six feet in diameter. Plan to water it during the summer if your location receives no summer rain.

Suitable Companions
Astragalus membranaceus, Milk Vetch, huáng qí
Carthamus tinctorius, Safflower, hóng huā

Flowering branch of the *Ziziphus jujuba* var. *spinosa* tree.

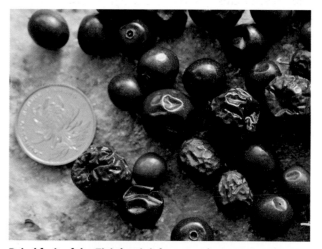

Dried fruit of the *Ziziphus jujuba* var. *spinosa* tree, suān zǎo rén. Photo by Nina Zhito.

Ephedra sinica, Ephedra, má huáng/má huáng gēn

Lycium chinense, Chinese Wolfberry, gǒu qǐ zǐ/dì gǔ pí

Salvia miltiorrhiza, S. przewalskii, S. bowleyana, Red Sage, dān shēn

Withania somnifera, Ashwagandha

Ziziphus jujuba, Chinese Date, dà zǎo

Field Production

Grow *Ziziphus jujuba* var. *spinosa* in full sun in at least somewhat well-drained soil on eight-foot centers. Drought tolerant and tough, they manage summer heat as well as winter cold. Deep watering is advised once or twice a season; as with many fruit trees, irrigation increases yield. *Ziziphus jujuba* var. *spinosa* is valued as a bee plant due to the high quantity of nectar production, and it is commonly used as a hedgerow component.[183]

Pests and Diseases

None.

Harvest and Yield

Harvest the small round fruit in the fall; I have not found yield information to pass on.

Notes

- A seed with a purplish-red, shiny surface and a yellowish interior denotes good quality.[184]
- *Ziziphus jujuba* var. *spinosa* is a wild form and is the rootstock onto which many *Ziziphus* cultivars are grafted.

Medicinal Uses of Suān zǎo rén

Suān zǎo rén is the seed of *Ziziphus jujuba* var. *spinosa*. Sweet and neutral, it nourishes the heart, calms the shen (spirits), and stops sweating. It is one of the most commonly used herbs for addressing insomnia and difficulty falling or staying asleep. It is also used to address issues such as palpitations, anxiety, irritability, dizziness, night sweats, and spontaneous sweats.

Suān zǎo rén is usually used in combination with other herbs. Common methods of administration include decoctions (crushed first), powders, concentrated granules, alcohol extracts, tablets, and pills. It is in formulas such as Suan Zao Ren Tang (*Ziziphus* Decoction), Gui Pi Tang (Restore the Spleen Decoction), Tian Wang Bu Xin Dan (Emperor of Heaven's Special Pill to Tonify the Heart), and Yang Xin Tang (Nourish the Heart Decoction).

Suān zǎo rén may be used either dried and unprocessed for insomnia with heat signs, or dry-fried for other types of insomnia.

Plant and Medicinal Name Cross-Reference Lists

Table A-1. Botanical Name Cross-Reference List

Botanical Name	Common Name	Pinyin
Acanthopanax gracilistylus		wǔ jiā shēn/pí
Achyranthes bidentata	Oxknee	huái niú xī
Agastache rugosa	Korean Mint	tǔ huò xiāng
Albizia julibrissin	Mimosa	hé huān pí/huā
Alisma plantago-aquatica subsp. *orientale*	Water Plantain	zé xiè
Allium macrostemon		xiè bái
Allium tuberosum	Garlic Chives	jiǔ cài zǐ
Andrographis paniculata	Kalmegh	chuān xīn lián
Anemarrhena asphodeloides		zhī mǔ
Angelica dahurica		bái zhǐ
Angelica pubescens		dú huó
Angelica sinensis	Dang Gui	dāng guī
Arctium lappa	Burdock	niú bàng zǐ
Artemisia annua	Sweet Annie	qīng hāo
Asparagus cochinchinensis		tiān mén dōng
Aster tataricus	Tartar Aster	zǐ wǎn
Astragalus membranaceus	Milk Vetch	huáng qí
Atractylodes macrocephala	Chinese Thistle Daisy	bái zhú
Bacopa monnieri	Brahmi	Brahmi
Belamcanda chinensis	Blackberry Lily	shè gān
Bupleurum chinense	Hare's Ear	chái hú
Carthamus tinctorius	Safflower	hóng huā
Celosia argentea		qīng xiāng zǐ
Celosia cristata	Cockscomb	jī guān huā
Centella asiatica	Gotu Kola	jī xuě cǎo
Chrysanthemum morifolium	Mum	jú huā
Clerodendrum trichotomum	Glorybower	chòu wú tóng
Codonopsis pilosula	Poor Man's Ginseng	dǎng shēn
Coix lacryma-jobi	Job's Tears	yì yǐ rén
Cornus officinalis	Dogwood	shān zhū yú
Crataegus pinnatifida	Chinese Hawthorn	shān zhā
Cyathula officinalis	Hookweed	chuān niú xī
Dianthus superbus	Fringed Pink	qú mài
Dioscorea opposita	Chinese Yam	shān yào
Dolichos lablab	Hyacinth Bean	bái biǎn dòu
Eclipta prostrata	Eclipta	mò hàn lián
Ephedra sinica	Ephedra	má huáng/má huáng gēn

Table A-1 *(continued)*

Botanical Name	Common Name	Pinyin
Eriobotrya japonica	Loquat	pí pá yè
Eucommia ulmoides	Hardy Rubber Tree	dù zhòng
Fallopia multiflora	Fo Ti	shǒu wū/yè jīao téng
Forsythia suspensa		lián qiào
Gentiana scabra		lóng dǎn cǎo
Gentiana straminea		qín jiāo
Ginkgo biloba	Ginkgo	bái guǒ
Glycyrrhiza uralensis	Chinese Licorice	gān cǎo
Gynostemma pentaphyllum	Sweet Tea Vine	jiǎo gǔ lán
Houttuynia cordata		yú xīng cǎo
Ligusticum jeholense	Chinese Lovage	gǎo běn
Ligustrum lucidum	Chinese Privet	nǚ zhēn zǐ
Lilium brownii	Lily	bǎi hé
Lilium lancifolium	Lily	bǎi hé
Lonicera japonica	Honeysuckle	jīn yín huā
Lycium chinense	Chinese Wolfberry	gǒu qǐ zǐ/dì gǔ pí
Magnolia denudata		xīn yí huā
Mentha haplocalyx	Field Mint	bò hé
Momordica charantia	Bitter Melon	kǔ guā
Ocimum sanctum	Sacred Basil	Tulsi
Ophiopogon japonicus	Lilyturf	mài mén dōng
Paeonia lactiflora	Chinese Peony	bái/chì sháo
Paeonia suffruticosa	Tree Peony	mǔ dān pí
Panax ginseng	Asian Ginseng	rén shēn
Panax quinquefolius	American Ginseng	xī yáng shēn
Pinellia ternata		bàn xià
Plantago asiatica	Plantain	chē qián zǐ
Platycodon grandiflorus	Balloon Flower	jié gěng
Prunella vulgaris	Heal All	xià kū cǎo
Rehmannia glutinosa	Chinese Foxglove	dì huáng
Rheum palmatum	Chinese Rhubarb	dà huáng
Salvia miltiorrhiza	Red Sage	dān shēn
Saposhnikovia divaricata	Siler	fáng fēng
Schisandra chinensis	Five Flavored Fruit	wǔ wèi zǐ
Schizonepeta tenuifolia	Japanese Catnip	jīng jiè
Scrophularia buergeriana	Figwort	běi xuán shēn
Scutellaria baicalensis	Baikal Skullcap	huáng qín
Scutellaria barbata	Barbat Skullcap	bàn zhī lián
Sophora flavescens		kǔ shēn
Trichosanthes kirilowii	Chinese Cucumber	guā lóu/tiān huā fěn
Withania somnifera	Ashwagandha	Ashwagandha
Ziziphus jujuba	Chinese Date	dà zǎo
Ziziphus jujuba var. *spinosa*		suān zǎo rén

Table A-2. Common Name Cross-Reference List

Common Name	Botanical Name	Pinyin
American Ginseng	*Panax quinquefolius*	xī yáng shēn
Ashwagandha	*Withania somnifera*	Ashwagandha
Asian Ginseng	*Panax ginseng*	rén shēn
Baikal Skullcap	*Scutellaria baicalensis*	huáng qín
Balloon Flower	*Platycodon grandiflorus*	jié gěng
Barbat Skullcap	*Scutellaria barbata*	bàn zhī lián
Bitter Melon	*Momordica charantia*	kŭ guā
Blackberry Lily	*Belamcanda chinensis*	shè gān
Brahmi	*Bacopa monnieri*	Brahmi
Burdock	*Arctium lappa*	niú bàng zǐ
Chinese Cucumber	*Trichosanthes kirilowii*	guā lóu/tiān huā fěn
Chinese Date	*Ziziphus jujuba*	dà zǎo
Chinese Foxglove	*Rehmannia glutinosa*	dì huáng
Chinese Hawthorn	*Crataegus pinnatifida*	shān zhā
Chinese Licorice	*Glycyrrhiza uralensis*	gān cǎo
Chinese Lovage	*Ligusticum jeholense*	gǎo běn
Chinese Peony	*Paeonia lactiflora*	bái/chì sháo
Chinese Privet	*Ligustrum lucidum*	nǚ zhēn zǐ
Chinese Rhubarb	*Rheum palmatum*	dà huáng
Chinese Thistle Daisy	*Atractylodes macrocephala*	bái zhú
Chinese Wolfberry	*Lycium chinense*	gǒu qǐ zǐ/dì gǔ pí
Chinese Yam	*Dioscorea opposita*	shān yào
Cockscomb	*Celosia cristata*	jī guān huā
Dang Gui	*Angelica sinensis*	dāng guī
Dogwood	*Cornus officinalis*	shān zhū yú
Eclipta	*Eclipta prostrata*	mò hàn lián
Ephedra	*Ephedra sinica*	má huáng/má huáng gēn
Field Mint	*Mentha haplocalyx*	bò hé
Figwort	*Scrophularia buergeriana*	běi xuán shēn
Five Flavored Fruit	*Schisandra chinensis*	wǔ wèi zǐ
Fo Ti	*Fallopia multiflora*	shǒu wū/yè jīao téng
Fringed Pink	*Dianthus superbus*	qú mài
Garlic Chives	*Allium tuberosum*	jiǔ cài zǐ
Ginkgo	*Ginkgo biloba*	bái guǒ
Glorybower	*Clerodendrum trichotomum*	chòu wú tóng
Gotu Kola	*Centella asiatica*	jī xuě cǎo
Hardy Rubber Tree	*Eucommia ulmoides*	dù zhòng
Hare's Ear	*Bupleurum chinense*	chái hú
Heal All	*Prunella vulgaris*	xià kū cǎo
Honeysuckle	*Lonicera japonica*	jīn yín huā

Table A-2 *(continued)*

Common Name	Botanical Name	Pinyin
Hookweed	*Cyathula officinalis*	chuān niú xī
Hyacinth Bean	*Dolichos lablab*	bái biǎn dòu
Japanese Catnip	*Schizonepeta tenuifolia*	jīng jiè
Job's Tears	*Coix lacryma-jobi*	yì yǐ rén
Kalmegh	*Andrographis paniculata*	chuān xīn lián
Korean Mint	*Agastache rugosa*	tǔ huò xiāng
Lily	*Lilium brownii*	bǎi hé
Lily	*Lilium lancifolium*	bǎi hé
Lilyturf	*Ophiopogon japonicus*	mài mén dōng
Loquat	*Eriobotrya japonica*	pí pá yè
Milk Vetch	*Astragalus membranaceus*	huáng qí
Mimosa	*Albizia julibrissin*	hé huān pí/huā
Mum	*Chrysanthemum morifolium*	jú huā
Oxknee	*Achyranthes bidentata*	huái niú xī
Plantain	*Plantago asiatica*	chē qián zǐ
Poor Man's Ginseng	*Codonopsis pilosula*	dǎng shēn
Red Sage	*Salvia miltiorrhiza*	dān shēn
Sacred Basil	*Ocimum sanctum*	Tulsi
Safflower	*Carthamus tinctorius*	hóng huā
Siler	*Saposhnikovia divaricata*	fáng fēng
Sweet Annie	*Artemisia annua*	qīng hāo
Sweet Tea Vine	*Gynostemma pentaphyllum*	jiǎo gǔ lán
Tartar Aster	*Aster tataricus*	zǐ wǎn
Tree Peony	*Paeonia suffruticosa*	mǔ dān pí
Water Plantain	*Alisma plantago-aquatica* subsp. *orientale*	zé xiè
	Acanthopanax gracilistylus	wǔ jiā shēn/pí
	Allium macrostemon	xiè bái
	Anemarrhena asphodeloides	zhī mǔ
	Angelica dahurica	bái zhǐ
	Angelica pubescens	dú huó
	Asparagus cochinchinensis	tiān mén dōng
	Celosia argentea	qīng xiāng zǐ
	Forsythia suspensa	lián qiào
	Gentiana scabra	lóng dǎn cǎo
	Gentiana straminea	qín jiāo
	Houttuynia cordata	yú xīng cǎo
	Magnolia denudata	xīn yí huā
	Pinellia ternata	bàn xià
	Sophora flavescens	kǔ shēn
	Ziziphus jujuba var. *spinosa*	suān zǎo rén

Table A-3. Pinyin/Hindi/Sanskrit Name Cross-Reference List

Pinyin	Botanical Name	Common Name
Ashwagandha	*Withania somnifera*	Ashwagandha
bái biǎn dòu	*Dolichos lablab*	Hyacinth Bean
bái guǒ	*Ginkgo biloba*	Ginkgo
bǎi hé	*Lilium brownii*	Lily
bǎi hé	*Lilium lancifolium*	Lily
bái/chì sháo	*Paeonia lactiflora*	Chinese Peony
bái zhǐ	*Angelica dahurica*	
bái zhú	*Atractylodes macrocephala*	Chinese Thistle Daisy
bàn xià	*Pinellia ternata*	
bàn zhī lián	*Scutellaria barbata*	Barbat Skullcap
běi xuán shēn	*Scrophularia buergeriana*	Figwort
bò hé	*Mentha haplocalyx*	Field Mint
Brahmi	*Bacopa monnieri*	Brahmi
chái hú	*Bupleurum chinense*	Hare's Ear
chē qián zǐ	*Plantago asiatica*	Plantain
chòu wú tóng	*Clerodendrum trichotomum*	Glorybower
chuān niú xī	*Cyathula officinalis*	Hookweed
chuān xīn lián	*Andrographis paniculata*	Kalmegh
dà huáng	*Rheum palmatum*	Chinese Rhubarb
dà zǎo	*Ziziphus jujuba*	Chinese Date
dān shēn	*Salvia miltiorrhiza*	Red Sage
dāng guī	*Angelica sinensis*	Dang Gui
dǎng shēn	*Codonopsis pilosula*	Poor Man's Ginseng
dì huáng	*Rehmannia glutinosa*	Chinese Foxglove
dú huó	*Angelica pubescens*	
dù zhòng	*Eucommia ulmoides*	Hardy Rubber Tree
fáng fēng	*Saposhnikovia divaricata*	Siler
gān cǎo	*Glycyrrhiza uralensis*	Chinese Licorice
gǎo běn	*Ligusticum jeholense*	Chinese Lovage
gǒu qǐ zǐ/dì gǔ pí	*Lycium chinense*	Chinese Wolfberry
guā lóu/tiān huā fěn	*Trichosanthes kirilowii*	Chinese Cucumber
hé huān pí/huā	*Albizia julibrissin*	Mimosa
hóng huā	*Carthamus tinctorius*	Safflower
huái niú xī	*Achyranthes bidentata*	Oxknee
huáng qí	*Astragalus membranaceus*	Milk Vetch
huáng qín	*Scutellaria baicalensis*	Baikal Skullcap
jī guān huā	*Celosia cristata*	Cockscomb
jī xuě cǎo	*Centella asiatica*	Gotu Kola
jiǎo gǔ lán	*Gynostemma pentaphyllum*	Sweet Tea Vine
jié gěng	*Platycodon grandiflorus*	Balloon Flower

Table A-3 *(continued)*

Pinyin	Botanical Name	Common Name
jīn yín huā	*Lonicera japonica*	Honeysuckle
jīng jiè	*Schizonepeta tenuifolia*	Japanese Catnip
jiŭ cài zĭ	*Allium tuberosum*	Garlic Chives
jú huā	*Chrysanthemum morifolium*	Mum
kŭ guā	*Momordica charantia*	Bitter Melon
kŭ shēn	*Sophora flavescens*	
lián qiào	*Forsythia suspensa*	
lóng dăn căo	*Gentiana scabra*	
má huáng/má huáng gēn	*Ephedra sinica*	Ephedra
mài mén dōng	*Ophiopogon japonicus*	Lilyturf
mò hàn lián	*Eclipta prostrata*	Eclipta
mŭ dān pí	*Paeonia suffruticosa*	Tree Peony
niú bàng zĭ	*Arctium lappa*	Burdock
nŭ zhēn zĭ	*Ligustrum lucidum*	Chinese Privet
pí pá yè	*Eriobotrya japonica*	Loquat
qín jiāo	*Gentiana straminea*	
qīng hāo	*Artemisia annua*	Sweet Annie
qīng xiāng zĭ	*Celosia argentea*	
qú mài	*Dianthus superbus*	Fringed Pink
rén shēn	*Panax ginseng*	Asian Ginseng
shān yào	*Dioscorea opposita*	Chinese Yam
shān zhā	*Crataegus pinnatifida*	Chinese Hawthorn
shān zhū yú	*Cornus officinalis*	Dogwood
shè gān	*Belamcanda chinensis*	Blackberry Lily
shŏu wū/yè jīao téng	*Fallopia multiflora*	Fo Ti
suān zăo rén	*Ziziphus jujuba* var. *spinosa*	
tiān mén dōng	*Asparagus cochinchinensis*	
tŭ huò xiāng	*Agastache rugosa*	Korean Mint
Tulsi	*Ocimum sanctum*	Sacred Basil
wŭ jiā shēn/pí	*Acanthopanax gracilistylus*	
wŭ wèi zĭ	*Schisandra chinensis*	Five Flavored Fruit
xī yáng shēn	*Panax quinquefolius*	American Ginseng
xià kū căo	*Prunella vulgaris*	Heal All
xiè bái	*Allium macrostemon*	
xīn yí huā	*Magnolia denudata*	
yì yĭ rén	*Coix lacryma-jobi*	Job's Tears
yú xīng căo	*Houttuynia cordata*	
zé xiè	*Alisma plantago-aquatica* subsp. *orientale*	Water Plantain
zhī mŭ	*Anemarrhena asphodeloides*	
zĭ wăn	*Aster tataricus*	Tartar Aster

Maps

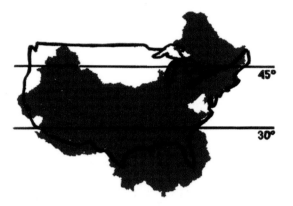

China–United States Latitude Overlay Map.

2006 arborday.org Hardiness Zones Map

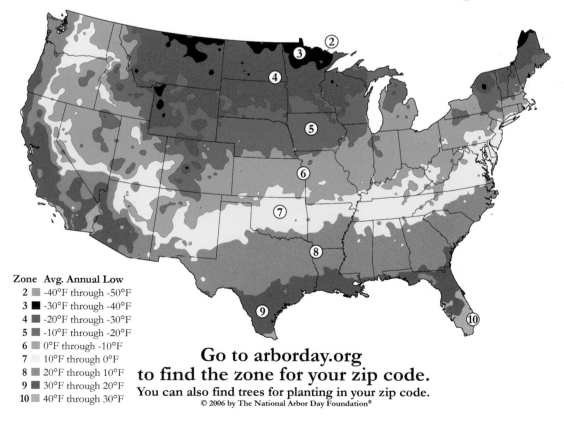

Zone	Avg. Annual Low
2	-40°F through -50°F
3	-30°F through -40°F
4	-20°F through -30°F
5	-10°F through -20°F
6	0°F through -10°F
7	10°F through 0°F
8	20°F through 10°F
9	30°F through 20°F
10	40°F through 30°F

**Go to arborday.org
to find the zone for your zip code.**
You can also find trees for planting in your zip code.

© 2006 by The National Arbor Day Foundation®

USDA Hardiness Zone Map. Map courtesy of Mark Derowitsch, ©2006 Mark Derowitsch.

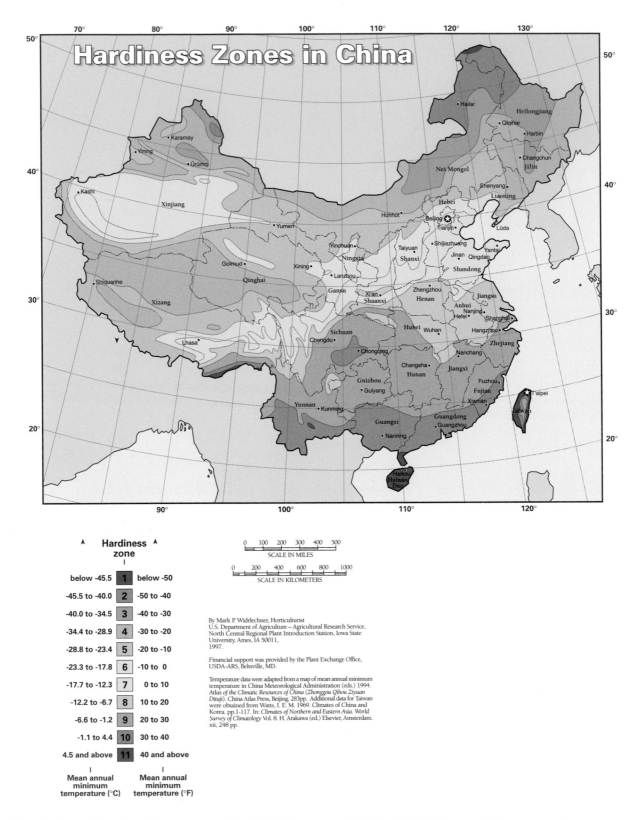

China Hardiness Zone Map. Map courtesy of Mark P. Widrlechner, ©1997 Mark P. Widrlechner (Color map, scale ca. 1:16,360,000). Iowa State University, Ames, Iowa.

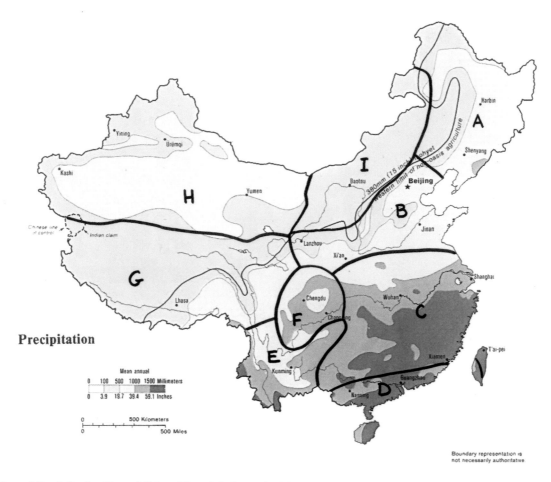

Climate and Precipitation Map of China. ©Peg Schafer and US Government. (Base map) 2011/2005.

	Zone	Summers	Winters	Indigenous Plant Cover
Climate Zone Map of China Key				
A	Temperate to cold temperate	warm	cold and dry	coniferous to mixed broadleaf forest
B	Warm temperate	hot and wet	cold and dry	mixed deciduous broadleaf forest
C	Temperate to subtropical	hot and wet	cold to cool and dry	evergreen broadleaf forest
D	Tropical	hot and wet	warm and dry	seasonal rainforest
E	Tropical to subtropical	warm and wet	cool and wet	high mountain and deep valley mixed alpine to rainforest
F	Subtropical to temperate	hot and wet	cool and overcast	high mountain and deep basin, distinct alpine to lowland meadow
G	Subtropical to temperate	cool and dry	cold and dry	high altitude vegetation
H	Temperate	hot and dry	cold and dry	desert
I	Temperate	cool and wet	cold and dry	grassland

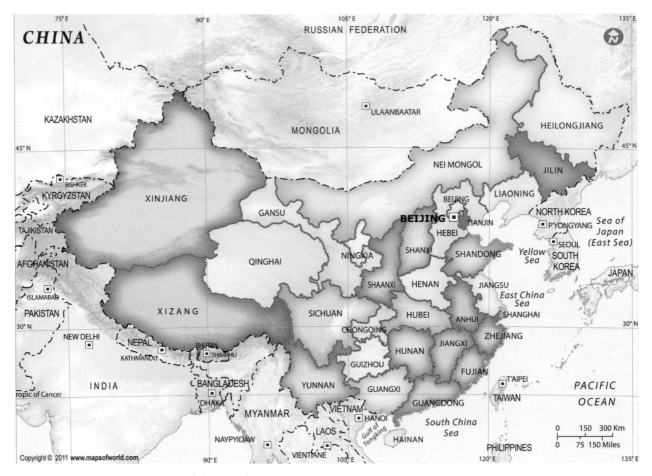

China Province Map. © 2011 Maps of the World.com.

Resources

SOURCES OF HERB SEEDS AND PLANTS

B & T World Seeds
Paguignan, 34210 Aigues-Vives, France
www.b-and-t-world-seeds.com/

Bountiful Gardens
18001 Shafter Road
Willits, CA 95490
(707) 459-6410
www.bountifulgardens.org

Chinese Medicinal Herb Farm
296 Wetmore Lane
Petaluma, CA 94952
(707) 765-9611
www.chinesemedicinalherbfarm.com
The Chinese Medicinal Herb Farm is a supplier of seed and fresh and dried herbs.

Companion Plants
7247 North Coolville Ridge Road
Athens, OH 45701
(614) 592-4643
www.companionplants.com

Crimson Sage
P.O. Box 83
Orleans, CA 95556
(530) 627-3457
www.crimsonsage.com

Forestfarm
990 Tethrow Road
Williams, OR 97544
(541) 846-7269
www.forestfarm.com

Goodwin Creek Gardens
P.O. Box 83
Williams, OR 97544
(800) 846-7357
www.goodwincreekgardens.com

Horizon Herbs
P.O. Box 69
Williams, OR 97544
(541) 846-6704
www.horizonherbs.com

J. L. Hudson, Seedsman
Box 337
La Honda, CA 94020
www.jlhudsonseeds.net

Johnny's Selected Seeds
184 Foss Hill Road
Albion, ME 04910
(877) 564-6697
www.johnnyseeds.com

Pacific Botanicals
4840 Fish Hatchery Road
Grants Pass, OR 97527
(541) 479-7777
www.pacificbotanicals.com
Pacific Botanicals is a supplier of fresh and dry medicinal plants.

Peaceful Valley Farm Supply
P.O. Box 2209
Grass Valley, CA 95945
(888) 784-1722
www.groworganic.com

Richters Herbs
357 Highway 47
Goodwood, ON L0C 1A0 Canada
(905) 640-6677
www.richters.com

Seed Savers Exchange
Flower and Herb Exchange
3094 North Winn Road
Decorah, IA 52101
(563) 382-5990
www.seedsavers.org

Seeds of Change
P.O. Box 15700
Santa Fe, NM 87504-5700
(888) 762-7333
www.seedsofchange.com

Territorial Seed Company
P.O. Box 157
Cottage Grove, OR 98424
(541) 942-0510
www.territorialseed.com

Turtle Tree Seed
Camphill Village
Copake, NY 12516
(888) 516-7797
www.turtletreeseeds.com

SOURCES OF FARM, NURSERY, AND GREENHOUSE SUPPLIES

A.M. Leonard, Inc.
P.O. Box 816
Piqua, OH 45356
(800) 543-8955
www.amleo.com

Charley's Greenhouse and Indoor Growing Supplies
17979 Star Route 536
Mount Vernon, WA 98723
(800) 322-4707
www.charleysgreenhouse.com

Conley's Greenhouse
4344 Mission Boulevard
Montclair, CA 91763
(800) 377-8441
www.conleys.com

FarmTek/TekSupply
1440 Field of Dreams Way
Dyersville, IA 52040
(800) 327-6835
www.farmtek.com

Harmony Farm Supply and Nursery
3244 Highway 116 North
Sebastopol, CA 95472
(707) 823-9125
www.harmonyfarm.com

McConkey Company
P.O. Box 1690
Sumner, WA 98390
(800) 426-8124
www.mcconkeyco.com

CONSERVATION ORGANIZATIONS

Convention on Biological Diversity
www.cbd.int
An international treaty to sustain the diversity of life on Earth

Convention on International Trade in Endangered Species of Wild Fauna and Flora (CITES) list
www.cites.org
An international agreement between governments. Its aim is to ensure that international trade in specimens of wild animals and plants does not threaten their survival.

Invasive Plant Atlas of the United States
www.invasive.org/weedus/index.html

Traffic International
219a Huntingdon Road
Cambridge CB3 ODL
United Kingdom
+44 (0) 1223 277427
www.traffic.org
Conservation of both animal- and plant-based Chinese herbs

The USDA Natural Resources Conservation Service
http://plants.usda.gov/java/noxiousDriver
Federal and state noxious weed lists

International Union for Conservation of Nature
1630 Connecticut Avenue
N.W. 3rd Floor
Washington D.C. 20009
(202) 387-4826
www.iucn.org

Recommended Reading

BOOKS

Chinese Herbal Medicine: Materia Medica, 3rd Edition
Dan Bensky, Steven Clavey, and Erich Stöger
Eastland Press

Chinese Medical Herbology and Pharmacology
John K. Chen and Tina T. Chen
Art of Medicine Press

The Complete Medicinal Herbal
Penelope Ody
DK Publishing

Food Plants of China
Shiu-ying Hu
The Chinese University Press
www.chineseupress.com
Very useful for giving valuable information about Chinese herbs and foodstuffs

Food Plants of the World
Ben-Erik van Wyk
Timber Press, Incorporated

Growing At-Risk Medicinal Herbs
Richo Cech
Horizon Herbs Publications
www.horizonherbs.com

Herbal Bounty: The Gentle Art of Herb Culture
Steven Foster
Gibbs Smith, Publisher

Herbal Emissaries, Bringing Herbs to the West: A Guide to Gardening, Herbal Wisdom, and Well-Being
Steven Foster and Yue Chongxi
Healing Arts Press

Herbal Renaissance
Steven Foster
Gibbs Smith, Publisher

Herbs
Lesley Bremness
DK Publishing

Herbs for Sale: Growing and Marketing
Lee Sturdivant
San Juan Naturals

Hortus III: A Concise Dictionary of Plants Cultivated in the U.S. and Canada
Staff of the L. H. Bailey Hortorium
Cornell University

Life in the Medicine: A Guide to Growing and Harvesting Herbs for Medicine Making
Leslie Gardner
Emerald Earth Publishing

The Medicinal Herb Grower
Richo Cech
Horizon Herbs Publications
www.horizonherbs.com

Medicinal Herbs in the Garden, Field, and Marketplace
Lee Sturdivant and Tim Blakley
San Juan Naturals

Mending the Web of Life
Elizabeth Call
www.mendingtheweb.com, www.redwingbooks.com/sku/MenWebLif.com

New Encyclopedia of Herbs and Their Uses
Deni Brown
DK Publishing

The One-Straw Revolution: An Introduction to Natural Farming
Masanobu Fukuoka
NYRB Classics

Practical Woody Plant Propagation for Nursery Growers
Bruce Macdonald
Timber Press

Reference Manual of Woody Plant Propagation
Michael Dirr and Charles Heuser
Varsity Press

Seed to Seed
Suzanne Ashworth
Seed Savers Exchange
www.seedsavers.org

Sunset Western Garden Book, 8th edition
Sunset Publishing
www.sunsetbooks.com

Test Your Soil With Plants! (Booklet #29)
John Beeby
Ecology Action

Weeds of the West, 9th Edition
Tom Whitson, Daniel A. Ball, David W. Cudney, Steven A Dewey, Clyde L. Elmore, Rodney G. Lynn, Don Morishita, Robert Parker, Dean G. Swan and Richard K. Zollinger.
Western Society of Weed Science

OTHER PUBLICATIONS

Acres USA
P.O. Box 91299
Austin, TX 78709
(800) 355-5313
www.acresusa.com
Acres has an interesting catalog of books.

The Herb Companion
201 East Fourth Street
Loveland, CO 80537
www.herbcompanion.com

The Herb Quarterly
1041 Shary Circle
Concord, CA 94518
(510) 668-0268
www.herbquarterly.com/support.html

HerbalGram
American Botanical Council
P.O. Box 144345
Austin, TX 78714
(512) 926-4900
www.herbalgram.org

HELPFUL WEBSITES AND ORGANIZATIONS

Alternative Farming Systems
Information Center
National Agricultural Library
Agricultural Research Service
U.S. Department of Agriculture
10301 Baltimore Avenue, Room 132
Beltsville, MD 20705
(301) 504-6559
www.nal.usda.gov/afsic

American Botanical Council
P.O. Box 144345
Austin, TX 78714
(512) 926-4900
www.herbalgram.org

American Herb Association
P.O. Box 1673
Nevada City, CA 95959
(530) 265-9552
www.ahaherb.com

American Herbalists Guild
P.O. Box 230741
Boston, MA 02123
(857) 350-3128
www.americanherbalistsguild.com

Asian Medicinal Herb Production and
Marketing (Chinese Medicinal Herb
Online Cultivation Workshop)
http://aces.nmsu.edu/medicinalherbs/
*Hours of free online lectures with Peg
Schafer and Jean Giblette*

ATTRA (National Sustainable
Agriculture Information Service)
Appropriate Technology Transfer for
Rural Areas
www.attra.ncat.org
*Offers free online publications on
specific agricultural topics*

Chinese Medicinal Herb Farm
296 Wetmore Lane
Petaluma, CA 94952
(707) 765-9611
 www.chinesemedicinalherbfarm.com
Author Peg Schafer's Website

Ecology Action
5798 Ridgewood Road
Willits, CA 95490
(707) 459-0150
www.growbiointensive.org

Flora of China
www.efloras.org
*The definitive key to specific plant
information*

GRIN Taxonomy for Plants
U.S. Agricultural Research Service
www.ars-grin.gov/cgi-bin/npgs/html
/index.pl

Herb Growing and Marketing Network
P.O. Box 245
Silver Spring, PA 17575
(717) 393-3295
www.herbnet.com

High Falls Gardens
P.O. Box 125
Philmont, NY 12565
(518) 672-7365
www.highfallsgardens.net
*Website of Jean Giblette, cofounder of
the Medicinal Herb Consortium and
Localherbs.org*

International Institute for Ecological
Agriculture
343 Soquel Avenue #191
Santa Cruz, CA 95062
(831) 688-8970
www.permaculture.com

International Trade Centre
Market News Service
www.intracen.org
*ITC's mission is to enable small
business export success in transition-
economy countries.*

Medicinal Herb Consortium
www.localherbs.org
*Chinese medicinal herb farmer-
consumer working group*

A Modern Herbal (electronic version)
www.botanical.com

Mountain Gardens
546 Shuford Creek Road
Burnsville, NC 28714
(828) 675-5664
joehollisherbs@gmail.com
http://www.mountaingardensherbs.com/

National Agricultural Library
www.nalusda.gov

The National Center for the Preservation
of Medicinal Herbs
33560 Beech Grove Road
Rutland, OH 45775
(740) 742-4401
www.ncpmh.org

Native Seeds/SEARCH
2509 North Campbell #325
Tucson, AZ 85719
www.nativeseeds.org

The Plant List
www.theplantlist.org
*A working list of accepted Latin plant
names*

Plants for a Future
www.pfaf.org

Seed Savers Exchange
3094 North Winn Road
Decorah, IA 52101
(563) 382-5990
www.seedsavers.org

Sonoma County Herb Association/
Sonoma County Herb Exchange
P.O. Box 2162
Sebastopol, CA 95473
(707) 861-0336
 www.sonomaherbs.org
*Fostering respect for the green world
and our community through the
responsible use and sustainable cultivation of herbs*

United Plant Savers
P.O. Box 400
East Barre, VT 05659
(802) 476-6467
www.unitedplantsavers.org

Glossary

HORTICULTURAL TERMS

Adventitious: Occurring in an unusual location. For example, roots forming on stem cuttings when placed into a cutting media.

Axil: The angle that forms between the stem and leaf.

Bipinnate: Leaves that are divided twice, from primary pinnae into secondary leaflets.

Bract: A modified or much-reduced leaf.

Calyx: The outer part of flowers that are usually green and leaflike.

Cambium: The thin layer of cells between xylem and phloem responsible for new growth.

Cordate: Heart-shaped, often applied to heart-shaped leaves.

Cortex: The skin tissue of a stem or root.

Corymb: An almost flat-topped flower blooming in an ascending pattern.

Crenate: Scalloped edges, commonly referred to with leaf margins.

Dentation: Sharply pointed, commonly referred to with leaf margins.

Dioecious: Male and female flowers on separate plants.

Emitter: Orifice for metered irrigation.

Faceted: Multifaced, as in a cut diamond or a seed with flattened sides.

Garble: Process of separating into parts.

Germplasm: Reproductive cells capable of growing into plants—seeds and cuttings are two simple examples.

Glaucous: A blue-green bloom or covering, an example being broccoli leaves.

Herbaceous: Nonwoody plant, usually referring to plants that die back to the ground at the end of the growing season.

Intercropping: Growing more than one type of crop in the same crop area.

Interplanting: Growing more than one type of plant in the same vicinity.

Lanceolate: Lance-shaped, usually referring to leaves longer than they are wide that taper to a point.

Landrace: An early, cultivated form of a crop evolved from a wild species.

Layering: A method of vegetative propagation involving plant stems rooting as a result of soil contact.

Multicycle Germinator: A seed that requires varying periods of moisture and/or temperature conditioning to break dormancy.

Node: The location where a leaf is attached to the stem, often the site of floral buds as well.

Obovate: Ovatelike in shape—as in a leaf, with the thickest part at the farthest end instead of the middle.

Opposite: An arrangement of leaves on a stem that occur in pairs on either sides of a node.

Ovate: Oval or egg-shaped, the most simple of leaf shapes.

Palmate: A leaf arrangement of leaflets in a compound leaf—shaped like a hand.

Panicle: A branching inflorescence.

Petiole: The stalk of a leaf that attaches the leaf to the stem of a plant.

Pinnate: A compound leaf with leaflets arranged featherlike on both sides of a mid rib.

Polyculture: A system of nature-based cultivation that consists of more than one type of plant in a planting area.

Pubescent: Fuzzy, as in leaves covered with soft hairs.

Raceme: An inflorescence in which the flowers are borne on unbranched stems.

Riddle, Riddling: To sift so as to separate different parts.

Scarify, Scarification: A method of scratching open the surface of a seed to start the germination process.

Serrate: Saw-toothed edge, usually in reference to a leaf margin.

Sessile: A position where flowers, leaves, or fruits are directly attached to a stem, without a stalk.

Simple: A leaf or a flower that is not divided or compound in shape.

Spatulate: Spoon-shaped, applied to a leaf that has a round end.

Stratification: The process of exposing seed to warm and/or cold conditions to break dormancy.

Terminal: Apical, or topmost; often applied to central flowers that often yield the largest seed.

Testa: The outer coat of a seed.

Trifoliate: Thrice divided, often referred to a leaf that is divided into three portions.

Umbel: An inflorescence, usually flat topped, that has the shape of an umbrella.

Venation: The arrangement of veins.

Wild-simulated, Wild-cultivated, Wild-quality: A method of cultivation that mimics nature.

MEDICINAL TERMS
By Sean Fannin

Ayurveda: The traditional medical system of India. Literally "the science of life" in Sanskrit.

Bi Syndrome: "Painful obstruction" syndrome, a TCM description of chronic arthritic or muscular pain.

Channels: The network of qi that carries specific qualities and functions throughout the body. There are twelve organ channels and eight extraordinary channels. Acupuncture points are concentrated areas or "points" along the channels.

Dampness: An accumulation of fluids that may refer to environmental conditions (humidity) or fluid accumulation within the body.

Decoction: A medicinal preparation made by bringing water to a boil and then simmering herbs in that water for an extended period of time.

Dosha: The three basic substances or elemental energies of the body within Ayurveda: Vata (Wind and Space), Pitta (Fire and Water), and Kapha (Water and Earth).

Essences: See Jing.

Fire: Extreme heat that typically affects a specific organ or function within the body (e.g., liver fire).

Heat: May refer to environmental heat (such as warm days in the summertime) or internal heat. Internal heat is characterized by overactive physiological and psychological activity, inflammation and fever, or a sensation of fever/heat.

Humor: The basic substances or elemental energies of the body, called doshas within Ayurveda.

Jing: Essences or essence. One of the fundamental substances of the body in TCM (along with qi, blood, fluids, and shen). Responsible for growth, development, reproduction, and regeneration within the body.

Kapha: One of the three doshas or elemental energies of the body within Ayurveda. Associated with water and earth.

Pitta: One of the three doshas or elemental energies of the body within Ayurveda. Associated with fire and water.

Qi: Vital energy, influence, function. Within the body qi is responsible for the proper functioning of the activities of life, specifically described as warmth, movement, transformation, containment, and defense.

Shen: Spirits or spirit. The most subtle manifestation of qi within the body, responsible for the organization and orchestration of life in concert with the jing. Characterized by mental clarity, appropriate emotional responses, acute sensory perception, and a healthy luster to the skin.

Stagnation (as in blood stagnation, qi stagnation): A localized accumulation of qi, blood, or fluids that disrupts the normal functioning of the affected area or organ.

Superior Herbs: A category of medicinal or food safe to use for long periods of time without side effects (versus inferior, which may have side effects).

Tonify: To strengthen or supplement.

Vata: One of the three doshas or elemental energies of the body within Ayurveda. Associated with wind and space.

Wind (as in wind heat, wind damp): Environmental wind that affects the surface of the body and is associated with colds, allergies, and muscle aches. It also may combine with other environmental factors such as heat or dampness and carry those factors into the body, disrupting the normal physiological processes and functions.

Yin and Yang: Yin and yang are a way to view and organize the changes and transformations that occur in nature and in the human body. Within the body yin refers to physical substances and the cooling, regulating, calming, and moistening processes. Yang refers to physiological/metabolic activities that include the warming, circulating, stimulating, and drying processes.

PINYIN TERMS

Bǎi: The color white, as in bǎi hé

Huáng: The color yellow, as in dà huáng

Hóng: The color red, as in hóng huā

Chì: The color of bright red, as in chì sháo

Jīn: The color gold, as in jīn yín huā

Yín: The color silver, as in jīn yín huā

Cǎo: Often, but not always, green herb, as in xià kū cǎo

Dòu: Seed, as in bái biǎn dòu

Gēn: Root, as in běi bǎn lán gēn

Guā: Fruit, as in guā lóu

Huā: Flower, as in xīn yí huā

Pí: Bark or skin, as in mǔ dān pí

Rén: Seed (or sometimes fruit), as in suān zǎo rén

Téng: Stem or caulis, as in yè jiāo téng

Yè: Leaf, as in pí pá yè

Zǐ: Seed, as in chē qián zǐ

Endnotes

Chapter 1

1 Bill Schoenbart, "High Performance Thin Layer Chromatographic (HPTLC) Analysis of Dān Shēn (Salvia miltiorrhiza) Roots Grown in Different Regions of the World," *California Journal of Oriental Medicine* 22, no. 1 (Spring/Summer 2011) 3.

2 Pei Shengji, Huai Huying, and Yang Lixin. *Important Plant Areas for Medicinal Plants in Chinese Himalaya: National Report of China*, 2005, 11.

3 Liu Xueyan. "Promoting Sustainable Use of Chinese Traditional Plant Medicine," *The State of Wildlife Trade in China* (2007): 8, http://www.traffic.org (March 15, 2011).

4 Dan Bensky, Steven Clavey, and Erich Stöger with Andrew Gamble, comp. and trans., *Chinese Herbal Medicine: Materia Medica, 3rd ed.* (Seattle: Eastland Press, 2004), 1145.

5 Christina Korpik, "Global Prices of Traditional Chinese Herbs Rising," *HerbalEgram* 8, no. 2 (2011), http://cms.herbalgram.org/heg/volume8/02February/TCMpricesrising.html (March 3, 2011).

6 Ibid.

Chapter 2

7 Dan Palevitch, "Agronomy Applied to Medicinal Plant Conservation," in *Conservation of Medicinal Plants*, ed. Olayiwola Akerele, Vernon Heywood, and Hugh Synge (Cambridge: Cambridge University Press, 1991), 168.

8 P. C. Leung and K. F. Cheng, "Good Agricultural Practice (GAP)—Does It Ensure a Perfect Supply of Medicinal Herbs for Research and Drug Development?" *International Journal of Applied Research in Natural Products* 1, no. 2 (2008), www.healthy-synergies.com.

9 Dan Bensky, Steven Clavey, and Erich Stöger with Andrew Gamble, comp. and trans., *Chinese Herbal Medicine: Materia Medica, 3rd ed*, xxii.

10 Liu Xueyan. "Promoting Sustainable Use of Chinese Traditional Plant Medicine," 10.

11 Ibid.

12 Andrew Shao, PhD, "US Dietary Supplement cGMPs and Ingredient Supplier Qualification," *Herbalgram* 89 (2011) 56.

13 "Development of a Framework for Good Agricultural Practices," Food and Agriculture Organization of the United Nations Committee on Agriculture, Seventeenth Session, Rome, March 31 to April 4, 2003 [http://www.fao.org/docrep/meeting/006/y8704e.htm] [date accessed November 20, 2010].

14 Bill Schoenbart, "High Performance Thin Layer Chromatographic (HPTLC) Analysis of Dān Shēn (Salvia miltiorrhiza) Roots Grown in Different Regions of the World," 3.

Chapter 4

15 Jean Giblette, "Local values," http://www.localherbs.org (April 30, 2011).

16 Botanical Raw Materials Committee of the American Herbal Products Association in cooperation with the American Herbal Pharmacopoeia, "Good Agricultural and Collection Practice for Herbal Raw Materials," 2006, http://www.ahpa.org/portals/0/pdfs/06_1208_AHPA-AHP_GACP.pdf, accessed February 13, 2011.

17 World Health Organization Guidelines on Good Agricultural and Collection Practices (GACP) for Medicinal Plants, 2003, http://whqlibdoc.who.int/publications/2003/9241546271.pdf, (February 13, 2011).

Chapter 5

18 "Sustainable Harvest of Medicinal Plants in India," *TRAFFIC* (2007), 1.

19 Liu Xueyan. "Promoting Sustainable Use of Chinese Traditional Plant Medicine," 9.

20 Liu Xueyan. "Promoting Sustainable Use of Chinese Traditional Plant Medicine," 10.

21 Liu Xueyan. "Promoting Sustainable Use of Chinese Traditional Plant Medicine," 8.

22 Ding ZiMian and Luo Zheng, ed. E. Leadley, "Role and Status of the Botanical Garden in the Process of Domestication of Medicinal Plants." Paper presented at 3rd Global Botanic Gardens Congress, Institute of Medicinal Plant Development, Beijing, April 2007.

23 Teresa Mulliken and Petra Crofton, "Review of the Status, Harvest, Trade and Management of Seven Asian CITES-listed Medicinal and Aromatic Plants Species," Bundesamt fur Naturschutz, http://cmsdata.iucn.org/downloads/review_of_the_status__harvest__trade_and_management_of_seven_asian_cites_listed_medic.pdf (March 3, 2011).

24 Courtney Cavaliere, "Bracing for Change," *World Conservation* 39, no. 1(2009):10.

25 Teresa Mulliken and Petra Crofton, "Review of the Status,

Harvest, Trade and Management of Seven Asian CITES-listed Medicinal and Aromatic Plants Species."

26 "Medicinal Plant Specialist Group, 2007. International Standard for Sustainable Wild Collection of Medicinal and Aromatic Plants (ISSC-MAP)," version 1.0, Bundesamt fur Naturschutz (BfN), MPSG/SSC/IUNC, WWF Germany, and TRAFFIC, Bonn, Gland, Frankfurt, and Cambridge (BfN-Skripten 195).

27 Teresa Mulliken and Petra Crofton, "Review of the Status, Harvest, Trade and Management of Seven Asian CITES-listed Medicinal and Aromatic Plants Species."

28 Ibid.

Part II

29 eFloras (2008), http://flora.huh.harvard.edu/china/PDF/PDF13/Eleutherococcus.pdf, Missouri Botanical Garden, St. Louis, MO, and Harvard University Herbaria, Cambridge, MA (accessed February 7, 2010).

30 Dan Bensky, Steven Clavey, and Erich Stöger with Andrew Gamble, comp. and trans., *Chinese Herbal Medicine: Materia Medica, 3rd ed.*, 938.

31 Ibid., 936.

32 eFloras (2008), http://flora.huh.harvard.edu/china/PDF/PDF23/Alisma.pdf, Missouri Botanical Garden, St. Louis, MO, and Harvard University Herbaria, Cambridge, MA (accessed December 19, 2010).

33 Dan Bensky, Steven Clavey, and Erich Stöger with Andrew Gamble, comp. and trans., *Chinese Herbal Medicine: Materia Medica, 3rd ed.*, 274.

34 eFloras (2008), http://www.efloras.org/florataxon.aspx?flora_id=2&taxon_id=200027501, Missouri Botanical Garden, St. Louis, MO, and Harvard University Herbaria, Cambridge, MA (accessed January 16, 2011).

35 eFloras (2008), http://www.efloras.org/florataxon.aspx?flora_id=3&taxon_id=200027461, Missouri Botanical Garden, St. Louis, MO, and Harvard University Herbaria, Cambridge, MA (accessed January 16, 2011).

36 Dan Bensky, Steven Clavey, and Erich Stöger with Andrew Gamble, comp. and trans., *Chinese Herbal Medicine: Materia Medica, 3rd ed.*, 542.

37 Ibid., 540.

38 Elizabeth M. Williamson, ed., Dabur Research Foundation and Dabur Ayurvet Limited, comp., *Major Herbs of Ayurveda* (London: Churchill Livingstone, 2002), 40.

39 Sabu, "Intraspecific Variation of Andrographis paniculata." (PhD thesis, University of Kerala, India, 2006), http://sabuthesis.thesciencenet.com/2006/11/discussion.html

40 Dan Bensky, Steven Clavey, and Erich Stöger with Andrew Gamble, comp. and trans., *Chinese Herbal Medicine: Materia Medica, 3rd ed.*, 183.

41 Dan Bensky and Andrew Gamble with Ted Kaptchuk, comp. and trans., *Chinese Herbal Medicine: Materia Medica, revised ed.*, (Seattle: Eastland Press, 1993), 92.

42 eFloras (2008), http://www.efloras.org/florataxon.

aspx?flora_id=2&taxon_id=200015358, Missouri Botanical Garden, St. Louis, MO, and Harvard University Herbaria, Cambridge, MA (accessed July 10, 2011).

43 Dan Bensky and Andrew Gamble with Ted Kaptchuk, comp. and trans., *Chinese Herbal Medicine: Materia Medica, revised ed.*, 34.

44 eFloras (2008), http://wwwefloras.org/florataxon.aspx?flora_id=3&taxon_id=200015353, Missouri Botanical Garden, St. Louis, MO, and Harvard University Herbaria, Cambridge, MA (accessed September 8, 2011).

45 eFloras (2008), http://wwwefloras.org/florataxon.aspx?flora_id=2&taxon_id=2000015389, Missouri Botanical Garden, St. Louis, MO, and Harvard University Herbaria, Cambridge, MA (accessed November 21, 2010).

46 Steven Foster and Yue Chongxi, *Herbal Emissaries: Bringing Chinese Herbs to the West* (Rochester, VT: Healing Arts Press, 1992), 70–71.

47 eFloras (2008), http://wwwefloras.org/florataxon.aspx?flora_id=2&taxon_id=2000015389, Missouri Botanical Garden, St. Louis, MO, and Harvard University Herbaria, Cambridge, MA (accessed November 21, 2010).

48 Lin Huilong, Zhuang Qiming, and Fu Hua. "Habitat Niche-Fitness and Radix Yield Prediction Models for Angelica sinensis Cultivated in the Alpine Area of the Southeastern Region of Gansu Province, China," *The Crop Science Society of Japan* 11, no. 1 (2008), http://ci.nii.ac.jp/els/110006546687.pdf?id=ART0008528643&type=pdf&lang=en&host=cinii&order_no=&ppv_type=0&lang_sw=&no=1295209005&cp.

49 Dan Bensky and Andrew Gamble with Ted Kaptchuk, comp. and trans., *Chinese Herbal Medicine: Materia Medica, revised ed.*, 221.

50 eFloras (2008), http://efloras.org/florataxon.aspx?flora_id=2&taxon_id=200027560, Missouri Botanical Garden, St. Louis, MO, and Harvard University Herbaria, Cambridge, MA (accessed December 20, 2010).

51 Dan Bensky and Andrew Gamble with Ted Kaptchuk, comp. and trans., *Chinese Herbal Medicine: Materia Medica, revised ed.*, 828.

52 Ibid., 441.

53 Ibid., 319.

54 Dan Bensky, Steven Clavey, and Erich Stöger with Andrew Gamble, comp. and trans., *Chinese Herbal Medicine: Materia Medica, 3rd ed.*, 722.

55 "Chinese Milkvetch, Astragalus," Otto Richter and Sons Limited, http:www.richters.com/progrow.cgi?search=Chinese_MilkvetchXX_Astragalus&cart_id (accessed January 4, 2005).

56 Dan Bensky and Andrew Gamble with Ted Kaptchuk, comp. and trans., *Chinese Herbal Medicine: Materia Medica, revised ed.*, 321.

57 eFloras (2008), http://www.efloras.org/florataxon.aspx?flora_id=3&taxon_id=200020622, Missouri Botanical Garden, St. Louis, MO, and Harvard University Herbaria, Cambridge, MA (accessed July 10, 2011).

58 Steven C. McCutcheon and Jerald L. Schnoor, eds.,

Phytoremediation: Transformation and Control of Contaminants (Hoboken, New Jersey: John Wiley & Sons, 2003), 898.

59 eFloras (2008), www.efloras.org/florataxon.aspx?flora_id=2&taxon_id=200028145, Missouri Botanical Garden, St. Louis, MO, and Harvard University Herbaria, Cambridge, MA (accessed January 21, 2011).

60 Dan Bensky, Steven Clavey, and Erich Stöger with Andrew Gamble, comp. and trans., *Chinese Herbal Medicine: Materia Medica, 3rd ed.*, 213.

61 eFloras (2008), http://wwwefloras.org/florataxon.aspx?flora_id=2&taxon_id=2000015417 Missouri Botanical Garden, St. Louis, MO, and Harvard University Herbaria, Cambridge, MA (accessed December 18, 2010).

62 Dan Bensky, Steven Clavey, and Erich Stöger with Andrew Gamble, comp. and trans., *Chinese Herbal Medicine: Materia Medica, 3rd ed.*, 77.

63 eFloras (2008), www.efloras.org/florataxon.aspx?flora_id=1&taxon_id=105754, Missouri Botanical Garden, St. Louis, MO, and Harvard University Herbaria, Cambridge, MA (accessed January 3, 2011).

64 eFloras (2008), www.efloras.org/florataxon.aspx?flora_id=2&taxon_id=200006992, Missouri Botanical Garden, St. Louis, MO, and Harvard University Herbaria, Cambridge, MA (accessed January 30, 2011).

65 Dan Bensky, Steven Clavey, and Erich Stöger with Andrew Gamble, comp. and trans., *Chinese Herbal Medicine: Materia Medica, 3rd ed.*, 114.

66 Ibid., 902.

67 eFloras (2008), http://www.efloras.org/florataxon.aspx?flora_id=1&taxon_id=200006993, Missouri Botanical Garden, St. Louis, MO, and Harvard University Herbaria, Cambridge, MA (accessed January 30, 2011).

68 eFloras (2008) http://www.efloras.org/florataxon.aspx?flora_id=3&taxon_id=200015478, Missouri Botanical Garden, St. Louis, MO, and Harvard University Herbaria, Cambridge, MA (accessed July 10, 2011).

69 Staff of the L. H. Bailey Hortorium, Cornell University, *Hortus Third: A Concise Dictionary of Plants Cultivated in the United States and Canada* (New York: Macmillan Publishing Company, 1976), 268.

70 eFloras (2008), www.efloras.org/florataxon.aspx?flora_id=2&taxon_id=200019352, Missouri Botanical Garden, St. Louis, MO, and Harvard University Herbaria, Cambridge, MA (accessed January 25, 2011).

71 Dan Bensky, Steven Clavey, and Erich Stöger with Andrew Gamble, comp. and trans., *Chinese Herbal Medicine: Materia Medica, 3rd ed.*, 360.

72 eFloras (2008), http://www.efloras.org/florataxon.aspx?flora_id=2&taxon_id=200022921, Missouri Botanical Garden, St. Louis, MO, and Harvard University Herbaria, Cambridge, MA (accessed July 10, 2011).

73 Steven Foster and Yue Chongxi, *Herbal Emissaries*, 64.

74 Dan Bensky, Steven Clavey, and Erich Stöger with Andrew Gamble, comp. and trans., *Chinese Herbal Medicine: Materia Medica, 3rd ed.*, 716.

75 eFloras (2008), http://www.efloras.org/florataxon.aspx?flora_id=2&taxon_id=200025080, Missouri Botanical Garden, St. Louis, MO, and Harvard University Herbaria, Cambridge, MA (accessed July 10, 2011).

76 Dan Bensky, Steven Clavey, and Erich Stöger with Andrew Gamble, comp. and trans., *Chinese Herbal Medicine: Materia Medica, 3rd ed.*, 277.

77 eFloras (2008), http://www.efloras.org/florataxon.aspx?flora_id=2&taxon_id=200016000, Missouri Botanical Garden, St. Louis, MO, and Harvard University Herbaria, Cambridge, MA (accessed January 11, 2011).

78 Dan Bensky, Steven Clavey, and Erich Stöger with Andrew Gamble, comp. and trans., *Chinese Herbal Medicine: Materia Medica, 3rd ed.*, 495.

79 eFloras (2008), http://www.efloras.org/florataxon.aspx?flora_id=2&taxon_id=200006998, Missouri Botanical Garden, St. Louis, MO, and Harvard University Herbaria, Cambridge, MA (accessed January 28, 2011).

80 Dan Bensky, Steven Clavey, and Erich Stöger with Andrew Gamble, comp. and trans., *Chinese Herbal Medicine: Materia Medica, 3rd ed.*, 641.

81 eFloras (2008), http://www.efloras.org/florataxon.aspx?flora_id=2&taxon_id=200007039, Missouri Botanical Garden, St. Louis, MO, and Harvard University Herbaria, Cambridge, MA (accessed January 29, 2011).

82 Steven Foster and Yue Chongxi, *Herbal Emissaries*, 184.

83 Dan Bensky, Steven Clavey, and Erich Stöger with Andrew Gamble, comp. and trans., *Chinese Herbal Medicine: Materia Medica, 3rd ed.*, 290.

84 Corey L. Gucker, "Dioscorea spp." in Fire Effects Information System, U.S. Department of Agriculture, Forest Service, Rocky Mountain Research Station, Fire Sciences Laboratory, 2009. http://www.fs.fed.us/database/feis/ (accessed December 18, 2010).

85 Zhengyi Y. Wu and Peter H. Raven, *Flora of China, Vol. 24* (St. Louis, Missouri: Botanical Garden Press, 2000), 293.

86 eFloras (2008), www.efloras.org/florataxon.aspx?flora_id=1&taxon_id=200023875, Missouri Botanical Garden, St. Louis, MO, and Harvard University Herbaria, Cambridge, MA (accessed January 26, 2011).

87 eFloras (2008), http://wwwefloras.org/florataxon.aspx?flora_id=2&taxon_id=200005521, Missouri Botanical Garden, St. Louis, MO, and Harvard University Herbaria, Cambridge, MA (accessed September 20, 2008).

88 Dan Bensky and Andrew Gamble with Ted Kaptchuk, comp. and trans., *Chinese Herbal Medicine: Materia Medica, revised ed.*, 28.

89 Dan Bensky Steven Clavey, and Erich Stöger with Andrew Gamble, comp. and trans., *Chinese Herbal Medicine: Materia Medica, 3rd ed.*, 8.

90 Dan Bensky and Andrew Gamble with Ted Kaptchuk, comp. and trans., *Chinese Herbal Medicine: Materia Medica, revised ed.*, 391.

91 Dan Bensky, Steven Clavey, and Erich Stöger with Andrew Gamble, comp. and trans., *Chinese Herbal Medicine: Materia Medica, 3rd ed.*, 897.

92 eFloras (2008), http://www.efloras.org/florataxon .aspx?flora_id=2&taxon_id=200010834, Missouri Botanical Garden, St. Louis, MO, and Harvard University Herbaria, Cambridge, MA (accessed January 21, 2011).

93 Ibid. (accessed January 19, 2011).

94 Steven Foster and Yue Chongxi, *Herbal Emissaries*, 253.

95 Ibid., 253.

96 Dan Bensky, Steven Clavey, and Erich Stöger with Andrew Gamble, comp. and trans., *Chinese Herbal Medicine: Materia Medica, 3rd ed.*, 792.

97 eFloras (2008), http://www.efloras.org/florataxon .aspx?flora_id=2&taxon_id=129162, Missouri Botanical Garden, St. Louis, MO, and Harvard University Herbaria, Cambridge, MA (accessed January 4, 2011).

98 Dan Bensky, Steven Clavey, and Erich Stöger with Andrew Gamble, comp. and trans., *Chinese Herbal Medicine: Materia Medica, 3rd ed.*, 940.

99 eFloras (2008), http://efloras.org/florataxon.aspx?flora_ id=2&taxon_id=200017769, Missouri Botanical Garden, St. Louis, MO, and Harvard University Herbaria, Cambridge, MA (accessed January 22, 2011).

100 Dan Bensky, Steven Clavey, and Erich Stöger with Andrew Gamble, comp. and trans., *Chinese Herbal Medicine: Materia Medica, 3rd ed.*, 155.

101 eFloras (2008), http://www.efloras.org/florataxon .aspx?flora_id=2&taxon_id=200018072 , Missouri Botanical Garden, St. Louis, MO, and Harvard University Herbaria, Cambridge, MA (accessed January 25, 2011).

102 Dan Bensky, Steven Clavey, and Erich Stöger with Andrew Gamble, comp. and trans., *Chinese Herbal Medicine: Materia Medica, 3rd ed.*, 144.

103 Sunset Books Editors, *Sunset Western Garden Book*, ed. Kathleen Norris Brenzel (Menlo Park, CA: Sunset Publishing Corp, 2007), 366.

104 Jim Jermyn, *The Himalayan Garden: Growing Plants from the Roof of the World* (Portland, OR: Timber Press, 2001), 184.

105 eFloras (2008), http://www.efloras.org/florataxon .aspx?flora_id=2&taxon_id=200018093, Missouri Botanical Garden, St. Louis, MO, and Harvard University Herbaria, Cambridge, MA (accessed January 19, 2011).

106 Dan Bensky, Steven Clavey, and Erich Stöger with Andrew Gamble, comp. and trans., *Chinese Herbal Medicine: Materia Medica, 3rd ed.*, 355.

107 Shiu-ying Hu, *Food Plants of China* (Hong Kong: The Chinese University Press, 2005), 100.

108 Dan Bensky, Steven Clavey, and Erich Stöger with Andrew Gamble, comp. and trans., *Chinese Herbal Medicine: Materia Medica, 3rd ed.*, 894.

109 Steven Foster and Yue Chongxi, *Herbal Emissaries*, 262.

110 Dan Bensky, Steven Clavey, and Erich Stöger with Andrew Gamble, comp. and trans., *Chinese Herbal Medicine: Materia Medica, 3rd ed.*, 732.

111 Francine Fevre and Georges Metailie, *Dictionnaire Ricci des plantes de Chine* (Paris, France: Association Ricci cerf., 2005) 230.

112 eFloras (2008), http://www.efloras.org/florataxon .aspx?flora_id=3&taxon_id=200022642, Missouri Botanical Garden, St. Louis, MO, and Harvard University Herbaria, Cambridge, MA (accessed July 10, 2011).

113 eFloras (2008), http://www.efloras.org/florataxon .aspx?flora_id=2&taxon_id=200005537 Missouri Botanical Garden, St. Louis, MO, andvHarvard University Herbaria, Cambridge, MA (accessed January 21, 2011).

114 eFloras (2008), http://www.efloras.org/florataxon .aspx?flora_id=2&taxon_id=118546, Missouri Botanical Garden, St. Louis, MO, and Harvard University Herbaria, Cambridge, MA (accessed January 22, 2011).

115 eFloras (2008), http://www.efloras.org/florataxon .aspx?flora_id=2&taxon_id=200015652, Missouri Botanical Garden, St. Louis, MO, and Harvard University Herbaria, Cambridge, MA (accessed January 22, 2011).

116 Dan Bensky and Andrew Gamble with Ted Kaptchuk, comp. and trans., *Chinese Herbal Medicine: Materia Medica, revised ed.*, 34.

117 Dan Bensky, Steven Clavey, and Erich Stöger with Andrew Gamble, comp. and trans., *Chinese Herbal Medicine: Materia Medica, 3rd ed.*, 23.

118 eFloras (2008), http://www.efloras.org/florataxon .aspx?flora_id=2&taxon_id=200017794, Missouri Botanical Garden, St. Louis, MO, and Harvard University Herbaria, Cambridge, MA (accessed January 23, 2011).

119 Michael A. Dirr and Charles W. Heuser, Jr., *The Reference Manual of Woody Plant Propagation: From Seed to Tissue Culture* (Athens, GA: Varsity Press, Inc., 1987), 147.

120 Dan Bensky, Steven Clavey, and Erich Stöger with Andrew Gamble, comp. and trans., *Chinese Herbal Medicine: Materia Medica, 3rd ed.*, 839.

121 eFloras (2008), www.efloras.org/florataxon.aspx?flora_ id=2&taxon_id=200027705, Missouri Botanical Garden, St. Louis, MO, and Harvard University Herbaria, Cambridge, MA (accessed December 26, 2010).

122 eFloras (2008), www.efloras.org/florataxon.aspx?flora_ id=1&taxon_id=200027720, Missouri Botanical Garden, St. Louis, MO, and Harvard University Herbaria, Cambridge, MA (accessed December 26, 2010).

123 Michael Jefferson-Brown, *The Gardner's Guide to Growing Lilies* (Portland, OR: Timber Press, Inc., 2002).

124 Dan Bensky, Steven Clavey, and Erich Stöger with Andrew Gamble, comp. and trans., *Chinese Herbal Medicine: Materia Medica, 3rd ed.*, 835.

125 Ibid., 150.

126 Ibid., 760.

127 Ibid., 223.

128 Ibid., 43.

129 eFloras (2008), http://www.efloras.org/florataxon .aspx?flora_id=2&taxon_id=210001261, Missouri Botanical Garden, St. Louis, MO, and Harvard University Herbaria, Cambridge, MA (accessed December 26, 2010).

130 eFloras (2008), http://www.efloras.org/florataxon .aspx?flora_id=3&taxon_id=200027794, Missouri

Botanical Garden, St. Louis, MO, and Harvard University Herbaria, Cambridge, MA (accessedJuly 10, 2011).

131 eFloras (2008), http://www.efloras.org/florataxon .aspx?flora_id=2&taxon_id=200008034. Missouri Botanical Garden, St. Louis, MO, and Harvard University Herbaria, Cambridge, MA (accessed January 8, 2011).

132 Dan Bensky and Andrew Gamble with Ted Kaptchuk, comp. and trans., *Chinese Herbal Medicine: Materia Medica, revised ed.*, 331.

133 Ibid., 755.

134 eFloras (2008), http://www.efloras.org/florataxon .aspx?flora_id=2&taxon_id=200008041, Missouri Botanical Garden, St. Louis, MO, and Harvard University Herbaria, Cambridge, MA (accessed July 10, 2011).

135 Dan Bensky and Andrew Gamble with Ted Kaptchuk, comp. and trans., *Chinese Herbal Medicine: Materia Medica, revised ed.*, 70.

136 Dan Bensky, Steven Clavey, and Erich Stöger with Andrew Gamble, comp. and trans., *Chinese Herbal Medicine: Materia Medica, 3rd ed.*, 128.

137 http://www.worldwildlife.org/wildworld/profiles/terres- trial/pa/pa0426_full.html, (accessed September 8, 2011).

138 Dan Bensky and Andrew Gamble with Ted Kaptchuk, comp. and trans., *Chinese Herbal Medicine: Materia Medica, revised ed.*, 314.

139 Dan Bensky, Steven Clavey, and Erich Stöger with Andrew Gamble, comp. and trans., *Chinese Herbal Medicine: Materia Medica, 3rd ed.*, 713.

140 http://www.cites.org/eng/cop/11/prop/54.pdf, (accessed December, 4, 2010).

141 Steven Foster and Yue Chongxi, *Herbal Emissaries*, 104.

142 Jackie Greenfield, M.S., and Jeanine M. Davis, PhD, *Medicinal Herb Production Guide*, 2.

143 Richo Cech. *Growing At-Risk Medicinal Herbs: Cultivation, Conservation and Ecology* (Williams, OR: Horizon Herbs, LLC, 2002), 75.

144 Jackie Greenfield, M.S., and Jeanine M. Davis, PhD, *Medicinal Herb Production Guide*, produced for the North Carolina Consortium on Natural Medicines and Public Health, 2004, www.naturalmedicinesofnc.org, 2.

145 Richo Cech. *Growing At-Risk Medicinal Herbs*, 75.

146 Ibid., 82.

147 Dan Bensky, Steven Clavey, and Erich Stöger with Andrew Gamble, comp. and trans., *Chinese Herbal Medicine: Materia Medica, 3rd ed.*, 822.

148 H. C. Harrison, J. L. Parke, E. A. Oelke, A. R. Kaminski, B. D. Hudelson, L. J. Martin, K. A. Kelling, and L. K. Binning, *Alternative Field Crops Manual: Ginseng*, University of Wisconsin-Extension, http://www.hort .purdue.edu/newcrop/afcm/ginseng.html (accessed December 9, 2010).

149 A. R. Harding, *Ginseng and Other Medicinal Plants: A Book of Valuable Information for Growers as Well as Collectors of Medicinal Roots, Barks, Leaves, Etc.* (Columbus, OH: A. R. Harding Publishing Co, 1966), 123.

150 eFloras (2008) http://www.efloras.org/florataxon

.aspx?flora_id=2&taxon_id=200015253, Missouri Botanical Garden, St. Louis, MO, and Harvard University Herbaria, Cambridge, MA (accessed December 9, 2010).

151 eFloras (2008), http://efloras.org/florataxon.aspx?flora_ id=3&taxon_id=200027299, Missouri Botanical Garden, St. Louis, MO, and Harvard University Herbaria, Cambridge, MA (accessed December 10, 2010).

152 Dan Bensky, Steven Clavey, and Erich Stöger with Andrew Gamble, comp. and trans., *Chinese Herbal Medicine: Materia Medica, 3rd ed.*, 280.

153 eFloras (2008), http://efloras.org/florataxon.aspx?flora_ id=120&taxon_id=200022990, Missouri Botanical Garden, St. Louis, MO, and Harvard University Herbaria, Cambridge, MA (accessed January 26, 2011).

154 Dan Bensky, Steven Clavey, and Erich Stöger with Andrew Gamble, comp. and trans., *Chinese Herbal Medicine: Materia Medica, 3rd ed.*, 431.

155 Ibid., 103.

156 eFloras (2008), http://wwwefloras.org/florataxon .aspx?flora_id=2&taxon_id=200021237, Missouri Botanical Garden, St. Louis, MO, and Harvard University Herbaria, Cambridge, MA (accessed September 10, 2008).

157 Dan Bensky, Steven Clavey, and Erich Stöger with Andrew Gamble, comp. and trans., *Chinese Herbal Medicine: Materia Medica, 3rd ed.*, 123.

158 eFloras (2008), http://www.efloras.org/florataxon .aspx?flora_id=2&taxon_id=200006744, Missouri Botanical Garden, St. Louis, MO, and Harvard University

- 159 Dan Bensky, Steven Clavey, and Erich Stöger with Andrew Gamble, comp. and trans., *Chinese Herbal Medicine: Materia Medica, 3rd ed.*, 239.

160 eFloras (2008), http://wwwefloras.org/florataxon .aspx?flora_id=3&taxon_id=200020230, Missouri Botanical Garden, St. Louis, MO, and Harvard University Herbaria, Cambridge, MA (accessed September 10, 2009).

161 Dan Bensky and Andrew Gamble with Ted Kaptchuk, comp. and trans., *Chinese Herbal Medicine: Materia Medica, revised ed.*, 604.

162 eFloras (2008), http://www.efloras.org/florataxon .aspx?flora_id=2&taxon_id=129162, Missouri Botanical Garden, St. Louis, MO, and Harvard University Herbaria, Cambridge, MA (accessed December 10, 2010).

163 Dan Bensky, Steven Clavey, and Erich Stöger with Andrew Gamble, comp. and trans., *Chinese Herbal Medicine: Materia Medica, 3rd ed.*, 19.

164 eFloras (2008), http://www.efloras.org/florataxon .aspx?flora_id=3&taxon_id=200008486, Missouri Botanical Garden, St. Louis, MO, and Harvard University Herbaria, Cambridge, MA (accessed July 10, 2011).

165 Steven Foster and Yue Chongxi, *Herbal Emissaries*, 151.

166 Dan Bensky, Steven Clavey, and Erich Stöger with Andrew Gamble, comp. and trans., *Chinese Herbal Medicine: Materia Medica, 3rd ed.*, 861.

167 Ibid., 16.

168 eFloras (2008), http://www.efloras.org/florataxon .aspx?flora_id=2&taxon_id=129905, Missouri Botanical

Garden, St. Louis, MO, and Harvard University Herbaria, Cambridge, MA (accessed January 14, 2011).

169 eFloras (2008), www.efloras.org/florataxon.aspx?flora_id=2&taxon_id=200020285, Missouri Botanical Garden, St. Louis, MO, and Harvard University Herbaria, Cambridge, MA (accessed December 12, 2010).

170 Dan Bensky, Steven Clavey, and Erich Stöger with Andrew Gamble, comp. and trans., *Chinese Herbal Medicine: Materia Medica, 3rd ed.*, 134.

171 Ibid., 134.

172 eFloras (2008), http://www.efloras.org/florataxon.aspx?flora_id=2&taxon_id=200020287, Missouri Botanical Garden, St. Louis, MO, and Harvard University Herbaria, Cambridge, MA (accessed July 10, 2011).

173 eFloras (2008), http://www.efloras.org/florataxon.aspx?flora_id=2&taxon_id=200012319, Missouri Botanical Garden, St. Louis, MO, and Harvard University Herbaria, Cambridge, MA (accessed January 24, 2011).

174 Dan Bensky, Steven Clavey, and Erich Stöger with Andrew Gamble, comp. and trans., *Chinese Herbal Medicine: Materia Medica, 3rd ed.*, 146.

175 Ibid., 385.

176 Ibid., 110.

177 eFloras (2008), http://www.efloras.org/florataxon.aspx?flora_id=2&taxon_id=200020616, Missouri Botanical Garden, St. Louis, MO, and Harvard University Herbaria, Cambridge, MA (accessed December 15, 2010).

178 eFloras (2008), http://www.efloras.org/florataxon.aspx?flora_id=2&taxon_id=200013464, Missouri Botanical Garden, St. Louis, MO, and Harvard University Herbaria, Cambridge, MA (accessed December 16, 2010).

179 Roger Meyer and Robert R. Chambers. *Jujube Primer and Source Book* (Fullerton, CA; California Rare Fruit Growers, Inc., The Fullerton Arboretum,1998), 7.

180 Dan Bensky, Steven Clavey, and Erich Stöger with Andrew Gamble, comp. and trans., *Chinese Herbal Medicine: Materia Medica, 3rd ed.*, 731.

181 Shiu-ying Hu, *Food Plants of China*, 88.

182 eFloras (2008), http://www.efloras.org/florataxon.aspx?flora_id=2&taxon_id=200013468, Missouri Botanical Garden, St. Louis, MO, and Harvard University Herbaria, Cambridge, MA (accessed December 17, 2010).

183 Ibid.

184 Dan Bensky and Andrew Gamble with Ted Kaptchuk, comp. and trans., *Chinese Herbal Medicine: Materia Medica, revised ed.*, 928.

Index

About the Author

Peg Schafer is recognized as one of the pioneers and leaders in the field of the cultivation of Asian herbs. After more than fifteen years

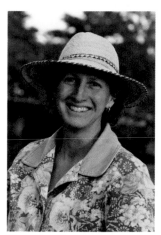

Photo by Nina Zhito

of commercial herb cultivation and research at the Chinese Medicinal Herb Farm in Petaluma, California, Schafer has distilled her findings into a guide for growers and practitioners of Chinese medicine. Schafer has played an influential role in establishing a network of organizations including Fu Tian Herbs, the first company in the United States to solely offer certified organic, domestically grown Chinese herbs (which she cofounded), the Sonoma County Herb Association, and the Medicinal Herb Consortium. Along with offering seed and field-grown herbs, Schafer's own Chinese Medicinal Herb Farm operates as an experimental farm to investigate herb cultivation and aid herb conservation. Its internship program gives people hands-on experience in all aspects of growing and harvesting Chinese herbs.

ABOUT THE FOREWORD AUTHOR

Author, photographer, and herbalist Steven Foster is the author of seventeen titles on medicinal plants, including two books on Chinese medicinal plants. He makes his home in the Arkansas Ozarks. More information is at www.stevenfoster.com.

ABOUT THE MEDICINAL USE DESCRIPTIONS AUTHOR

Sean Fannin, CH, Dipl.CEM practices traditional Chinese herbal medicine and medical qigong at the Center for Traditional Health Arts in Petaluma, California, and is cofounder of Fu Tian Herbs. He has worked in a clinical practice that is based on the Chinese medical and philosophical classics since 1992. Sean's primary interest is in classical Asian philosophy and its practical applications to modern life. This has formed the basis for his clinical practice, teaching, and writing. He lives in Petaluma, California, with his family.

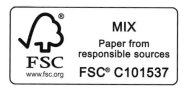

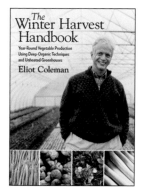
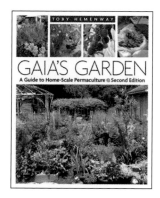
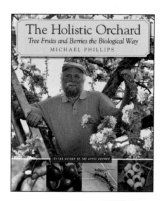
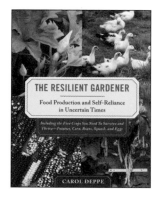
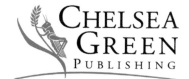

the politics and practice of sustainable living

CHELSEA GREEN PUBLISHING

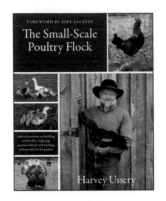

THE SMALL-SCALE POULTRY FLOCK
*An All-Natural Approach to Raising Chickens
and Other Fowl for Home and Market Growers*
HARVEY USSERY
9781603582902
Paperback • $39.95

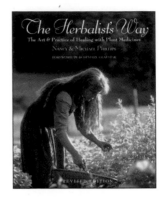

THE HERBALIST'S WAY
*The Art and Practice of Healing
with Plant Medicines*
NANCY PHILLIPS and MICHAEL PHILLIPS
9781931498760
Paperback • $30.00

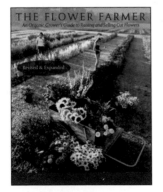

THE FLOWER FARMER, REVISED AND EXPANDED
*An Organic Grower's Guide to
Raising and Selling Cut Flowers*
LYNN BYCZYNSKI
9781933392653
Paperback • $35.00

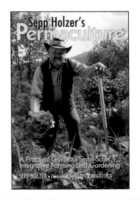

SEPP HOLZER'S PERMACULTURE
*A Practical Guide to Small-Scale,
Integrative Farming and Gardening*
SEPP HOLZER
9781603583701
Paperback • $29.95

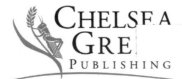

CHELSEA
GREEN
PUBLISHING

the politics and practice of sustainable living

31901051068734

...rmation or to request a catalog,
...vw.chelseagreen.com or
call toll-free **(800) 639-4099**.